The Achilles Tendon

The Achilles Tendon

Samuel B. Adams

Editor

The Achilles Tendon

Pathology, Treatment and Rehabilitation

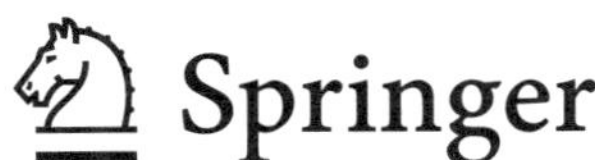 Springer

Editor
Samuel B. Adams
Department of Orthopaedic Surgery
Duke University Medical Center
Durham, NC, USA

ISBN 978-3-031-45596-4   ISBN 978-3-031-45594-0   (eBook)
https://doi.org/10.1007/978-3-031-45594-0

This Springer imprint is published by the registered company Springer Nature Switzerland AG
The registered company address is: Gewerbestrasse 11, 6330 Cham, Switzerland

Paper in this product is recyclable.

Contents

About the Book

In the ever-evolving landscape of orthopedic surgery, the treatment of Achilles tendon injuries continues to be a dynamic and challenging area. This textbook aims to provide a comprehensive and up-to-date guide to Achilles tendon surgery, covering a wide spectrum from diagnosis to post-operative rehabilitation. This textbook serves as a valuable resource for orthopedic surgeons, physical therapists, and medical professionals involved in the care and treatment of Achilles tendon injuries. We hope that this comprehensive guide will contribute to the continued advancement of knowledge in the field and ultimately enhance patient outcomes.

Part I

General Considerations for the Achilles Tendon

Anatomy and Pathology of the Achilles Tendon: Tendonitis, Tendinitis, or Tendinopathy, Which Is It?

Albert T. Anastasio, Amanda N. Fletcher, Baofu Wei, and Annunziato Amendola

Anatomy

Introduction

To serve as an introduction to this textbook, this chapter will discuss the anatomy of the Achilles tendon and will include a brief discussion of the terminology and concepts related to common pathologies affecting the Achilles tendon. The Achilles tendon is a conjoined tendon composed of the two heads of the gastrocnemius and the soleus muscles (the "gastroc-soleus complex") and variably the plantaris tendon. It is the strongest and largest tendon in the human body [1], capable of withstanding extreme forces during sprinting, jumping, and lifting movements. The Achilles tendon, therefore, is susceptible to the development of both acute injuries from high force magnitude insults and chronic pathologic progression from tendon overuse. The discussion will begin with the anatomy of the Achilles tendon, including details of the tendon microstructure, and then proceed to gross anatomy.

Microstructure

Tendons consist of collagen fibrils embedded in a proteoglycan matrix with relatively few cellular structures within. A predominance of Type I collagen fibrils is interspersed by tenoblasts and tenocytes—cells with elongated, spindle-shaped bodies that are arranged in rows between fibrils and act to continually produce and turn over the extracellular matrix proteins [2]. A collagen fiber is created from the cross-linking of tropocollagen molecules, which are aggregated into microfibrils and further combined to form fibrils [3]. Fibrils then accumulate to create the functional unit of a tendon, the collagen fiber [2].

Individual collagen fibers are organized by connective tissue that consists of three distinct components: endotenon, epitenon, and paratenon. The endotenon is a fine sheath of connective tissue that surrounds collagen fiber bundles, binding them together. The endotenon facilitates the gliding of fiber groups to allow for tendon motion and provides neural, vascular, and lymphatic access channels to the Achilles [1]. The epitenon is a fine connective tissue sheath that is continuous through the inner surface of the endotenon and surrounds the whole tendon [4]. The Achilles tendon lacks a true synovial tendon sheath—

A. T. Anastasio · A. N. Fletcher
Department of Orthopaedic Surgery, Duke University Hospital, Duke University, Durham, NC, USA
e-mail: Albert.anastasio@duke.edu;
Amanda.fletcher@duke.edu

B. Wei
Shandong Provincial Hospital, Affiliated to Shandong First Medical University,
Jinan, Shandong Province, China

A. Amendola (✉)
Division of Sports Medicine, Duke University Hospital, Durham, NC, USA
e-mail: Ned.amendola@duke.edu

rather, the tendon is encompassed by a paratenon. The paratenon is the outermost layer surrounding the tendon and is composed of loose, fatty, areolar tissue that allows the tendon to glide freely against the surrounding tissues [5]. Both nerves and blood vessels travel in the paratenon, and the paratenon functions by providing the main blood supply to the middle portion of the tendon. These distinct tendinous support structures can undergo their own pathologic changes, such as paratenonitis, or inflammation of the paratenon [6].

Gross Anatomy

Together, the gastroc-soleus complex and the plantaris muscle comprise the superficial posterior compartment of the leg. These muscles are innervated from the first and second sacral roots through the tibial nerve and obtain their blood supply from the posterior tibial and peroneal arteries [1]. The discussion will begin with the muscular anatomy of the gastroc-soleus complex and the plantaris muscle, proceed to the surrounding tendinous and osseous anatomy, and finally consider the vascularity and innervation of the Achilles tendon complex in greater detail (Image 1.1).

Gastrocnemius

The gastrocnemius muscle spans three joints: the knee, ankle, and subtalar joint. It acts to flex the knee, plantar flex the ankle, and invert the subtalar joint. The gastrocnemius contains two heads, which arise from the posterior aspect of the femur, just proximal to the medial and lateral femoral condyles [7]. It also attaches to the oblique popliteal ligament to form a confluence with the knee joint capsule [7]. The muscle fibers from the two heads then run distally in an oblique fashion to join together at the midline raphe, which broadens to form a thick aponeurosis on the anterior surface of the muscle. The gastrocnemius aponeurosis ultimately narrows to unite with the soleus tendon to form the Achilles tendon.

Soleus

The soleus serves as the primary plantar flexor of the ankle joint [8] and originates on the posterior surface of the fibular head, the proximal 25% of the posterior surface of the fibula, and the posteromedial border of the tibia. It is a pennate muscle with fascicles attaching obliquely to its tendon and is wider than the gastrocnemius. The soleus consists of an anterior and a posterior aponeurosis, which contain the majority of the muscle fibers within. Fibers arising from the anterior aponeurosis travel more distally than the fibers of the gastrocnemius to insert on the posterior aponeurosis, which is located directly anterior to the gastrocnemius aponeurosis. Here, these fibrous tissues unite to form the Achilles tendon, with the soleus typically contributing more fibers to the Achilles tendon than the gastrocnemius. The presence of an accessory soleus muscle is noted in 0.7% to 6% of specimens [9, 10]. The proximal origin of the accessory soleus is most commonly found on the distal posterior aspect of the tibia, and the muscle typically inserts anteromedial to the Achilles tendon insertion via a separate tendon on the calcaneus [11]. The accessory soleus muscle has been identified as a potential source of posteromedial ankle pain thought to result from a localized, exertional compartment syndrome [11].

Plantaris

The plantaris originates on the distal aspect of the linea aspera of the posterior femur and on the oblique popliteal ligament of the posterolateral knee joint capsule [12]. The thin, fusiform muscle belly of the plantaris crosses obliquely between the gastrocnemius and soleus muscles and runs parallel to the medial aspect of the Achilles tendon to insert onto the posteromedial part of the calcaneal tuberosity. The plantaris tendon has been found to join with the medial aspect of the Achilles tendon and form a common tendinous insertion in 22% of cadaveric specimens [13]. The plantaris is absent in up to 10% of individuals [13]. While considered vestigial and

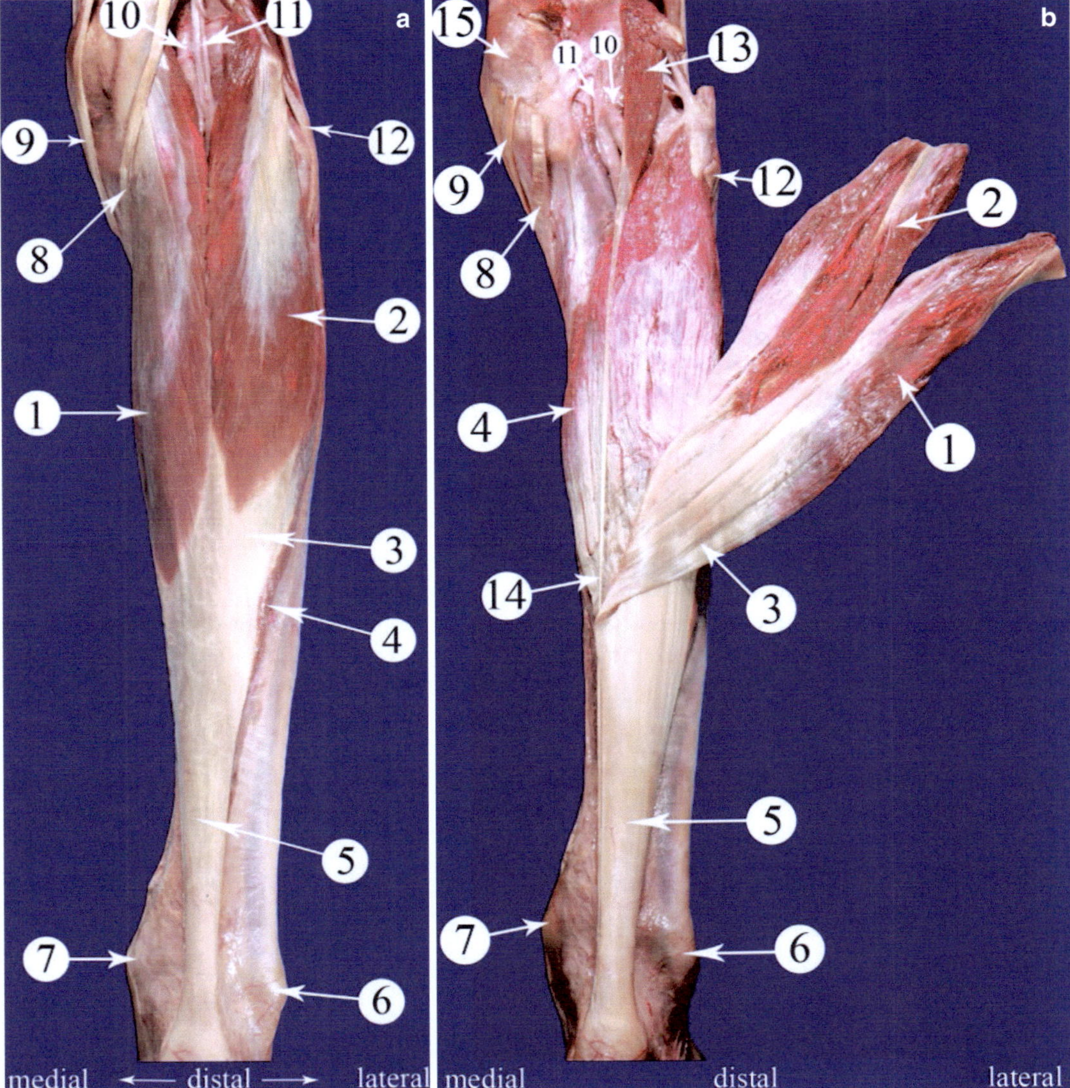

Image 1.1 The gross anatomy of the Achilles tendon and the surrounding musculature. (**a**) Posterior aspect of the leg. (**b**) Gastrocnemius muscle reflected to expose the soleus muscle. (1) Medial gastrocnemius. (2) Lateral gastrocnemius. (3) Aponeurosis of gastrocnemius. (4) Soleus muscle. (5) Achilles tendon. (6) Lateral malleolus. (7) Medial malleolus. (8) Semitendinosus muscle. (9) Semimembranosus muscle. (10) Popliteal artery. (11) Tibial nerve. (12) Common peroneal nerve. (13) Plantaris muscle. (14) Plantaris tendon. (15) Medial condyle

lacking a strong functional contribution, the plantaris may serve to aid in proprioception of the foot and to weakly flex the knee joint and plantar flex the ankle joint. The anatomical variation of the plantaris tendon morphology has been implicated in both insertional and non-insertional Achilles tendinopathy.

Achilles Tendon

The tendons of the gastrocnemius, soleus, and variably plantaris muscles combine to form the Achilles tendon. The length of the Achilles tendon complex is approximately 10–15 cm [12], and the thickness varies by age, from roughly

4.6 mm in childhood to an average of 6.9 mm after 30 years of age [14]. The contribution of fibers from the gastrocnemius and soleus to the Achilles tendon is variable, but in most individuals, the soleus contributes more fibers than the gastrocnemius [12]. The tendon is broad and flat at its proximal origin at the confluence of the gastrocnemius and soleus muscles. As it travels distally, it becomes progressively more ovoid before flattening out again just prior to inserting on the middle third of the posterior surface of the calcaneal tuberosity [12]. The fibers of the Achilles tendon internally rotate 90 degrees in a spiral manner as they descend (Image 1.2). This phenomenon allows for elongation and elastic recoil within the tendon to contribute to the release of stored energy during the appropriate phase of gait [15]. This stored energy permits greater instantaneous muscle power than could be achieved by the contraction of the gastrocnemius and soleus muscles alone [15] but also accounts for the large force magnitudes that the Achilles tendon must withstand. The Achilles tendon inserts approximately 1 cm distal to the most superior border of the calcaneus with an average area of insertion of roughly 19.8 mm in length with a width of 24 mm proximally and 31 mm distally [16]. At its insertion, the Achilles tendon displays the typical structure of a fibrocartilaginous enthesis with the presence of four distinct zones of tissue: dense fibrous connective tissue, uncalcified fibrocartilage, calcified fibrocartilage, and bone [17].

Kager's Triangle

The space created from the Achilles tendon posteriorly and the tibia anteriorly is known as Kager's triangle and is occupied by a mass of adipose tissue called Kager's fat pad. This seemingly innocuous structure functions importantly in a number of ways. Given a high density of sensory nerve endings, Kager's fat pad likely contributes to proprioception [18]. It functions

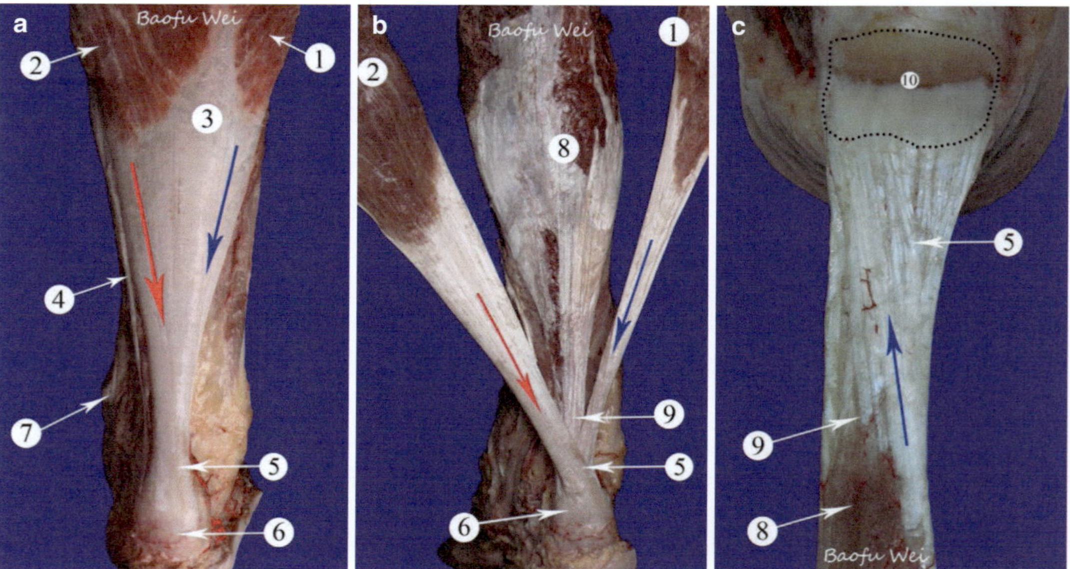

Image 1.2 (**a**) The torsion of the fibers of the Achilles tendon. (**b**) The fibers of the Achilles tendon cross over as demonstrated. (**c**) Reverse view of fiber rotation. (1) Lateral head of the gastrocnemius muscle. (2) Medial head of the gastrocnemius muscle. (3) Aponeurosis of the gastrocnemius muscle. (4) Plantaris tendon. (5) Achilles tendon. (6) Insertion of Achilles tendon. (7) Medial malleolus. (8) Soleus muscle. (9) The central fascicles of the Achilles tendon. (10) Retrocalcaneal bursa. Blue arrow: direction of the lateral fascicles. Red arrow: direction of the medial fascicles

mechanically to reduce friction between the Achilles tendon and the tibia. Additionally, it fills an otherwise potential space, serving to prevent the buildup of negative pressure in the bursa during plantarflexion and to prevent kinking of the tendon during plantarflexion [19]. It also protects nutrient vessels that course through the fat pad to supply the tendon.

Retrocalcaneal Bursa

There are two bursae located at the posterior heel which function to lubricate and protect the Achilles tendon by reducing friction between the tendon and adjacent tissues (Image 1.3). The bursa located posterior to the Achilles tendon between the Achilles tendon and the skin is termed the superficial or subcutaneous Achilles bursa. The second bursa, the retrocalcaneal bursa, is located between the Achilles tendon insertion and the posterosuperior aspect of the calcaneus. The retrocalcaneal bursa is horseshoe shaped and has two arms that extend medially and laterally on either edge of the tendon. It largely consists of highly mobile synovial projections that undergo shape alterations throughout the range of motion of the ankle to enable smooth motion of the tendon and bone [20]. The portion of the retrocalcaneal bursa that lies adjacent to the anterior surface

of the Achilles tendon contains dense sesamoid fibrocartilage, which allows for the resistance of compressive loading of the tendon during dorsiflexion as the tendinous tissue comes in contact with the posterior-superior calcaneal bone [20]. Inflammation of these bursae, termed retrocalcaneal bursitis or subcutaneous Achilles bursitis, can cause pain at the posterior heel and is implicated in a constellation of pathologies involved in insertional Achilles tendinopathy.

Vascularity of the Achilles Tendon

The blood supply of the Achilles tendon is complex and arises from the intrinsic vascular system at the myotendinous junction and the osteotendinous junction as well as from the extrinsic segmental vascular system which courses through the paratenon [1] (Image 1.4). The majority of the blood supply to the Achilles tendon arises from the posterior tibial artery delivered via the paratenon

on the anterior surface of the tendon [21]. Additionally, the tendon receives blood from endotenon-penetrating arteries at the myotendinous junction [22]. Further proximal blood supply arises from a recurrent branch of the posterior tibial artery and a vascular complex known as the rete arteriosum calcaneum (formed by branches

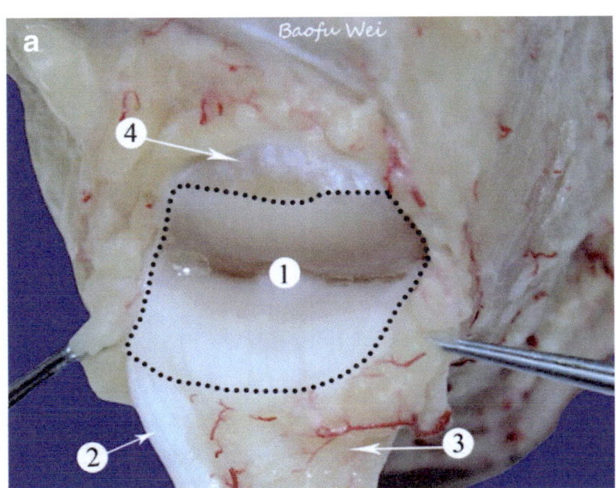

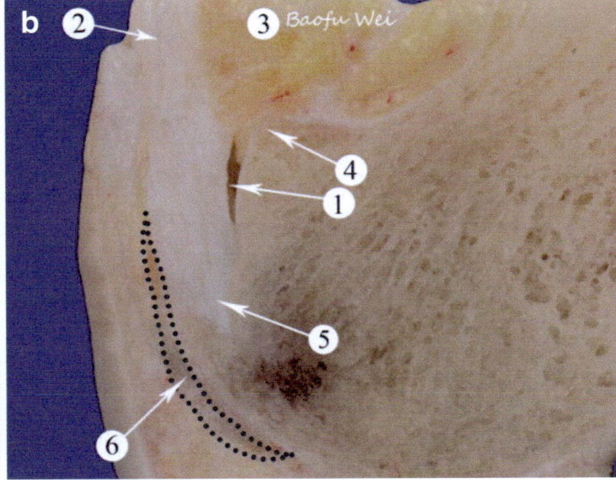

Image 1.3 The gross anatomy of the retrocalcaneal bursa. (**a**) The gross anatomy of the retrocalcaneal bursa. (**b**) Sagittal view of the retrocalcaneal bursa. (1) Retrocalcaneal bursa. (2) Achilles tendon. (3) Fat tissue. (4) Posterior superior tubercle of calcaneus. (5) Insertion of Achilles tendon. (6) Subcutaneous calcaneal bursa

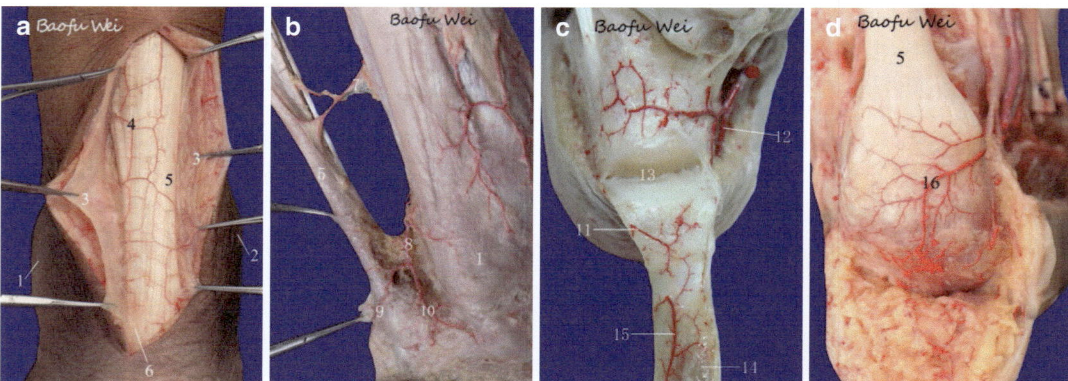

Image 1.4 The supplying arteries of the Achilles tendon. (a) The superficial artery network. (b) The lateral artery at the insertion of the Achilles tendon. (c) The deep artery network of the Achilles tendon. (d) The medial artery of the insertion of the Achilles tendon. (1) Lateral malleolus. (2) Medial malleolus. (3) Paratendon (opened). (4) Artery network. (5) Achilles tendon. (6) Epitendon. (7) Supplying artery of Achilles tendon. (8) Terminal branch of the peroneal artery. (9) Lateral artery of the insertion of Achilles tendon. (10) Lateral calcaneal artery. (11) Lateral artery of the insertion of the Achilles tendon. (12) Medial calcaneal artery. (13) Retrocalcaneal bursa. (14) Soleus muscle. (15) Supplying artery of Achilles tendon. (16) Medial artery of the insertion of Achilles tendon

of the posterior tibial, peroneal, and lateral plantar arteries), which contributes substantially to the distal blood supply [23]. While there is considerable heterogeneity among reports regarding vascular distribution [24–26], it is generally agreed upon that the midsection of the tendon is the most poorly supplied, specifically between 3 and 6 cm proximal to the tendon insertion [27]. It is this area of relative hypoperfusion that correlates with the most common site of Achilles tendon rupture [27], either through direct reduction of tendon tensile strength or through poor healing of chronic processes. leading to degenerative change.

Innervation of the Achilles Tendon

The gastrocnemius and soleus muscles are innervated from the first and second sacral roots through the tibial nerve. The Achilles tendon receives its innervation from the nerves, supplying the gastrocnemius and soleus, as well as from small fasciculi from the sural nerve and other cutaneous nerves [28]. Tendinous structures contain a relative paucity of nerve fibers and nerve endings compared to other mesoder-

mal structures. Still, the Achilles tendon transmits sensory and proprioceptive input through numerous receptors located throughout the tendon proper and the paratenon [1, 28]. The sural nerve, as the primary cutaneous nerve supplying the Achilles tendon, deserves special mention, especially given that it is the primary neurovascular structure at risk when operating on the Achilles tendon. It is a purely sensory nerve, providing sensation to the lateral border of the foot. The sural nerve arises from the confluence of the peroneal communicating branch (off the lateral sural cutaneous nerve which divides from the common peroneal nerve) and the medial cutaneous branch of the tibial nerve [28]. Small branches arising from the sural nerve combine to form the longitudinal plexus supplying the Achilles tendon. These nerves enter the tendon properly by way of the endotenon, or they pass from the paratenon through the epitenon to reach the surface of the tendon or to pierce internally [29].

With regard to the anatomic course of the sural nerve, after descending distally through the medial and lateral heads of the gastrocnemius, the nerve angles laterally and takes a highly variable path as it travels distally into the lateral heel. At the level of the gastroc-soleus junction, the sural nerve may be found superficial or deep to the muscle fascia [28], and it lies approximately 46 mm lateral to the medial border of the gastrocnemius tendon [28] or 12 mm medial to the lateral border [30]. The nerve then crosses the lateral border of the Achilles tendon, an average of 9.83 cm proximal to the tendon insertion before continuing to course distally and laterally [31]. Special care should be maintained when performing gastrocnemius recession (Strayer procedure) given an approximately 10% reported risk of the sural nerve being directly adhered to the gastrocnemius tendon [28]. When operating in and around the Achilles tendon, the proximal extent of the sural nerve as it crosses over the lateral border of the Achilles should always be considered to avoid damaging this important structure.

Pathophysiology

The Achilles tendon undergoes pathophysiologic processes similar to those that affect other tendinous structures, such as the patellar tendon and the rotator cuff. There have been inconsistencies and confusion regarding the lexicon utilized to describe the pathologies that can affect the Achilles tendon [32]. Thus, the brief discussion of terminology below will allow for the consistent use of these terms throughout this text.

Tendinosis

Tendinosis refers to the histopathological diagnosis of intratendinous degeneration and disorganization of collagen fibers without clinical or histological signs of intratendinous inflammation [33]. In overuse clinical conditions involving tendons, frank inflammation is infrequent. Instead, acute inflammation is mostly associated with tendon ruptures occurring after a high-magnitude eccentric load. Tendinosis does not always manifest clinically as "tendinopathy."

Tendinopathy

Tendinopathy refers to the general clinical condition characterized by pain, swelling, and functional limitation of a tendon and the surrounding anatomical structures [34]. The description "partial tear" of a tendon often refers to the progression of the degenerative tendinopathic process [32].

Tendinitis

Tendonitis refers to the histopathological diagnosis of inflammatory features within the tendon proper [32]. The term "Achilles tendonitis" is commonly used by athletes and coaches to describe the clinical entity that is more properly termed "Achilles tendinopathy," given a lack of findings of acute inflammation in histological specimens, and potentially belying the chronic nature of Achilles tendon degenerative change.

Paratenonitis

Paratenonitis refers to inflammation of the paratenon surrounding the tendon. It includes the following terms: peritendinitis, tenosynovitis, and tenovaginitis [35]. Paratenonitis is characterized by diffuse infiltration of inflammatory cells and is often accompanied by the production of a fibrinous exudate that fills the tendon sheath [32]. As previously mentioned, the Achilles tendon is not a sheathed tendon (as is the posterior tibial tendon, for example), and thus "paratenonitis" is a more appropriate term in relation to conditions causing inflammation in the structures surrounding the Achilles tendon than is "tenosynovitis" (referring to inflammation of the tendon sheath).

Etiology of Achilles Pathology

The pathology of Achilles injuries includes both acute and chronic (degenerative) processes. Acute Achilles tendon rupture is commonly seen in patients with preexisting intratendinous degeneration [36], and thus these entities are often linked. The etiology of Achilles tendon pathologies involves both intrinsic and extrinsic factors. Generally, Achilles tendon injuries are thought to arise from exposure to an extrinsic factor in an already predisposed individual with intrinsic etiological factors [33].

Intrinsic Factors

Intrinsic factors, or factors innate to an individual that predispose to the development of chronic Achilles tendinopathy, include anatomic features, age-related factors, and systemic factors. Anatomic variants that affect the Achilles tendon include alignment issues in the hindfoot, muscle/tendon inflexibility and weakness, and postural imbalance issues. A cavus foot, for example, results in a more vertical calcaneus and subsequent equinus contracture and/or impingement of the Achilles tendon and the surrounding soft tissues. In regard to age-related factors, there is a higher likelihood of tendon degeneration with increased age. This is thought to be consequent to a decreasing tendinous healing response, decreased vascularity, and increased tendon stiffness with mucopolysaccharide degradation and progenitor cell scarcity [33]. Tendon vascularity has been shown to decrease with age in vivo [37], and while tendon mechanical properties do not appear to be altered due to age during homeostasis, the healing potential is significantly altered due to impairments in matrix production [38]. Lastly, systemic factors contribute to Achilles tendinopathy, with obesity, smoking, diabetes mellitus, and inflammatory enthesopathies being commonly implicated in the development of this condition [39]. Imbalances in hormones, such as leptin, that are associated with obesity and the development of metabolic syndrome are thought to contribute to a chronic, low-grade inflammatory state, which may predispose to tendinous pathology [33]. Likewise, nicotine upregulates apoptotic cells and decreases tenocyte density, leading to poor tendon healing from microtrauma and a predisposition to tendinopathy [40].

Extrinsic Factors

Tendinous mechanical overload can be categorized as resulting either from repetitive microtrauma to the tendon or from an abrupt large magnitude of load [33]. Activities such as long-distance running are thought to involve numerous microtrauma events to the tendon. Chronic degenerative changes develop when such activity is followed by an inadequate rest period or the individual has predisposing intrinsic factors that do not allow for interval tendinous healing. Large eccentric loading is thought to be the primary cause leading to acute tendon rupture in a younger person, whereas cyclic loading in a tendon exhibiting degradative tendinosis is primarily responsible for tendon rupture in an older person.

Tendinopathy Classification

Achilles tendinopathy can be broadly divided into "insertional Achilles tendinopathy" and "noninsertional Achilles tendinopathy." Both of these entities will be described in significantly greater detail in the chapters to follow. As a brief overview, Achilles tendinopathy is a general term for pain in the Achilles tendon. It comprises a spectrum of acute and chronic insults and changes involving the Achilles tendon and its surrounding tissues. Degenerative changes within the tendon occur and result in a constellation of histopathologic, radiographic, and clinical signs and symptoms presenting as a painful Achilles tendon. Insertional Achilles tendinopathy, and the name infers, is a tendinopathy of the distal Achilles tendon located at the tendinous insertion onto the calcaneus. Noninsertional Achilles tendinopathy affects the tendon more proximally within the Achilles tendon proper and the surrounding tissues. Nonoperative management is the mainstay of treatment for both pathologies and includes rest, activity modification, stretching, eccentric strengthening, heel lifts, and nonsteroidal anti-inflammatories. Operative management is reserved for patients with symptoms refractory to these conservative modalities. Operative techniques continue to be developed and refined, and typically positive outcomes and high patient satisfaction result.

References

 1. Paavola M, Kannus P, Järvinen TA, Khan K, Józsa L, Järvinen M. Achilles tendinopathy. J Bone Joint Surg Am. 2002;84(11):2062–76.
 2. Maffulli N, Longo UG, Maffulli GD, Rabitti C, Khanna A, Denaro V. Marked pathological changes proximal and distal to the site of rupture in acute Achilles tendon ruptures. Knee Surg Sports Traumatol Arthrosc. 2011;19(4):680–7.
 3. Magnusson SP, Qvortrup K, Larsen JO, et al. Collagen fibril size and crimp morphology in ruptured and intact Achilles tendons. Matrix Biol. 2002;21(4):369–77.
 4. O'Brien M. Anatomy of tendons. In: Maffulli N, Renström P, Leadbetter WB, editors. Tendon injuries: basic science and clinical medicine. London: Springer; 2005. p. 3–13.
 5. Sun YL, Yang C, Amadio PC, Zhao C, Zobitz ME, An KN. Reducing friction by chemically modifying the surface of extrasynovial tendon grafts. J Orthop Res. 2004;22(5):984–9.
 6. Stecco A, Busoni F, Stecco C, et al. Comparative ultrasonographic evaluation of the Achilles paratenon in symptomatic and asymptomatic subjects: an imaging study. Surg Radiol Anat. 2015;37(3):281–5.
 7. DiGiovanni CW, Kuo R, Tejwani N, et al. Isolated gastrocnemius tightness. J Bone Joint Surg Am. 2002;84(6):962–70.
 8. Kvist M. Achilles tendon injuries in athletes. Sports Med. 1994;18(3):173–201.
 9. Kendi TK, Erakar A, Oktay O, Yildiz HY, Saglik Y. Accessory soleus muscle. J Am Podiatr Med Assoc. 2004;94(6):587–9.
10. Palaniappan M, Rajesh A, Rickett A, Kershaw CJ. Accessory soleus muscle: a case report and review of the literature. Pediatr Radiol. 1999;29(8):610–2.
11. Brodie JT, Dormans JP, Gregg JR, Davidson RS. Accessory soleus muscle. A report of 4 cases and review of literature. Clin Orthop Relat Res. 1997;337:180–6.
12. Cummins EJ, Anson BJ, et al. The structure of the calcaneal tendon (of Achilles) in relation to orthopedic surgery, with additional observations on the plantaris muscle. Surg Gynecol Obstet. 1946;83:107–16.
13. Olewnik Ł, Wysiadecki G, Podgórski M, Polguj M, Topol M. The plantaris muscle tendon and its relationship with the Achilles tendinopathy. Biomed Res Int. 2018;2018:9623579.
14. Koivunen-Niemelä T, Parkkola K. Anatomy of the Achilles tendon (tendo calcaneus) with respect to tendon thickness measurements. Surg Radiol Anat. 1995;17(3):263–8.
15. Alexander RM, Bennet-Clark HC. Storage of elastic strain energy in muscle and other tissues. Nature. 1977;265(5590):114–7.
16. Chao W, Deland JT, Bates JE, Kenneally SM. Achilles tendon insertion: an in vitro anatomic study. Foot Ankle Int. 1997;18(2):81–4.
17. Shaw HM, Benjamin M. Structure-function relationships of entheses in relation to mechanical load and exercise. Scand J Med Sci Sports. 2007;17(4):303–15.
18. Bjur D, Alfredson H, Forsgren S. The innervation pattern of the human Achilles tendon: studies of the normal and tendinosis tendon with markers for general and sensory innervation. Cell Tissue Res. 2005;320(1):201–6.
19. Theobald P, Bydder G, Dent C, Nokes L, Pugh N, Benjamin M. The functional anatomy of Kager's fat pad in relation to retrocalcaneal problems and other hindfoot disorders. J Anat. 2006;208(1):91–7.
20. Rufai A, Ralphs JR, Benjamin M. Structure and histopathology of the insertional region of the human Achilles tendon. J Orthop Res. 1995;13(4):585–93.
21. Ahmed IM, Lagopoulos M, McConnell P, Soames RW, Sefton GK. Blood supply of the Achilles tendon. J Orthop Res. 1998;16(5):591–6.
22. Kvist M, Hurme T, Kannus P, et al. Vascular density at the myotendinous junction of the rat gastrocnemius muscle after immobilization and remobilization. Am J Sports Med. 1995;23(3):359–64.
23. Sanz-Hospital FJ, Martín CM, Escalera J, Llanos LF. Achilleo-calcaneal vascular network. Foot Ankle Int. 1997;18(8):506–9.
24. Theobald P, Benjamin M, Nokes L, Pugh N. Review of the vascularisation of the human Achilles tendon. Injury. 2005;36(11):1267–72.
25. Aström M, Westlin N. Blood flow in the human Achilles tendon assessed by laser Doppler flowmetry. J Orthop Res. 1994;12(2):246–52.
26. Aström M. Laser Doppler flowmetry in the assessment of tendon blood flow. Scand J Med Sci Sports. 2000;10(6):365–7.
27. Zantop T, Tillmann B, Petersen W. Quantitative assessment of blood vessels of the human Achilles tendon: an immunohistochemical cadaver study. Arch Orthop Trauma Surg. 2003;123(9):501–4.
28. Stilwell DL Jr. The innervation of tendons and aponeuroses. Am J Anat. 1957;100(3):289–317.
29. Arnoczky SP. Human tendons. Anatomy, physiology, and pathology. László G. Józsa and Pekka Kannus. Champaign, Illinois, Human Kinetics, 1997. $79.00, 573 pp. JBJS. 1999;81(1):148.
30. Tashjian RZ, Appel AJ, Banerjee R, DiGiovanni CW. Anatomic study of the gastrocnemius-soleus junction and its relationship to the sural nerve. Foot Ankle Int. 2003;24(6):473–6.
31. Webb J, Moorjani N, Radford M. Anatomy of the sural nerve and its relation to the Achilles tendon. Foot Ankle Int. 2000;21(6):475–7.
32. Maffulli N, Khan KM, Puddu G. Overuse tendon conditions: time to change a confusing terminology. Arthroscopy. 1998;14(8):840–3.

33. Federer AE, Steele JR, Dekker TJ, Liles JL, Adams SB. Tendonitis and tendinopathy: what are they and how do they evolve? Foot Ankle Clin. 2017;22(4):665–76.
34. Loiacono C, Palermi S, Massa B, et al. Tendinopathy: pathophysiology, therapeutic options, and role of nutraceutics. A narrative literature review. Medicina. 2019;55(8):447.
35. Aström M, Rausing A. Chronic Achilles tendinopathy. A survey of surgical and histopathologic findings. Clin Orthop Relat Res. 1995;316:151–64.
36. Park SH, Lee HS, Young KW, Seo SG. Treatment of acute achilles tendon rupture. Clin Orthop Surg. 2020;12(1):1–8.
37. Adler RS, Fealy S, Rudzki JR, et al. Rotator cuff in asymptomatic volunteers: contrast-enhanced US depiction of intratendinous and peritendinous vascularity. Radiology. 2008;248(3):954–61.
38. Ackerman JE, Bah I, Jonason JH, Buckley MR, Loiselle AE. Aging does not alter tendon mechanical properties during homeostasis, but does impair flexor tendon healing. J Orthop Res. 2017;35(12):2716–24.
39. van der Vlist AC, Breda SJ, Oei EHG, Verhaar JAN, de Vos R-J. Clinical risk factors for Achilles tendinopathy: a systematic review. Br J Sports Med. 2019;53(21):1352–61.
40. Duygulu F, Karaoğlu S, Zeybek ND, Kaymaz FF, Güneş T. The effect of subcutaneously injected nicotine on achilles tendon healing in rabbits. Knee Surg Sports Traumatol Arthrosc. 2006;14(8):756–61.

Physical Examination and Imaging of the Achilles Tendon

Brandon A. Haghverdian, Dan Prat, and Daniel C. Farber

Physical Examination

Despite recent advances in imaging technology, the mainstay in the diagnosis of Achilles tendon disease and injury remains a comprehensive history and physical examination. A detailed examination of the tendon is paramount as up to 25% of Achilles tendon ruptures are missed. An examination also allows for a focused differential diagnosis, guides further diagnostic assessments, and directs initial treatment [1, 2]. As with other clinical evaluations, a physical assessment of the Achilles tendon begins with inspection and palpation, which may signal the exact nature and location of the pathology, followed by range of motion testing, strength testing, gait assessment, and, lastly, provocative maneuvers [3]. Because Achilles tendinopathy represents a broad spectrum of disease, knowledge of tendon anatomy and the classic manifestations of Achilles tendon pathology will allow the diagnostician to categorize the pathology as insertional or noninser-

tional tendinopathy, adjacent soft tissue pathology, muscle pathology, or tendon rupture. Pain with examination of other large and small joints may indicate a systemic cause, including inflammatory arthritis, connective tissue disorders, metabolic disease, or infection.

Inspection and Palpation

Examination of the Achilles tendon is best achieved with both legs fully exposed above the knee with any constrictive clothing removed. External manifestations of Achilles tendonitis and rupture frequently include soft tissue edema and bogginess and less frequently erythema of the overlying skin. The tendon may exhibit fusiform thickening, which begins approximately 4 cm proximal to its insertion and tapers to a normal width as it tracks distally. The extent of swelling may also cause the medial and lateral borders of the tendon to become indistinct and confluent with the surrounding soft tissue. In cases of chronic rupture of the tendon, disuse atrophy of the posterior calf musculature may also be observed when compared to the contralateral extremity. Further inspection may allow for more subtle findings, including the examination of the skin for previous surgical incisions, the use of orthotics or heel lifts in the patient's shoes, and the resting position of the foot while the patient is seated on the examination table, wherein a less plantarflexed foot compared to the other leg may indicate tendon rupture.

B. A. Haghverdian
Orthopaedic Specialty Institute, Orange, CA, USA
e-mail: Bhaghverdian@osiortho.com

D. Prat
Department of Orthopaedic Surgery, Chaim Sheba Medical Center, Affiliated with the Sackler Faculty of Medicine, Tel Aviv University, Ramat Gan, Israel
e-mail: Dan.Prat@sheba.health.gov.il

D. C. Farber (✉)
Department of Orthopaedic Surgery, Hospital of the University of Pennsylvania, Philadelphia, PA, USA
e-mail: Daniel.Farber@pennmedicine.upenn.edu

Focused palpation of the entire tendon is essential in determining the precise location of tendon pain. In noninsertional tendinopathy, palpation of the tendon will yield tenderness referred to the substance of the tendon in a region approximately 2–6 cm above its insertion, most severe in the region of fusiform swelling. The pain and swelling will typically migrate with tendon movement (painful arc sign) and will often be relieved when the tendon is put under tension with maximal active ankle dorsiflexion (Royal London Hospital test) [4, 5]. In contrast, pathologic inflammation of the paratenon, termed *paratenonitis*, will cause a diffuse but fixed, nonmigratory pain that is unrelieved by tension.

Pain localized to the posterior eminence of the calcaneus is more consistent with insertional tendinopathy, with pain usually worsening with active and passive hindfoot motion. This condition is difficult to distinguish from other causes of posterior heel pain, such as retrocalcaneal bursitis, calcaneal stress fractures, and *Sever's disease* (calcaneal traction apophysitis) by examination alone. In these cases, radiographs and advanced imaging may be necessary for an accurate diagnosis if initial conservative treatment has failed to relieve the patient's symptoms. In addition, pain from retrocalcaneal bursitis is best elicited with a two-finger squeeze of the tissue proximal and anterior to the tendon insertion. With all conditions, associated crepitation and warmth of the tendon and adjacent soft tissue are nonspecific but nevertheless helpful, physical examination signs and should therefore be recorded. Discrete nodularity within the tendon substance is a common finding and suggests a chronic inflammatory process resulting in thickening and scarring in damaged areas of the tendon.

With a rupture of the Achilles tendon, tenderness of the tendon with palpation may not be a significant complaint, particularly with subacute and chronic tears [6]. In these instances, the presence of a tendon "gap" may also be masked by surrounding swelling and herniated fat in acute tears and by organized hematoma and healing tendon tissue in chronic tears [7]. Therefore, a number of provocative maneuvers have been described in the diagnosis of Achilles tendon rupture, which will be detailed in a later section.

Range of Motion, Motor, and Gait

The range of motion of the involved ankle is frequently diminished in the presence of Achilles tendinopathy, particularly in dorsiflexion, with respect to the contralateral ankle. Normal ankle range of motion is approximately 20–25° of dorsiflexion, and 50° of plantarflexion, although significant variability exists depending on age, gender, and ethnicity [8]. As a result, the range of motion of the involved ankle should be compared to the contralateral, uninvolved ankle (in cases of unilateral disease). Insertional tendinopathy typically results in a significant diminution in the range of dorsiflexion, whereas noninsertional tendinopathy exhibits a preserved, though painful, arc of motion [5, 9]. Contractures of the Achilles tendon can be distinguished from other causes of ankle stiffness using the Silfverskiöld test, in which ankle dorsiflexion is measured with the knee flexed to 90°, then again with the knee fully extended. If the cause of stiffness is primarily tightness of the gastrocnemius musculature, ankle dorsiflexion will improve with knee flexion, whereas contractures of the soleus or combined (triceps surae) contractures will result in equal dorsiflexion in both positions. Finally, in cases of acute or chronic tendon rupture, dorsiflexion may be increased in the injured ankle owing to the absence of opposing tension by the Achilles tendon.

Motor testing is also performed to assess residual plantarflexion strength. In the setting of Achilles tendinopathy, accurate strength testing is difficult to evaluate, secondary to pain and patient effort. Classically, acute tendon ruptures result in diminished push-off strength; however, the recruitment of accessory muscles (tibialis posterior, digital flexor, peroneal, and intrinsic musculature) may compensate for the loss in power. Patients with Achilles tendon ruptures may therefore exhibit relatively normal gait patterns but typically have difficulty in performing a single-limb heel rise. Ambulation in patients with Achilles tendinopathy is frequently limited by pain, resulting in an antalgic gait in which the mid-stance and terminal stance phases are shortened so as to avoid recruitment of the diseased tendon. Gait assessment should be performed without footwear or orthotics as heel padding or lifting may cloak Achilles-related heel pain and allow for normal-appearing gait.

Special Testing

Numerous provocative tests have been described to assist in the diagnosis of Achilles tendinopathy or rupture. In the setting of Achilles tendinopathy, commonly used maneuvers include the Arc sign, Royal London Hospital test, and Hop test [4, 10]. In the Arc sign, the patient is asked to dorsiflex and plantarflex the ankle; a positive finding is suggested when there is tenderness to palpation within the substance of the tendon which migrates with ankle motion. In the Royal London Hospital test, tenderness over the distal 2–6 cm of the Achilles tendon which diminishes or resolves with maximal ankle dorsiflexion is considered a positive finding correlating with tendinopathy. Hop testing is positive if the patient endorses pain when hopping forward over a line marked on the floor using the involved leg. Additionally, patients may endorse pain with single-limb heel rise (on either upward or downward movement), as well as during a forward lunge stretch with the involved leg pointing forward and toes pointing straight.

The calf-squeeze test, first described by Simmonds in 1957 and later by Thompson in 1962, describes a maneuver in which the patient lies prone with ankles extending beyond the end of the table or with the knees at 90° of flexion (Fig. 2.1) [11, 12]. The examiner then squeezes the proximal calf musculature, causing a bowstringing effect on the triceps surae muscles. With an intact Achilles tendon, this will cause the foot to plantarflex; however, with a complete tendon rupture, this effect will be diminished or absent. Additional maneuvers include the Matles test, in which the patient again lies prone with the

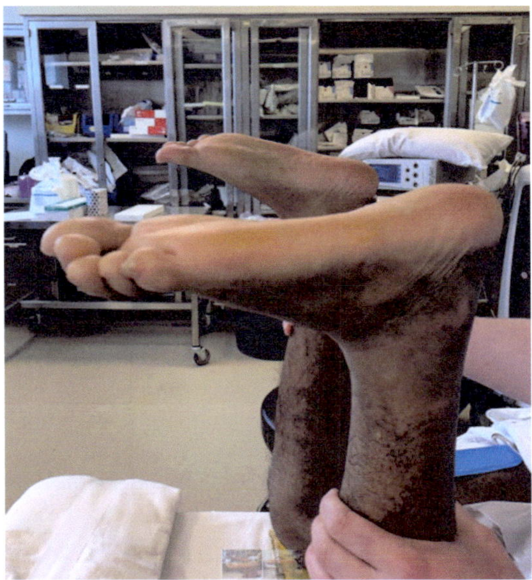

Fig. 2.1 Thompson test for Achilles tendon rupture. With the patient lying prone, the knees are flexed to 90°. The calf muscles are then compressed, yielding ankle plantarflexion when the tendon is intact (left ankle). In a ruptured tendon, the ankle remains dorsiflexed (right ankle). The test may also be performed with the knees straight and the ankle extending beyond the end of the table

knees flexed to 90°, indicating tendon rupture when the foot on the affected side falls into neutral or dorsiflexion compared to the contralateral foot (Fig. 2.2). The O'Brien test involves the placement of a needle (21–25 gauge) in region 10 cm proximal to the superior portion of the calcaneus, just medial to the midline, so that the tip is within the substance of the tendons [13]. Continuity of the tendon is confirmed if passive foot motion leads to the swiveling of the needle. Finally, in the Copeland test, a blood pressure cuff is applied to the mid-calf with the patient prone and then inflated to 100 mmHg. In a normal ankle, the pressure is expected to rise by up to 40 mmHg when the ankle is passively dorsiflexed by the examiner. In the setting of a tendon rupture, this elevation is absent [14].

Multiple studies have been performed to investigate the utility of special testing in the diagnosis of Achilles tendon ruptures. Reiman and colleagues performed a systematic review, including three studies assessing the diagnostic accuracy of both subjective and objective clini-

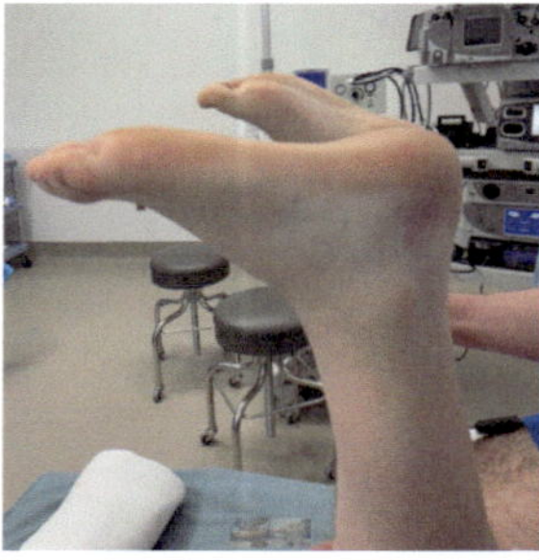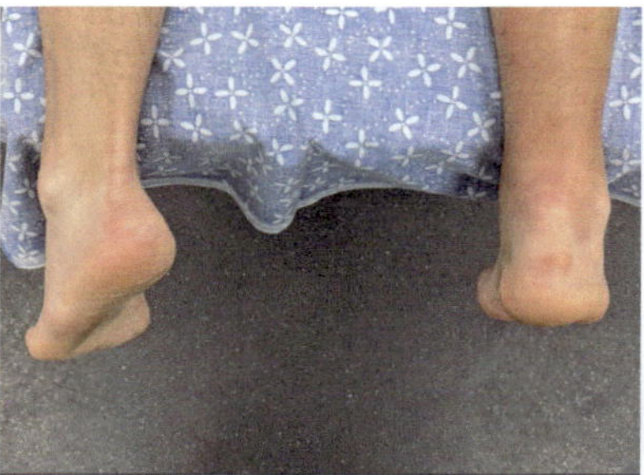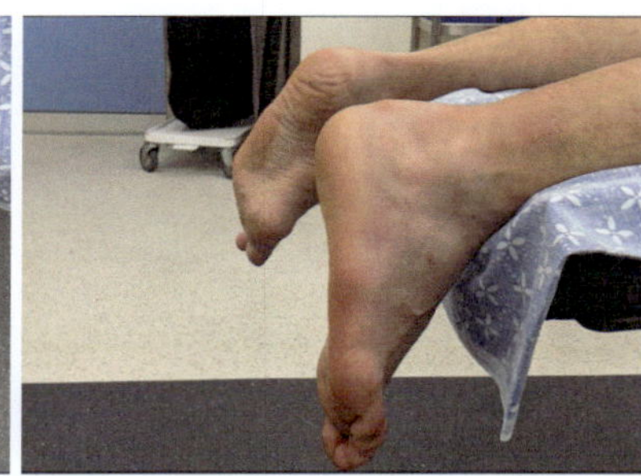

Fig. 2.2 Matles test for Achilles tendon rupture. The patient is positioned in a similar fashion as in the Thompson test. (Left) Tendon rupture is indicated by a relatively dorsiflexed resting angle in the injured extrem-

ity (right ankle) compared to the contralateral extremity). (Middle, right) Similar findings are observed in a separate patient when the legs are extended off the edge of the examination table

cal measures for Achilles tendon pathology [15]. Among these, the calf-squeeze test demonstrated the strongest sensitivity, specificity, and positive and negative likelihood ratios in the diagnosis of Achilles tendon rupture. For Achilles tendinopathy, the authors conclude that most clinical tests demonstrate strong specificity but poor sensitivity, rendering them valuable as diagnostic but not screening tools. Maffulli et al. found, in a comprehensive review of 202 patients, that at least two tests (among palpation, calf squeeze, Matles, Copeland, and O'Brien tests) were positive in all patients with an Achilles tendon rupture [7]. As such, the clinical examiner may call upon several testing methods to arrive at an accurate diagnosis.

Imaging

Several imaging modalities are available for use in the diagnosis of Achilles tendon pathology and rupture, including plain radiographs, magnetic resonance imaging (MRI), and ultrasound. While clinical examination may alone suffice in obtaining an initial diagnosis, conventional and advanced imaging techniques are helpful in borderline presentations and cases recalcitrant to conservative treatment. It is therefore recommended to obtain advanced imaging whenever the diagnosis is unclear and surgical intervention is being considered. Further, advanced imaging can be helpful for surgical planning.

Conventional Radiographs

Although limited in its ability to depict soft tissue structures, plain radiography is frequently obtained as part of the routine assessment of patients with foot and ankle pain owing to its accessibility and relatively low cost. Of the available projections, a lateral weight-bearing view of the foot and an axial view of the calcaneus provide the most valuable information in the assessment of posterior heel pain [16]. On the lateral view, the Achilles tendon is typically a well-visualized structure, exhibiting a sharp contrast between the contours of its anterior surface and the pre-Achilles (Kager's) fat pad. The blurring of this interface is consistent with Achilles tendinopathy, whereas partial opacification and obliteration of the fat pad suggest rupture of the tendon (Fig. 2.3). Ossification or calcification within the tendon substance or its insertion is also found with many pathologic disorders of the Achilles tendon as well as chronic rupture (Fig. 2.4). Haglund's deformity, also known as a "pump bump," is defined radiologically by the presence of insertional exostoses which lie superior to a pitch line that parallels the plantar surface of the anterior slope of the calcaneus (Fig. 2.5) [17]. With tendon rupture, the Achilles may also demonstrate a pathologic anterior curvature (termed Arner's sign), and the angle subtended by the posterior heel skin as it curves over the calcaneus is reduced below 150° (Toygar's angle) (Fig. 2.3)

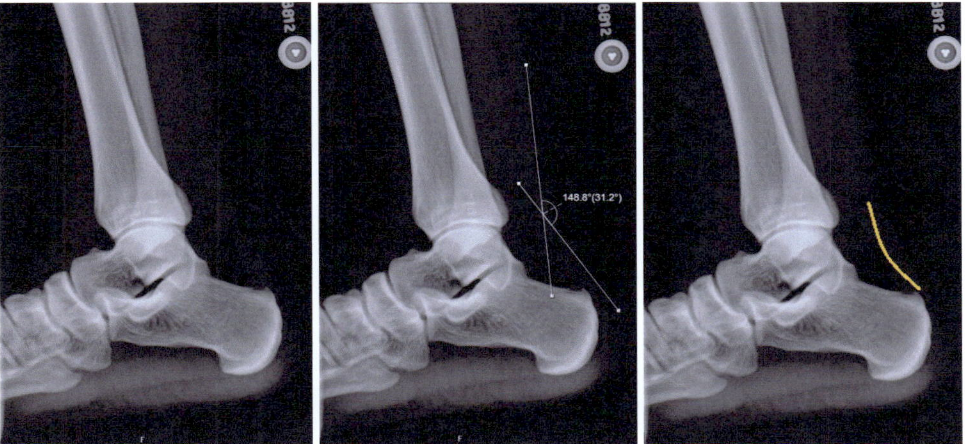

Fig. 2.3 Acute Achilles tendon rupture, indicated by the (left) blurring of the tendon-fat pad border at the rupture site, (middle) reduction in Toygar's angle <150°, (right) positive Arner's sign (pathologic anterior curvature of the tendon)

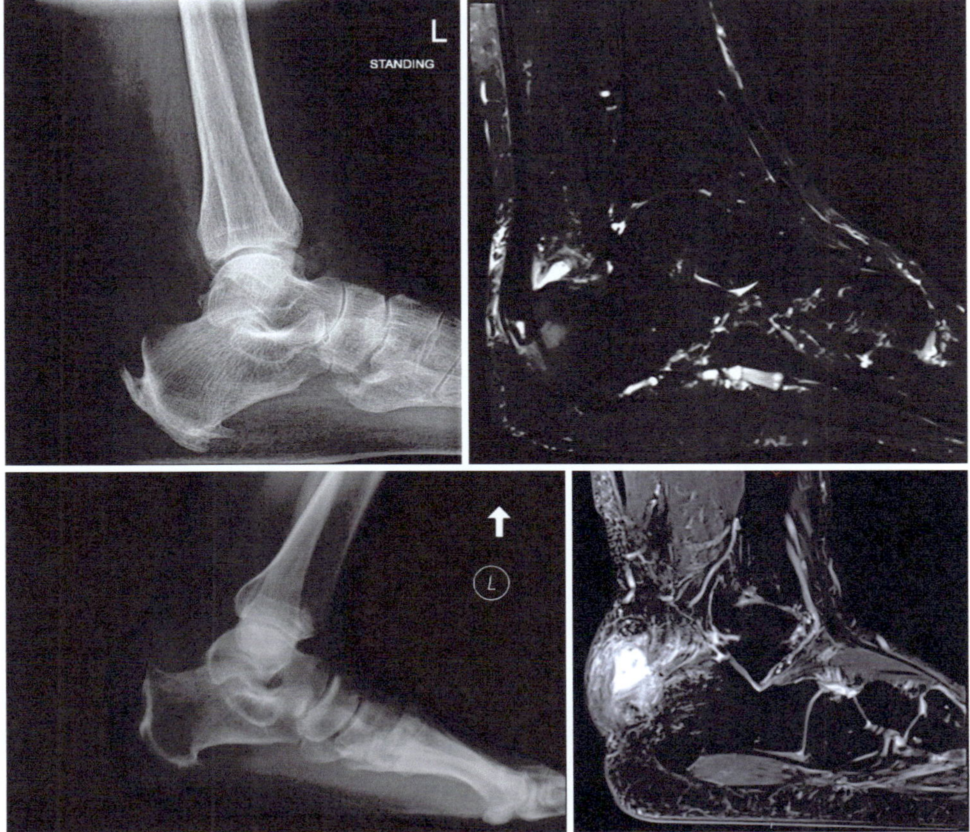

Fig. 2.4 (Top left) Large bony spurs formed on the calcaneal insertion site of the Achilles tendon, consistent with traction enthesitis and insertional tendinopathy. (Top right) T2-weighted MRI demonstrating calcaneal enthesophyte formation with associated reactive signal changes and abnormal thickening of the tendon insertion. (Bottom left, bottom right) Similar findings are observed in a separate patient with marked peri-tendinous tissue signal intensity and edema consistent with chronic insertional tendinopathy

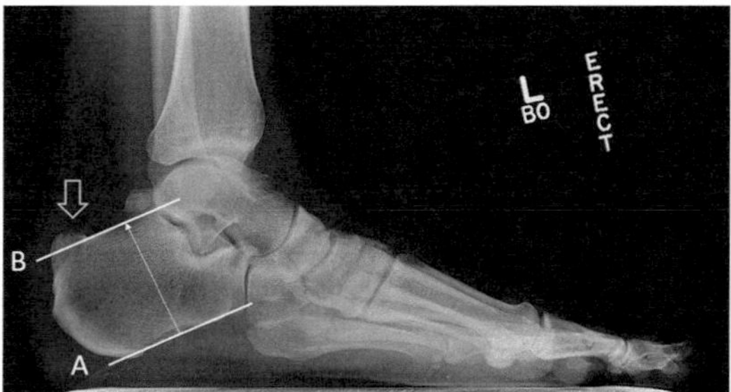

Fig. 2.5 Haglund's deformity. A bony protuberance at the superior posterior margin of the calcaneus is seen, known as Haglund's deformity. A line is first drawn along the plantar surface of the anterior process to the medial tubercle (line A). A parallel pitch line is then drawn along the posterior facet of the calcaneus (line B). Haglund's deformity exists when the bony protuberance peaks above this parallel pitch line

[18, 19]. Additionally, radiographs will reveal the presence of an avulsion fracture or posterior tuberosity fracture that can mimic an Achilles tendon rupture and will certainly affect the patient's treatment plan.

MRI

Although MRI is a less available and more costly modality, it provides exceptional soft tissue detail and offers the ability to differentiate between the various etiologies of posterior heel pain [16]. Owing to its low water content, a normal Achilles tendon displays low signal and appears relatively uniform in arrangement as it tapers to its insertion on the calcaneus. In a diseased tendon, there are regions of irregular, fusiform thickening, nodularity, mucoid degeneration, and increased signal enhancement on T1-weighted, T2-weighted, and sagittal short tau inversion recovery (STIR) sequences. Notably, these findings may be coincidentally found in asymptomatic patients, and as such, their presence should be correlated with clinical findings. Contrast enhancement, when performed, may introduce additional signals within the tendon or paratenon, consistent with the increased blood flow delivery to diseased tissue. Acute rupture of the tendon causes a focally increased signal at the rupture site with fraying and retraction of the tendon edges (Fig. 2.6). In cases of chronic rupture, MRI

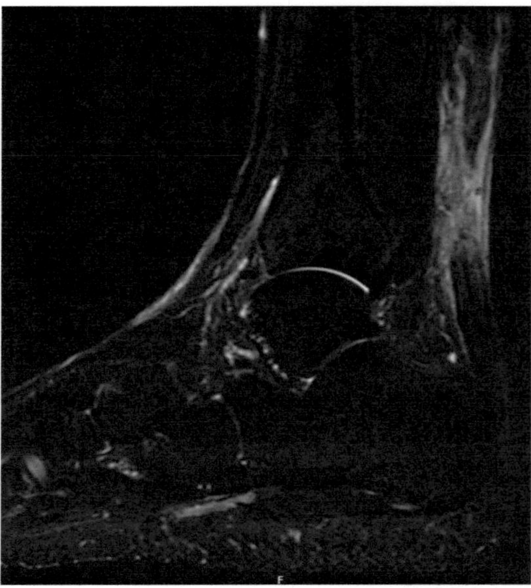

Fig. 2.6 Sagittal STIR sequence MR imaging of acute Achilles tendon rupture. There is a 2.5 cm gap within the substance of the tendon, with associated retraction and fraying of the tendon edges. Signal uptake within the edges and the surrounding soft tissue may obscure the gap and lead to overestimation of the tendon gap

can be helpful in assessing the tendon gap, although due to its sensitivity to fluid, it may overestimate the extent of the diseased tendon.

MRI has high sensitivity and accuracy in the diagnosis of tendon rupture, ranging from 91 to 95% [20, 21]. Despite this, the current American Academy of Orthopaedic Surgeons (AAOS) clinical practice guideline grades the recommendation to routinely obtain MRI to confirm the diagnosis of acute tendon rupture as "Inconclusive" [22]. Garras and colleagues found that clinical diagnosis could sufficiently be achieved by physical examination alone, which was more sensitive and less time-consuming or costly than MRI [20]. Nevertheless, they suggest that MRI should be employed for vague presentations, in the case of subacute or chronic injuries, and when physical examination did not reveal the classic findings of tendon rupture.

Ultrasound

In recent decades, the use of ultrasound has emerged as a clinically valuable tool in a variety of musculoskeletal conditions [23–25]. In com-

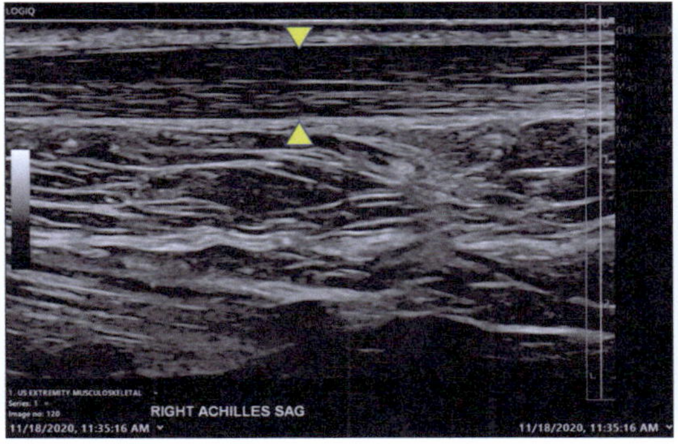

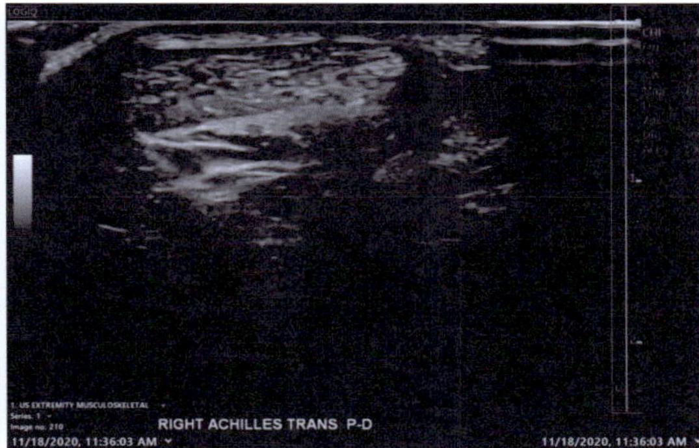

Fig. 2.7 (Left) Longitudinal grayscale ultrasound image of a normal Achilles tendon (yellow arrowhead) depicted at the mid portion of the tendon. The tendon fibers are white echogenic lines parallel aligned along the long axis and tightly packed like a "pile of lumber." (Right) Short-axis grayscale ultrasound image of a normal Achilles tendon. The tendon is oval shaped and well defined. The fibers are homogenous in distribution and appear like a "brush on end"

parison to MRI, it is relatively affordable, available, and accurate in the diagnosis of Achilles tendinopathy [26, 27]. Ultrasound also provides dynamic images and, in many instances, can be used therapeutically to assist in the treatment of various Achilles tendon disorders. The normal Achilles tendon demonstrates well-defined echogenic fibers surrounded by retrocalcaneal and subcutaneous bursae (Fig. 2.7) [16]. With tendon disease, the tendon appears less uniform, with irregular hypoechoic regions and abnormal thickening [28]. The color Doppler function may be also used to visualize increased blood flow in diseased areas of the tendon (Fig. 2.8) [29]. By comparison, paratenonitis may be demonstrated by the presence of peritendinous fluid as well as thick adhesions surrounding the tendon edge. In the setting of acute tendon rupture, ultrasound may exhibit a hypoechoic void between the tendon edges (Fig. 2.9). Dynamic movement of the foot, or alternatively the calf squeeze test, confirms the diagnosis by demonstrating approximation of the tendon edges and collapse of the gap. As with MRI, imaging

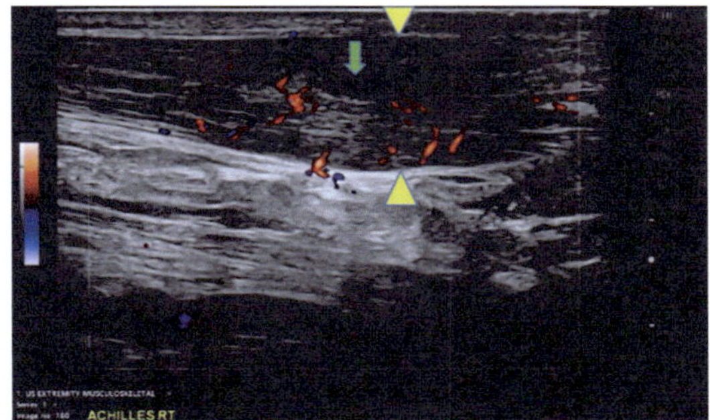

Fig. 2.8 Longitudinal color Doppler ultrasound image of the mid to proximal Achilles tendon. The tendon demonstrates fusiform thickening (yellow arrowheads) with heterogenous echogenicity and focal elongated clefts of hypoechogenicity (green arrow), indicating tendinopathy with interstitial tear. There is increased, abnormal intratendinous vascularity demonstrated by color Doppler imaging (red and blue markings overlying the tendon), indicating hyperemia of the tendon and consistent with acute tendinopathy

findings may be present in patients without clinical symptoms; therefore, imaging findings should not be used exclusively in the diagnosis of these clinical conditions [30].

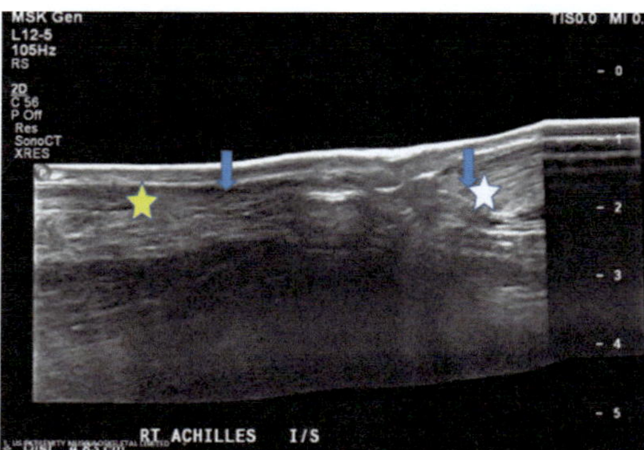

Fig. 2.9 Longitudinal grayscale ultrasound image of the Achilles tendon. There is complete disruption of the normal fibrillary pattern of the Achilles tendon. The proximal (yellow star) and distal (white star) tendon fibers end abruptly and have retracted. There is a gap of 4–5 cm in between the tendon fibers with herniation of fat from Kager's fat pad into the defect (blue arrows)

Conclusion

A comprehensive evaluation of the Achilles tendon allows for a distinction between various tendon-related disorders, including insertional tendinopathy, noninsertional tendinopathy, paratenonitis, and acute or chronic tendon rupture. Physical examination will demonstrate differences in heel and ankle appearance, alterations in range of motion, loss of motor strength, and tenderness in distinct locations within and around the tendon. Various imaging studies are available and offer a valuable supplement to the examination, of which MRI and ultrasound provide the finest detail, sensitivity, and specificity. An awareness of these techniques and modalities may thus improve the clinician's diagnostic accuracy and, as a result, the likelihood of treatment success.

Acknowledgment The authors thank our colleague, Antje Greenfield, MD, for providing original ultrasound images.

References

1. Ballas MT, Tytko J, Mannarino F. Commonly missed orthopedic problems. Am Fam Physician. 1998;57(2):267–74.
2. Inglis AE, Scott WN, Sculco TP, Patterson AH. Ruptures of the tendo achillis. An objective assessment of surgical and non-surgical treatment. J Bone Joint Surg Am. 1976;58(7):990–3.
3. Longo UG, Ronga M, Maffulli N. Achilles tendinopathy. Sports Med Arthrosc Rev. 2018;26(1):16–30.
4. Maffulli N, Kenward MG, Testa V, Capasso G, Regine R, King JB. Clinical diagnosis of Achilles tendinopathy with tendinosis. Clin J Sport Med. 2003;13(1):11–5.
5. Maffulli N, Longo UG, Kadakia A, Spiezia F. Achilles tendinopathy. Foot Ankle Surg. 2020;26(3):240–9.
6. Kauwe M. Acute achilles tendon rupture: clinical evaluation, conservative management, and early active rehabilitation. Clin Podiatr Med Surg. 2017;34(2):229–43.
7. Maffulli N. The clinical diagnosis of subcutaneous tear of the Achilles tendon. A prospective study in 174 patients. Am J Sports Med. 1998;26(2):266–70.
8. Sepic SB, Murray MP, Mollinger LA, Spurr GB, Gardner GM. Strength and range of motion in the ankle in two age groups of men and women. Am J Phys Med. 1986;65(2):75–84.
9. Philandrianos C, Moullot P, Gay AM, Bertrand B, Legré R, Kerfant N, et al. Soft tissue coverage in distal lower extremity open fractures: comparison of free anterolateral thigh and free latissimus dorsi flaps. J Reconstr Microsurg. 2018;34(2):121–9.
10. Hutchison A-M, Evans R, Bodger O, Pallister I, Topliss C, Williams P, et al. What is the best clinical test for Achilles tendinopathy? Foot Ankle Surg. 2013;19(2):112–7.
11. Simmonds FA. The diagnosis of the ruptured Achilles tendon. Practitioner. 1957;179(1069):56–8.
12. Thompson TC, Doherty JH. Spontaneous rupture of tendon of Achilles: a new clinical diagnostic test. J Trauma. 1962;2:126–9.
13. Matles AL. Rupture of the tendo achilles: another diagnostic sign. Bull Hosp Joint Dis. 1975;36(1):48–51.
14. Copeland SA. Rupture of the Achilles tendon: a new clinical test. Ann R Coll Surg Engl. 1990;72(4):270–1.
15. Reiman M, Burgi C, Strube E, Prue K, Ray K, Elliott A, et al. The utility of clinical measures for the diagnosis of achilles tendon injuries: a systematic review with meta-analysis. J Athl Train. 2014;49(6):820–9.
16. Wijesekera NT, Calder JD, Lee JC. Imaging in the assessment and management of Achilles tendinopathy and paratendinitis. Semin Musculoskelet Radiol. 2011;15(1):89–100.
17. Pavlov H, Heneghan MA, Hersh A, Goldman AB, Vigorita V. The Haglund syndrome: initial and differential diagnosis. Radiology. 1982;144(1):83–8.
18. Toygar O. Subcutaneous rupture of the Achilles tendon (diagnosis and treatment results). Helv Chir Acta. 1947;14(3):209–31.
19. Arner O, Lindholm A, Orell SR. Histologic changes in subcutaneous rupture of the Achilles tendon; a study of 74 cases. Acta Chir Scand. 1959;116(5–6):484–90.
20. Garras DN, Raikin SM, Bhat SB, Taweel N, Karanjia H. MRI is unnecessary for diagnosing acute Achilles

tendon ruptures: clinical diagnostic criteria. Clin Orthop Relat Res. 2012;470(8):2268–73.

21. Reddy SS, Pedowitz DI, Parekh SG, Omar IM, Wapner KL. Surgical treatment for chronic disease and disorders of the achilles tendon. J Am Acad Orthop Surg. 2009;17(1):3–14.

22. Chiodo CP, Glazebrook M, Bluman EM, Cohen BE, Femino JE, Giza E, et al. Diagnosis and treatment of acute Achilles tendon rupture. J Am Acad Orthop Surg. 2010;18(8):503–10.

23. Hullfish TJ, Baxter JR. A reliable method for quantification of tendon structure using B-mode ultrasound. J Ultrasound Med. 2018;37(10):2419–24.

24. van Schie HTM, de Vos RJ, de Jonge S, Bakker EM, Heijboer MP, Verhaar JAN, et al. Ultrasonographic tissue characterisation of human Achilles tendons: quantification of tendon structure through a novel non-invasive approach. Br J Sports Med. 2010;44(16):1153–9.

25. Wezenbeek E, Mahieu N, Willems TM, Van Tiggelen D, De Muynck M, De Clercq D, et al. What does normal tendon structure look like? New insights into tissue characterization in the Achilles tendon. Scand J Med Sci Sports. 2017;27(7):746–53.

26. Alfredson H, Spang C. Clinical presentation and surgical management of chronic Achilles tendon disorders - a retrospective observation on a set of consecutive patients being operated by the same orthopedic surgeon. Foot Ankle Surg. 2018;24(6):490–4.

27. Ehiwe E, Ohuegbe CI, Arogundade R. Ultrasound evaluation of achilles tendinopathy. J Med Imaging Radiat Sci. 2010;41(3):133–6.

28. Matthews W, Ellis R, Furness J, Hing W. Classification of tendon matrix change using ultrasound imaging: a systematic review and meta-analysis. Ultrasound Med Biol. 2018;44(10):2059–80.

29. Mitchell AWM, Lee JC, Healy JC. The use of ultrasound in the assessment and treatment of Achilles tendinosis. J Bone Joint Surg Br. 2009;91(11):1405–9.

30. Noback PC, Freibott CE, Tantigate D, Jang E, Greisberg JK, Wong T, et al. Prevalence of asymptomatic Achilles tendinosis. Foot Ankle Int. 2018;39(10):1205–9.

The Effect of the Plantaris Tendon on Achilles Tendinopathy

Stefan Wever, Jarrod Antflick, and James Calder

Introduction

The role of plantaris longus in midportion Achilles tendinopathy has evolved over the last 2 decades with more interest in this vestigial muscle. Steenstra and van Dijk were the first to publish on the possible role this tendon plays in medially located midportion Achilles tendon pain [1]. Midportion Achilles tendinopathy can be a debilitating condition, common in athletes, with potentially devastating effects on their careers [2]. The annual incidence of plantaris injuries in athletes has been shown to be between 3.9% and 9.3%, with associated Achilles midportion tendinopathy in up to 74% [3]. This highlights the important association between these two structures and the subsequent pathological conditions. Even though plantaris problems are more common in younger age groups, there seems to be a correlation between increased age and associated Achilles tendon pathology, explaining the bimodal distribution [3–5]. The plantaris has been reported to be absent in 8–20% of cases; however, more recent evidence refutes this, stating that it is present in 98–100%, often missed when adhered distally to the Achilles tendon [6–9].

Anatomy and Function

The plantaris consists of a small muscle belly ranging between 7 and 13 cm with a long thin tendon ranging from 24 to 37 cm in length [10–12]. The plantaris can have multiple variations in both the muscle and tendon course; however, it originates most commonly from the lateral supracondylar line of the femur (Fig. 3.1), passing superior and medial to the lateral head of the gastrocnemius muscle often attaching to the oblique popliteal ligament in the posterior knee [13]. The muscle belly continues down between the popliteus anteriorly and the lateral head of the gastrocnemius before becoming tendinous approximately at the level of the soleus muscle. Perhaps change to "It may play a role in knee instability and is frquently injured in anterior cruciate ligament ruptures [14, 15]. The elongated tendon passes between the gastrocnemius and soleus posteriorly, often curving around the medial border of the Achilles tendon with various anatomical insertions. Cadaver studies report the insertion of the tendon to be variable, with the most common (66%) being wide and fan shaped onto the calcaneal tuberosity on the medial side of the Achilles tendon. Olewnik et al. described five different insertion types of the plantaris with two variants

S. Wever · J. Antflick
Fortius Clinic, London, UK
e-mail: Stefan.Wever@fortiusclinic.com;
jarrod.antflick@fortiusclinic.com

J. Calder (✉)
Fortius Clinic, London, UK

Department of Bioengineering, Imperial College London, London, UK
e-mail: james.calder@fortiusclinic.com

S. B. Adams (ed.), *The Achilles Tendon*, https://doi.org/10.1007/978-3-031-45594-0_3

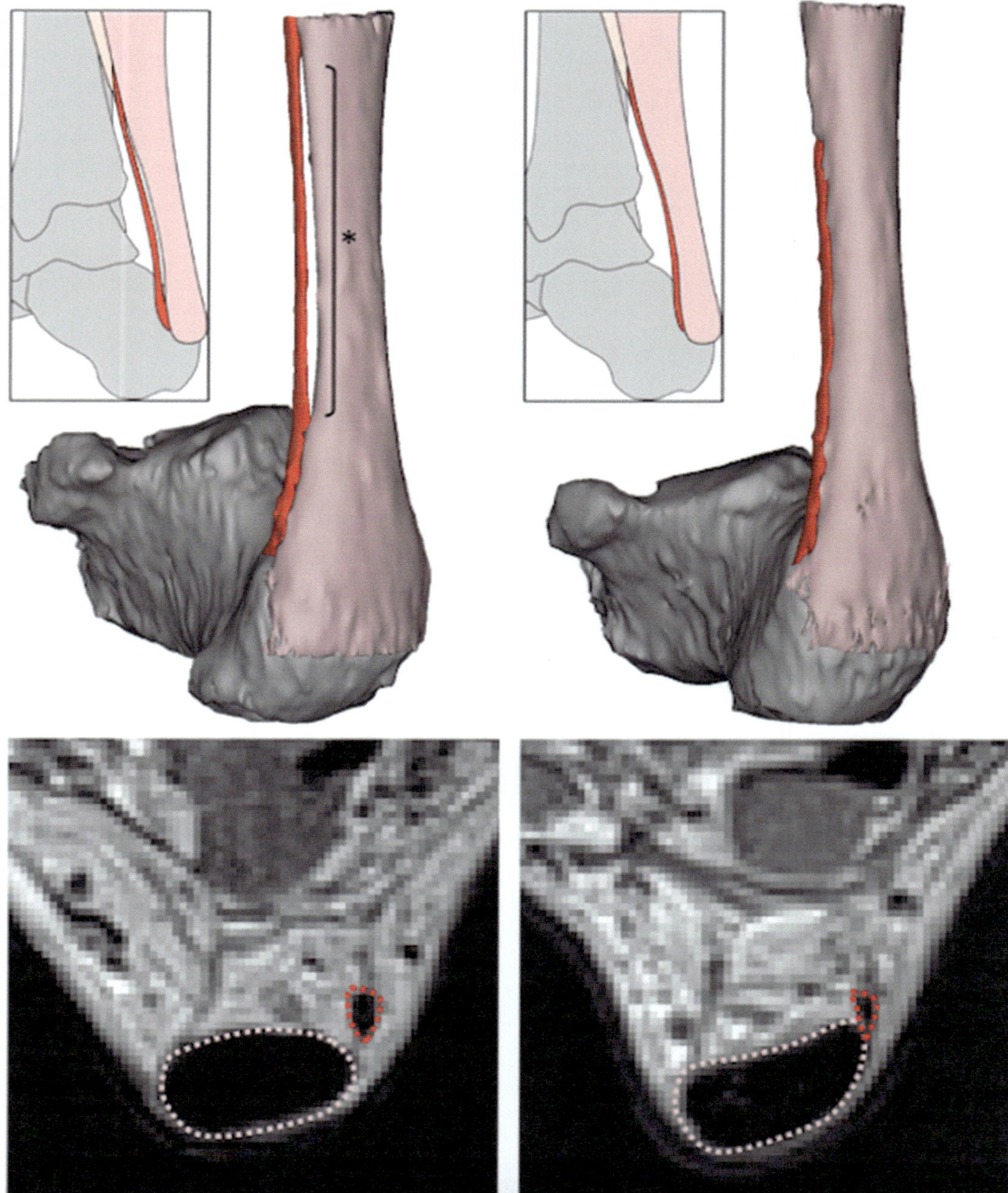

Fig. 3.1 3D MRI reconstructed image: a spectrum of gaps between the Achilles tendon and plantaris tendon was found within type 1 plantaris tendons. This gap related to the Achilles tendon (pink) and the plantaris tendon (red) can differ even when they have similar insertions

related to the Achilles tendon. 84% were variant A where the tendon entered the space between the gastrocnemius muscle and soleus muscle before passing down the medial side of the leg. Variant B initially follows a similar course but then passes anteromedially [16]. The plantaris muscle is thought to play a role in both the proprioception function and the plantar flexor of the lower limb;

however, with a 1% relative strength percentage, it is 50 times weaker than the gastro-soleus complex combined [17]. It has further been shown that the resection of this structure does not seem to affect the overall power in the lower limb [3].

Role of Plantaris in Causing Midportion Achilles Tendinopathy

Tendons are dynamic structures with a constant turnover of the extracellular matrix (ECM), which is the substrate holding cells together. Disruption in the normal remodelling and turnover of the ECM is thought to be one of the intrinsic causes of tendinopathy [18]. A mismatch in the Young's modulus of the plantaris and Achilles tendons also play a role in its mechanical aetiology. The plantaris is a tri-articulate structure that is stiffer than the bi-articulate Achilles tendon, explaining why simultaneous Achilles and plantaris tendon ruptures are rare, with isolated plantaris rupture being described in the literature [3, 19–21]. Due to this mismatch, a painful frictional syndrome can result in an inflammatory change around the interface, potentially triggering subsequent Achilles intratendinous pathology [22]. This compression/frictional theory has been confirmed in studies showing a higher incidence in endurance runners and track athletes, specifically bend sprinters, who are affected four times more frequently on the right side [21, 23]. Another proposed mechanism is that the insertion of the plantaris into the medial edge of the Achilles tendon leads to a differential traction on the tendon, subsequently causing tendinopathy.

It has been suggested that similar to midportion Achilles tendinopathy, plantaris problems often have intrinsic degeneration; however, in a study of 16 patients treated surgically, 13 tendons had histologically normal tissue characteristics. This feature was confirmed on magnetic resonance imaging and ultrasound scans. Three patients with abnormal plantaris tendons showed morphologically abnormal tenocytes with rounded and widened cells on histology. In all the patients, the plantaris tendon was in close proximity or adhered (also termed 'invaginated') to

the medial border of the Achilles tendon with surrounding richly vascularised fatty tissue and mild tendinopathic changes in the Achilles tendon [24]. This would support the biomechanical theory as an underlying cause for the midportion Achilles tendinopathy.

Clinical Presentation

Pain in the medial aspect 2–6 cm proximal to the Achilles tendon insertion is often the main complaint. The patient may report extrinsic factors such as a change in exercise intensity and duration, shoe wear or running on cambered surfaces. Intrinsic causes include abnormalities in biomechanics, such as decreased ankle dorsiflexion, leg length discrepancy and malalignment, pes cavus and lateral ankle instability [25–28]. The classic presentation is focal medial-sided pain with careful palpation of the lateral, medial and central areas of the Achilles tendon. The tendon body will often feel normal but will have a specific point tenderness, with a nodule of thickened tissue (Fig. 3.2) posterome-

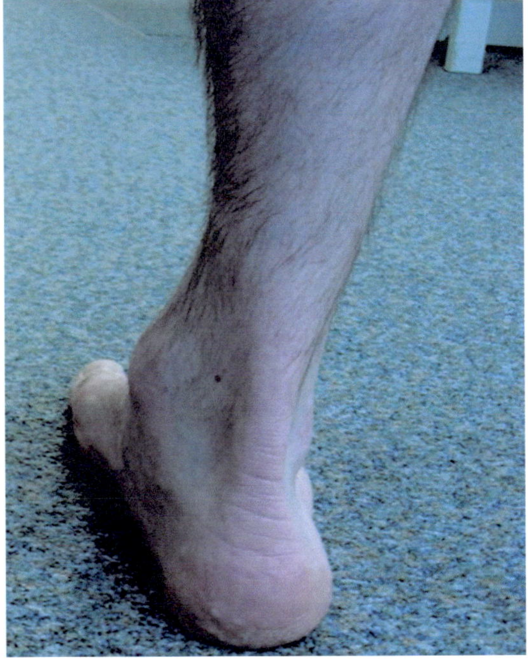

Fig. 3.2 Clinical picture of subtle medial swelling

dial representing the interface between plantaris and the Achilles [29]. With careful palpation, a plantaris tendon can be felt deep and medial to the Achilles tendon.

Diagnosis

Greyscale ultrasound and colour Doppler is commonly used showing medial sided hypoechoic changes and localised increased blood flow with high correlation to patient symptoms, however in recent years the use of ultrasound tissue characterisation (UTC) has been introduced to better visualise and quantify the structure of the Achilles tendon (Fig. 3.3)

[30]. This imaging modality uses transverse ultrasound images to form a three-dimensional data block. Making use of specific algorithms, the tendon matrix quality can be classified into four different echo types. Type 1 (green) and type 2 (blue) represent an organised matrix, whereas type 3 (red) and type 4 (black) represent a disorganised tendon matrix. This modality also has the ability to indirectly detect a plantaris tendon located close to the medial border of the Achilles [31–34]. Magnetic resonance imaging (Fig. 3.4) is also useful to visualise tendinopathic changes in both the plantaris and Achilles tendons, excluding other possible causes of pain; however, in many instances, this might not be necessary [34, 35].

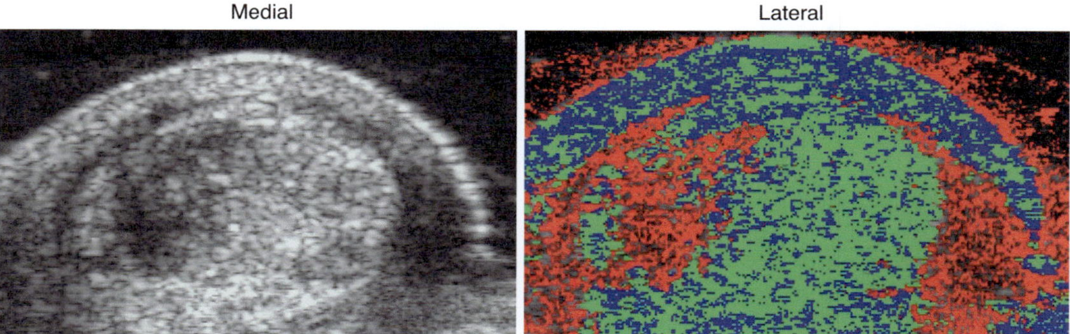

Fig. 3.3 Picture of greyscale, UTC and 3D coronal image

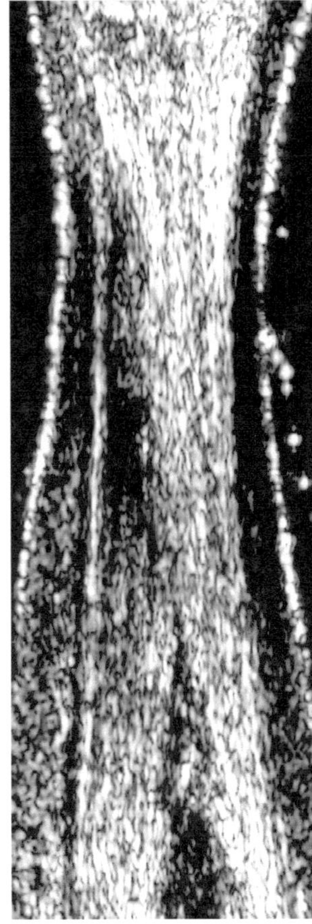

Fig. 3.4 T2 MRI axial slice showing plantaris and Achilles tendon

Treatment Options

Even if the plantaris is thought to be the culprit, initial treatment is similar to midportion Achilles tendinosis. It is imperative to exhaust conservative treatment options, including relative unloading, modification of training regimes and specific exercises. Special attention should also be given to correcting underlying limb malalignment with the use of orthoses, although the efficacy and benefit have been brought into question with recent studies [36, 37].

Tendon loading programmes are the first line of treatment with eccentric exercises (ECC) historically being used [38]. The exact mechanism is not clearly understood, but studies using ultrasound have shown a reduction in neovascular tissue, improved tendon structure and matrix, as the tendon is stretched. Heavy slow resistance (HSR) training compared to eccentric exercises has shown higher patient satisfaction rates and compliance [39]. It is proposed that the bent knee component of the HSR programme reduces the compression and irritation of the Achilles by bringing the origin and insertion of the plantaris tendon closer together, thereby increasing slack in the tendon [5, 40]. Furthermore, high-magnitude loading exercises cause both morphological and material property changes in tendons rather than muscle contraction type [36, 41–44]. However, a recent randomized controlled trial (RCT) has found no difference in clinical outcome and tendon structure at 1 year between moderate and heavy-loading exercise programmes [45]. In the literature, loading programmes typically last 8–12 weeks and have been shown to induce adaptive tendon changes; however, programmes with longer duration (>12 weeks) seem to be more effective [44].

Although repetitive low-energy shock-wave therapy (ESWT) combined with tendon-loading exercises has been shown to have good clinical results, in midportion Achilles tendinopathy, results are less satisfactory in the plantaris-related tendinopathy [38]. ESWT seems to work by selectively affecting sensory nerve endings as well as initiating a tissue healing response [46, 47].

High-volume image-guided injection (HVIGI) mechanism of action is by stretching and breaking the neovascular ingrowth. These injections target either the interface between Kager's fat pad and the Achilles tendon or the plantaris tendon and the Achilles. Denervation, as the paratenon is released from the Achilles and/or plantaris tendon, is thought to be the main reason for pain relief [48]. The initial technique described used a combination of bupivacaine hydrochloride, hydrocortisone and normal saline with short- to medium-term success in up to 70% [48]. Nielsen et al. in a chort with an average age of 45 years (16–63) recently reported that only 33% showed improvement 1 year after a single HVIGI. with an average age of 45 years (16–63).

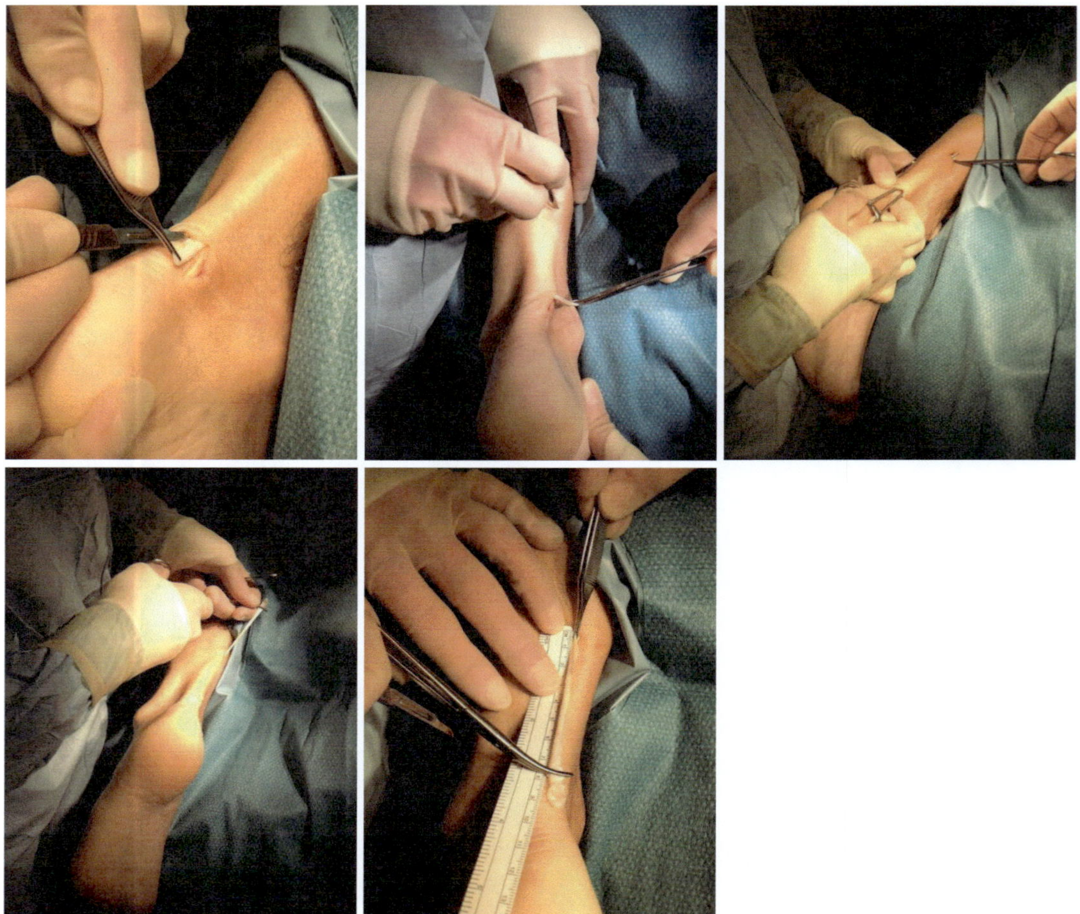

Fig. 3.5 Photo of medial incision technique and stripping with resection of PT

This in turn could be explained by the fact that paratendinous adhesions are removed but the plantaris tendon as a contributing factor was not addressed. In a recent randomised control trial, HVI with corticosteroid showed improved short-term but similar medium-term outcomes compared to HVI without corticosteroid [49].

Hyaluronic acid (HA) is another modality used, occurring naturally in synovial fluid. It is manufactured using a fermentation process and works, as shown in in vitro studies, by increasing collagen type 1 production and tenocyte viability [50, 51]. Another proposed mechanism is a decrease in gliding resistance due to HA's visco-elastic properties [52]. Various studies have shown a benefit of HA injections over placebo

and steroids and ECWT regarding pain relief and functional improvements in both short- and long-term follow-ups [53–56].

In patients who have failed a trial of conservative treatment, surgical scraping of the ventral surface with the removal of the inflamed tissue and plantaris excision can be considered (Fig. 3.5). Although endoscopic release and plantaris tenotomy have been described with acceptable outcomes, there is a risk of recurrence due to reattachment of the plantaris tendon. For this reason, it is recommended that a medial mini incision with resection of at least 8–10 cm of the plantaris tendon using a separate proximal incision be performed [29, 57]. Favourable outcomes following this procedure have been reported to be between 85 and 94%, with less consistent results in the nonathletic population [58–60]. Structural improvement of the Achilles tendon has also been shown following plantaris resection using UTC [59, 61]. A novel minimally invasive outpatient technique of ultrasound-guided plantaris tendon release (UPTR) has recently been described with promising results; however, further clinical trials are needed [62].

Conclusion

The plantaris tendon is an important intrinsic cause of midportion Achilles tendinopathy with an incidence of associated Achilles tendinopathy in 74% of cases. The majority of patients will improve with a plantaris-focused conservative treatment programme alone; however, some recalcitrant cases will need surgical intervention. Plantaris resection seems to have superior results in younger athletic patients with minimal to no Achilles tendinopathy, compared to older sedentary patients with more advanced changes.

References

1. Steenstra F, van Dijk CN. Achilles tendoscopy. Foot Ankle Clin. 2006;11(2):429–38, viii.
2. Lysholm J, Wiklander J. Injuries in runners. Am J Sports Med. 1987;15(2):168–71.
3. Pollock N, Dijkstra P, Calder J, Chakraverty R. Plantaris injuries in elite UK track and field athletes over a 4-year period: a retrospective cohort study. Knee Surg Sports Traumatol Arthrosc. 2016;24(7):2287–92.
4. Taunton JE, Ryan MB, Clement D, McKenzie DC, Lloyd-Smith D, Zumbo B. A retrospective case-control analysis of 2002 running injuries. Br J Sports Med. 2002;36(2):95–101.
5. Ames PRJ, Longo UG, Denaro V, Maffulli N. Achilles tendon problems: not just an orthopaedic issue. Disabil Rehabil. 2008;30(20-22):1646–50.
6. Freeman AJ, Jacobson NA, Fogg QA. Anatomical variations of the plantaris muscle and a potential role in patellofemoral pain syndrome. Clin Anat. 2008;21(2):178–81.
7. Harvey FJ, Chu G, Harvey PM. Surgical availability of the plantaris tendon. J Hand Surg Am. 1983;8(3):243–7.
8. Saxena A, Bareither D. Magnetic resonance and cadaveric findings of the incidence of plantaris tendon. Foot Ankle Int. 2000;21(7):570–2.
9. van Sterkenburg MN, Kerkhoffs GM, Kleipool RP, Niek van Dijk C. The plantaris tendon and a potential role in mid-portion Achilles tendinopathy: an observational anatomical study. J Anat. 2011;218(3):336–41.
10. Moore KL, Dalley AF. Clinically oriented anatomy. Gurugram: Wolters Kluwer India Pvt Ltd; 2018.
11. Wehbé MA. Tendon graft donor sites. J Hand Surg Am. 1992;17(6):1130–2.
12. Nayak SR, Krishnamurthy A, Ramanathan L, Ranade AV, Prabhu LV, Jiji P, et al. Anatomy of plantaris muscle: a study in adult Indians. Clin Ter. 2010;161(3):249–52.
13. Delgado GJ, Chung CB, Lektrakul N, Azocar P, Botte MJ, Coria D, et al. Tennis leg: clinical US study of 141 patients and anatomic investigation of four cadavers with MR imaging and US. Radiology. 2002;224(1):112–9.
14. Gopinath T, Jagdish J, Krishnakiran K, Shaji P. Rupture of plantaris muscle-A mimic: MRI findings. J Clin Imaging Sci. 2012;2:19.
15. Helms CA, Fritz RC, Garvin GJ. Plantaris muscle injury: evaluation with MR imaging. Radiology. 1995;195(1):201–3.
16. Olewnik Ł, Wysiadecki G, Podgórski M, Polguj M, Topol M. The plantaris muscle tendon and its relationship with the achilles tendinopathy. Biomed Res Int. 2018;2018:9623579.
17. Silver R, De La Garza J, Rang M. The myth of muscle balance. A study of relative strengths and excursions of normal muscles about the foot and ankle. J Bone Joint Surg. 1985;67(3):432–7.
18. Modesti A, Oliva F. All is around ECM of tendons!? Muscles Ligaments Tendons J. 2013;3(1):1.
19. Lintz F, Higgs A, Millett M, Barton T, Raghuvanshi M, Adams M, et al. The role of Plantaris Longus in Achilles tendinopathy: a biomechanical study. Foot Ankle Surg. 2011;17(4):252–5.
20. Allard JC, Bancroft J, Porter G. Imaging of plantaris muscle rupture. Clin Imaging. 1992;16(1):55–8.
21. Pollock N, Calder J, Dijkstra P, Chakraverty R. 80 Plantaris injuries in elite UK track and field athletes from 2009 to 2013. Knee Surg Sports Traumatol Arthrosc. 2016;24(7):2287–92.
22. Cook JL, Purdam C. Is compressive load a factor in the development of tendinopathy? Br J Sports Med. 2012;46(3):163–8.
23. Chang Y-H, Kram R. Limitations to maximum running speed on flat curves. J Exp Biol. 2007;210(6):971–82.
24. Calder JD, Stephen JM, van Dijk CN. Plantaris excision reduces pain in midportion Achilles tendinopathy even in the absence of plantaris tendinosis. Orthop J Sports Med. 2016;4(12):2325967116673978.
25. Volpi P. Arthroscopy and sport injuries: applications in high-level athletes. Cham: Springer; 2016.
26. Waldecker U, Hofmann G, Drewitz S. Epidemiologic investigation of 1394 feet: coincidence of hindfoot

malalignment and Achilles tendon disorders. Foot Ankle Surg. 2012;18(2):119–23.

27. Rabin A, Kozol Z, Finestone AS. Limited ankle dorsiflexion increases the risk for mid-portion Achilles tendinopathy in infantry recruits: a prospective cohort study. J Foot Ankle Res. 2014;7(1):1–7.

28. Longo UG, Ronga M, Maffulli N. Achilles tendinopathy. Sports Med Arthrosc Rev. 2018;26(1):16–30.

29. Pearce CJ, Carmichael J, Calder JD. Achilles tendinoscopy and plantaris tendon release and division in the treatment of non-insertional Achilles tendinopathy. Foot Ankle Surg. 2012;18(2):124–7.

30. Warden SJ, Kiss ZS, Malara FA, Ooi AB, Cook JL, Crossley KM. Comparative accuracy of magnetic resonance imaging and ultrasonography in confirming clinically diagnosed patellar tendinopathy. Am J Sports Med. 2007;35(3):427–36.

31. Wijesekera NT, Chew NS, Lee JC, Mitchell AW, Calder JD, Healy JC. Ultrasound-guided treatments for chronic Achilles tendinopathy: an update and current status. Skelet Radiol. 2010;39(5):425–34.

32. Van Schie H, de Vos R-J, de Jonge S, Bakker E, Heijboer M, Verhaar J, et al. Ultrasonographic tissue characterisation of human Achilles tendons: quantification of tendon structure through a novel non-invasive approach. Br J Sports Med. 2010;44(16):1153–9.

33. Rosengarten SD, Cook JL, Bryant AL, Cordy JT, Daffy J, Docking SI. Australian football players' Achilles tendons respond to game loads within 2 days: an ultrasound tissue characterisation (UTC) study. Br J Sports Med. 2015;49(3):183–7.

34. Masci L, Spang C, van Schie HT, Alfredson H. How to diagnose plantaris tendon involvement in midportion Achilles tendinopathy-clinical and imaging findings. BMC Musculoskelet Disord. 2016;17(1):1–6.

35. Pearce CJ, Tan A. Non-insertional Achilles tendinopathy. EFORT Open Rev. 2016;1(11):383–90.

36. Alfredson H, Pietilä T, Jonsson P, Lorentzon R. Heavy-load eccentric calf muscle training for the treatment of chronic Achilles tendinosis. Am J Sports Med. 1998;26(3):360–6.

37. Crago D, Bishop C, Arnold JB. The effect of foot orthoses and insoles on running economy and performance in distance runners: a systematic review and meta-analysis. J Sports Sci. 2019;37(22):2613–24.

38. Rompe JD, Furia J, Maffulli N. Eccentric loading versus eccentric loading plus shock-wave treatment for midportion achilles tendinopathy: a randomized controlled trial. Am J Sports Med. 2009;37(3):463–70.

39. Beyer R, Kongsgaard M, Hougs Kjær B, Øhlenschlæger T, Kjær M, Magnusson SP. Heavy slow resistance versus eccentric training as treatment for Achilles tendinopathy: a randomized controlled trial. Am J Sports Med. 2015;43(7):1704–11.

40. Nunes JP, Costa BD, Kassiano W, Kunevaliki G, Castro-e-Souza P, Rodacki AL, et al. Different foot positioning during calf training to induce portion-specific gastrocnemius muscle hypertrophy. J Strength Cond Res. 2020;34(8):2347–51.

41. Ishigaki T, Kubo K. Effects of eccentric training with different training frequencies on blood circulation, collagen fiber orientation, and mechanical properties of human Achilles tendons in vivo. Eur J Appl Physiol. 2018;118(12):2617–26.

42. Roche A, Calder J. Achilles tendinopathy: a review of the current concepts of treatment. Bone Joint J. 2013;95(10):1299–307.

43. Maganaris CN, Chatzistergos P, Reeves ND, Narici MV. Quantification of internal stress-strain fields in human tendon: unraveling the mechanisms that underlie regional tendon adaptations and mal-adaptations to mechanical loading and the effectiveness of therapeutic eccentric exercise. Front Physiol. 2017;8:91.

44. Bohm S, Mersmann F, Arampatzis A. Human tendon adaptation in response to mechanical loading: a systematic review and meta-analysis of exercise intervention studies on healthy adults. Sports Med Open. 2015;1(1):1–18.

45. Agergaard A-S, Svensson RB, Malmgaard-Clausen NM, Couppé C, Hjortshoej MH, Doessing S, et al. Clinical outcomes, structure, and function improve with both heavy and moderate loads in the treatment of patellar tendinopathy: a randomized clinical trial. Am J Sports Med. 2021;2021:363546520988741.

46. Rompe JD, Furia JP, Maffulli N. Mid-portion Achilles tendinopathy–current options for treatment. Disabil Rehabil. 2008;30(20-22):1666–76.

47. Han SH, Lee JW, Guyton GP, Parks BG, Courneya J-P, Schon LC. J. Leonard Goldner Award 2008: effect of extracorporeal shock wave therapy on cultured tenocytes. Foot Ankle Int. 2009;30(2):93–8.

48. Chan O, O'Dowd D, Padhiar N, Morrissey D, King J, Jalan R, et al. High volume image guided injections in chronic Achilles tendinopathy. Disabil Rehabil. 2008;30(20-22):1697–708.

49. Boesen AP, Langberg H, Hansen R, Malliaras P, Boesen MI. High volume injection with and without corticosteroid in chronic midportion achilles tendinopathy. Scand J Med Sci Sports. 2019;29(8):1223–31.

50. Abate M, Schiavone C, Salini V. The use of hyaluronic acid after tendon surgery and in tendinopathies. Biomed Res Int. 2014;2014:783632.

51. Wiig M, Abrahamsson S-O, Lundborg G. Effects of hyaluronan on cell proliferation and collagen synthesis: a study of rabbit flexor tendons in vitro. J Hand Surg Am. 1996;21(4):599–604.

52. Kolodzinskyi MN, Zhao C, Sun Y-L, An K-N, Thoreson AR, Amadio PC, et al. The effects of hylan gf 20 surface modification on gliding of extrasynovial canine tendon grafts in vitro. J Hand Surg Am. 2013;38(2):231–6.

53. Frizziero A, Oliva F, Vittadini F, Vetrano M, Bernetti A, Giordan N, et al. Efficacy of ultrasound-guided hyaluronic acid injections in achilles and patellar tendinopathies: a prospective multicentric clinical trial. Muscles Ligaments Tendons J. 2019;9(3):305–13.

54. Lynen N, De Vroey T, Spiegel I, Van Ongeval F, Hendrickx N-J, Stassijns G. Comparison of peri-

tendinous hyaluronan injections versus extracorporeal shock wave therapy in the treatment of painful achilles' tendinopathy: a randomized clinical efficacy and safety study. Arch Phys Med Rehabil. 2017;98(1):64–71.

55. Ayyaswamy B, Vaghela M, Alderton E, Majeed H, Limaye R. Early outcome of a single peri-tendinous hyaluronic acid injection for mid-portion non-insertional achilles tendinopathy-a pilot study. Foot. 2020;2020:101738.

56. Gervasi M, Barbieri E, Capparucci I, Annibalini G, Sisti D, Amatori S, et al. Treatment of achilles tendinopathy in recreational runners with peritendinous hyaluronic acid injections: a viscoelastometric, functional, and biochemical pilot study. J Clin Med. 2021;10(7):1397.

57. van Sterkenburg MN, Kerkhoffs GM, van Dijk CN. Good outcome after stripping the plantaris tendon in patients with chronic mid-portion Achilles tendinopathy. Knee Surg Sports Traumatol Arthrosc. 2011;19(8):1362–6.

58. Jowett CR, Richmond A, Bedi HS. Paratendinous scraping and excision of plantaris for achilles tendinopathy. Techniques Foot Ankle Surg. 2018;17(1):27–30.

59. Bedi HS, Jowett C, Ristanis S, Docking S, Cook J. Plantaris excision and ventral paratendinous scraping for Achilles tendinopathy in an athletic population. Foot Ankle Int. 2016;37(4):386–93.

60. Calder JD, Freeman R, Pollock N. Plantaris excision in the treatment of non-insertional Achilles tendinopathy in elite athletes. Br J Sports Med. 2015;49(23):1532–4.

61. Masci L, Spang C, van Schie HT, Alfredson H. Achilles tendinopathy—do plantaris tendon removal and Achilles tendon scraping improve tendon structure? A prospective study using ultrasound tissue characterisation. BMJ Open Sport Exerc Med. 2015;1(1):e000005.

62. Hickey B, Lee J, Stephen J, Antflick J, Calder J. It is possible to release the plantaris tendon under ultrasound guidance: a technical description of ultrasound guided plantaris tendon release (UPTR) in the treatment of non-insertional Achilles tendinopathy. Knee Surg Sports Traumatol Arthrosc. 2019;27(9):2858–62.

4

Summary of Data Comparing Nonoperative, Open, and Minimally Invasive Treatment of Achilles Tendon Tears

Andrew E. Hanselman

Introduction

The management of acute Achilles tendon ruptures remains a highly debated topic. Whether it is determining the best treatment option, the most appropriate rehab protocol, or the best surgical technique, there is no shortage of discussion among foot and ankle surgeons. Every year, there is more literature published on the topic, sometimes helping to make sense of the difficult questions and other times making it more complicated. This chapter serves as a brief review of the recent literature recent literature for the management of acute Achilles tendon ruptures.

Tendon Gap Measurement

Traditionally, nonoperative management for Achilles tendon rupture was reserved for elderly patients, low-demand patients, and those with surgical contraindications. There was concern that nonoperative treatment may lead to higher complication rates, including tendon rerupture [1]. Recently, those studies have undergone scrutiny, and there are many surgeons who believe that nonoperative treatment can produce similar patient outcomes while limiting the risks

of surgery. In this regard, the amount of tendinous gap between the two rupture tendon ends and the impact this distance has on patient outcomes have become an increasingly popular area of study for patients undergoing nonoperative management. In a prospective cohort study, Lawrence et al. evaluated 38 patients with acute (<2 weeks) Achilles tendon ruptures. They used dynamic ultrasound to both confirm the diagnosis and measure the tendon gap distance. Patients were treated with 8 weeks of sequential casting, from plantarflexion to neutral, followed by physical therapy. The outcome measures were dynamometric plantarflexion testing and the Achilles Tendon Total Rupture Score (ATRS). Patients were grouped into <10 mm gap or ≥10 mm gap cohorts. Patients in the ≥10 mm gap group demonstrated greater peak torque deficit compared to the <10 mm group. There was no difference in the ATRS [2]. This study promotes the idea of a 10 mm gap threshold and its potential impact on patient outcomes. Unfortunately, patients in this study were immobilized for 8 weeks; therefore, the impact of early mobilization was not evaluated. Another study by Hufner et al. looked retrospectively at the long-term results of Achilles tendon ruptures in patients treated nonoperatively with a functional rehab program. In their practice, patients were treated nonoperatively if they had <10 mm gap at neutral and were able to achieve complete apposition of the tendon edges with 20 degrees of plantarflexion. Patients had their gap

A. E. Hanselman (✉)
Department of Orthopaedic Surgery, Duke University, Durham, NC, USA
e-mail: andrew.hanselman@duke.edu

© The Author(s), under exclusive license to Springer Nature Switzerland AG 2023
S. B. Adams (ed.), *The Achilles Tendon*, https://doi.org/10.1007/978-3-031-45594-0_4

measured using ultrasound at the initial injury and then confirmed complete apposition again 2–5 days after injury. The study included 168 patients with a mean follow-up of 5.5 years. Patients reported 73.5% good/excellent subjective outcomes with only a 6.4% rerupture rate [3]. A prospective cohort study by Kotnis et al. used similar standards to divide patients into operative and nonoperative treatment groups. Using dynamic ultrasound at the time of injury, patients with an intertendinous gap of less than 5 mm were treated nonoperatively using a functional rehab protocol. Sixty-seven patients in the operative group and 58 in the nonoperative group were evaluated and showed no statistical difference in regard to the rerupture rate, chronic pain, numbness, wound infection, or deep vein thrombosis (DVT). No subjective outcomes were measured [4]. Using a similar threshold of 5 mm, Westin et al. retrospectively evaluated 45 patients who underwent either operative or nonoperative management of acute midsubstance Achilles tendon ruptures. All patients underwent ultrasound evaluation at the time of injury and were separated into three cohorts: ≤5 mm diastasis, >5 and ≤10 mm diastasis, and >10 mm diastasis. Of note, three out of four nonoperative patients in the >10 mm diastasis group had a rerupture. When comparing clinical and functional outcomes, patients treated nonoperatively in the ≤5 mm group had a higher mean ATRS and a higher mean heel raise height at 12 months compared to patients with >5 mm diastasis [5]. One of the more recent studies by Yassin et al. evaluated the size of the tendon gap in regard to patient-reported outcomes for patients treated nonoperatively with functional rehabilitation. Eighty-two patients were evaluated using dynamic ultrasound to measure the tendon gap in maximal plantarflexion and treated nonoperatively using a function rehabilitation protocol. Mean follow-up was 20 months, and they showed an inverse relationship between gap size and ATRS outcomes. Gaps >5 mm had a lower mean ATRS compared to gaps ≤5 mm. Gaps >10 mm had the lowest mean ATRS. The rerupture rate was 1.5% among all groups [6]. Overall, these studies may be helpful for surgeons treating acute Achilles ruptures conservatively by proposing a 5–10 mm tendon gap threshold as a marker for success.

Early Weight-Bearing

Historically, patients have been treated with prolonged immobilization and delayed weight-bearing (i.e., 6–8 weeks), regardless of operative or nonoperative treatment. Numerous studies have challenged these traditional weight-bearing limitations by evaluating their impact on patient outcomes and healing. Patel et al. retrospectively evaluated 52 patients after percutaneous Achilles tendon repair. Patients were treated with 2 weeks of non-weight-bearing in a cast, followed by immediate weight-bearing in a boot. Over the next 6 weeks, patients were weaned down from their heel wedges and transitioned into a flat regular shoe. At final follow-up, they reported only a 3.8% rate of wound dehiscence and no cases of rerupture [7]. Costa et al. performed a randomized controlled study comparing traditional non-weight-bearing to early weight-bearing protocols. Patients treated both operatively and nonoperatively were randomized into one of the two postop weight-bearing protocol groups. Patients were shown to have no difference in rerupture rate between the two groups; however, those in the early weight-bearing groups had improved "time to normal walking" rates and improved stair climbing ability [8]. In another study by Suchak et al., patients who underwent surgical repair for acute Achilles tendon ruptures were treated initially with non-weight-bearing for 2 weeks and then randomized to begin weight-bearing at 2 weeks or kept non-weight-bearing for another 4 weeks. The early weight-bearing group had improved functional outcomes at 6 weeks; however, that benefit showed no difference by 6 months. There were, however, no reruptures in either group [9]. Okoroha et al. performed a randomized controlled study evaluating tendon elongation between traditional and accelerated weight-bearing after undergoing acute Achilles rupture repair. Patients were randomized into either a traditional protocol (no weight-bearing until 6 weeks postop) or an accelerated protocol (graduated weight-bearing beginning at 2 weeks). Postoperative tendon elongation was measured using radiostereometric beads placed during surgery. Eighteen patients were included in the study, and they found that all patients had significant tendon lengthening (mean 15.9 mm) with no differences between the two groups. The greatest amount of lengthening occurred between 2 and 6 weeks and the least amount of lengthening between 6 and 12 weeks. There were no differences in ankle ROM or patient outcome scores (ATRS) [10]. Maempel et al. performed a single-center, randomized, nonblinded study evaluating 140 patients treated nonoperatively for acute Achilles tendon ruptures. Patients were allocated into one of two groups: non-weight-bearing in a cast, with a subsequent reduction in equinus, for 8 weeks after injury versus immediate full weight-bearing in a walking boot, with subsequent reduction in equinus, for 8 weeks. At 6 months follow-up, patients in the early weight-bearing group had statistically significantly improved Short Musculoskeletal Function Assessment (SFMA) dysfunction index, SMFA bother index, ATRS, and Foot and Ankle Questionnaire core score. There was no significant difference in rerupture, DVT, or return-to-work time. There was a higher rate of skin problems in the early weight-bearing group [11]. Brumann et al. conducted a systematic review of randomized controlled trials that evaluated patients with acute, isolated Achilles tendon rupture treated with operative repair. Three of the studies evaluated early weight-bearing. Patients treated with early weight-bearing had higher satisfaction scores, less use of rehabilitation resources, earlier return to preinjury activities, increased calf muscle strength, reduced muscle atrophy, and reduced tendon elongation. There was no difference in rerupture rate [12]. Costa et al. conducted a multicenter, randomized controlled study evaluating patients treated nonoperatively for acute Achilles tendon rupture. Patients were allocated to either a traditional plaster cast protocol (subsequent decrease in equinus casting until plantigrade with non-weight-bearing until plantigrade) or early weight-bearing protocol (immediate weight-bearing in boot walker with heel wedges with the subsequent removal of wedges). Both groups were removed from their immobilization at 8 weeks and started in therapy. Five hundred and twenty-seven patients were included in the analysis. At 9 months postinjury, there was no difference between groups in ATRS and no difference in rerupture rate, and the early weight-bearing group had a lower mean total health and personal social care cost [13]. A recent systematic study by Jamjoom reviewed 18 publications (either randomized controlled trials or prospective cohort studies) encompassing 1068 patients who underwent nonoperative treatment for acute Achilles tendon ruptures. In comparing early weight-bearing patients to late weight-bearing patients, the early weight-bearing patients had significantly lower rates of DVT, earlier return to work, and improved ATRS. There was no difference between patients in regard to rerupture rate or return to sport [14].

Early Motion

Similar to the use of traditional weight-bearing restrictions after injury, strict immobilization has also been used to promote the healing of the ruptured tendon ends, regardless of the treatment type. Fortunately, this treatment mentality has also been challenged recently by numerous studies in the literature, although it can be difficult to evaluate studies that specifically focus on motion while controlling for weight-bearing. Kangas et al. evaluated 50 patients treated with operative management of acute ruptures and randomized them into two groups. In the control group, patients were immobilized postoperatively in a cast for 6 weeks. In the study group, patients were placed into a brace that allowed plantarflexion motion for the first 6 weeks. Both groups were allowed to commence weight-bearing at 3 weeks. The primary outcome measure was tendon elongation using radiographic markers. At the final follow-up (mean 60 weeks), there was no difference in tendon elongation between the two groups with a trend toward less elongation in the early motion group [15]. Barfod et al. conducted a randomized controlled study evaluating the benefit of early controlled motion (ECM) in patients treated nonoperatively for acute Achilles tendon ruptures. For both groups, patients were initially placed in a plantarflexed cast for the first 2 weeks. After 2 weeks, all patients were placed into a walking boot with a 1.5 cm heel lift, and full weight-bearing was allowed. In the control group, patients were instructed to remain in the boot at all times. In the study group, patients were instructed to perform daily ankle range of motion (ROM) exercises five times per day from postinjury weeks 3 to 8. At the end of week 8, patients in both groups were weaned from the boot and enrolled in a similar rehabilitation protocol. One hundred and thirty patients were included in the study. At 1-year follow-up, there was no difference in ATRS, no difference in heel-rise work test (HRW), no difference in rerupture rate, and no difference in tendon elongation [16]. Using the same data, the previous authors also compared the risk of DVT between the two groups. Overall, they had a 47.7% deep vein thrombosis rate with no difference between the ECM group and the immobilization group [17]. In the systematic review cited earlier by Jamjoom, nonoperative patients were also compared in regard to early controlled range of motion. The ECM group had lower rates of rerupture, earlier return to work, and improved ATRS. There was no difference in DVT or return to sport [14].

Surgical Incision Location

Surgical incision location is another debated topic, with the two most common approaches being a posterior midline approach versus a posteromedial approach. The superficial location of the Achilles tendon makes surgeons concerned about its susceptibility to wound healing complications compared to other orthopedic issues. Yepes et al. performed a classic cadaveric study using angiography to map out the angiosomes of the posterior soft tissues of the heel. They identified three main vascular zones: medial, lateral, and posterior. The medial zone had the richest blood supply, the lateral zone was considered "good" but less robust than the medial zone, and the posterior zone showed the poorest blood supply. They concluded that medial-based or lateral-based incisions may have better chances of adequate wound healing, given the increased blood supply [18]. In contrast, Highlander et al. performed a systematic review of 38 studies evaluating the surgical approach for the Achilles tendon. Specifically, they evaluated studies that involved a posterior midline incision and studies involving a posteromedial incision. They found that the wound complication rate among both groups was 8.2%. There was no significant difference between the posterior midline and posteromedial approaches (7.0% and 8.3%, respectively). They determined that comorbidities, such as age, delayed surgical intervention, prior surgery, female sex, and postoperative protocols, had a more substantial impact on wound complications than the location of the incision [19]. Likewise, Hippensteel et al. retrospectively evaluated 125 patients who underwent Achilles tendon surgery using either a longitudinal posterior midline incision, a longitudinal posteromedial incision, or an L-shaped posteromedial incision. Surgeries for both acute rupture repairs and Achilles tendinopathy were included. According to the authors, L-shaped incision was only used for certain patients undergoing Achilles tendinopathy based on surgeon preference. The average follow-up was 10.3 months, and there were no significant differences in regard to sural nerve injury, superficial infection, or deep wound infection. There was, however, a significantly higher rate of wound complications in the posteromedial group when an L-shaped incision was used for Achilles tendinopathy debridement [20].

Standard Open Repair Versus Minimally Invasive Repair

Another area of debate is the type of surgical technique when treating acute midsubstance Achilles ruptures operatively. Advocates of a standard open repair report better visualization of the zone of injury, which allows for adequate debridement of the tendon ends and the ability to provide secure fixation while avoiding injury to the sural nerve. Advocates of less-invasive techniques report a lower rate of wound complications and the ability to expedite the rehabilitation process. For the purpose of this chapter, these less-invasive techniques will encompass percutaneous, minimally invasive, and limited-open repairs.

In regard to wound complications, Bruggeman et al., in 2004, retrospectively reviewed 164 patients after undergoing standard open Achilles tendon repair. Their overall wound complication rate was 10.4%, higher than most orthopedic surgeries. They also showed that there was a significantly higher rate of complications among tobacco users, chronic steroid users, and female patients [21]. Likewise, van Maele et al. retrospectively evaluated 105 patients undergoing standard open acute Achilles tendon rupture repair and demonstrated a high wound healing complication rate of 28% [22]. Other studies in the literature have confirmed similar findings of elevated wound healing complications in standard open Achilles tendon repairs compared to other orthopedic procedures. As a result, percutaneous and minimally invasive techniques have been developed, with their popularity increasing. Ma and Griffith, in 1977, were one of the first to report their results using a percutaneous technique. They had 18 patients who underwent surgical intervention with no reported wound complications [23]. Stavenuiter et al. retrospectively evaluated postoperative complications in 615 patients who underwent acute Achilles tendon rupture repair utilizing either a standard open repair or a minimally invasive repair. Overall, the wound complication rate between both groups was 5.2%; however, there was no statistical difference between the two techniques [24]. Recently, Akoh et al. reported on a novel limited open Achilles tendon repair without the use of an instrumented guide. Retrospectively, the evaluated 33 patients demonstrated no wound complications at a median follow-up of 3.7 years [25]. In 2015, Hsu et al. retrospectively compared 270 patients who underwent acute Achilles tendon rupture repair utilizing either open repair (5–8 cm

posteromedial incision with FiberWire in a Krackow fashion) or percutaneous repair (2 cm transverse incision with the Arthrex PARS system). They reported an overall superficial wound dehiscence rate of 3.7% and a superficial wound infection rate of 1.1%, with no statistical difference between groups [26].

In addition to wound complications, several larger studies have compared the different surgical techniques in regard to clinical outcomes, rerupture rates, and sural nerve injuries. In 2014, Del Buono et al. performed a systematic review of 12 studies (six retrospective studies, five randomized controlled studies, and one prospective cohort study) comparing standard open and minimally invasive techniques. A total of 781 patients were included in the review, with 375 undergoing standard open repair and 406 undergoing minimally invasive surgery. Ankle range of motion was better in the minimally invasive group in two studies but similar in seven other studies. Gait analysis, AOFAS hindfoot scores, and calf circumference were similar among most studies. There was a trend toward lower complication rates in the minimally invasive group in regard to rerupture, infection, wound complications, and scarring. There was, however, a higher rate of nerve injury in the minimally invasive group [27]. In 2018, Grassi et al. performed a meta-analysis of eight studies comparing minimally invasive repair to standard open repair. One-hundred and eighty-two patients were included in the minimally invasive group and 176 in the standard open group. They demonstrated a significantly decreased risk ratio for both overall complications and wound infection in the minimally invasive group. They demonstrated no significant differences between the groups in regard to rerupture, sural nerve injury, return to preinjury activity level, return-to-work time, and ankle range of motion [28]. In 2019, Wu et al. performed a meta-analysis of randomized controlled trials that evaluated different management methods for acute Achilles tendon ruptures. Twenty-nine studies were included in the analysis with 2060 patients separated into one of six groups: nonsurgical with accelerated rehab (NS + AR), minimally invasive with accelerated rehab (MIS

+ AR), standard open with accelerated rehab (OS + AR), nonsurgical with early immobilization (NS + EI), minimally invasive with early immobilization (MIS + EI), or standard open with early immobilization (OS + EI). The authors found that minimally invasive surgical treatment with accelerated rehab had the lowest risk of DVT, deep infection, and tendon rerupture [29]. In 2021, Gatz et al. performed a meta-analysis comparing minimally invasive and standard open techniques for acute Achilles tendon ruptures. Twenty-five articles were included in the study, with 1055 open procedures and 1168 minimally invasive procedures compared. There was no statistical difference in rerupture rate between the two groups. The open group had a lower rate of sural nerve palsy. The minimally invasive group had a lower rate of postoperative wound necrosis and scarring, as well as lower rates of superficial and deep infections [30].

Nonoperative Versus Operative Repair

Perhaps the most controversial debate when discussing the best treatment for acute Achilles tendon ruptures is between the use of operative and nonoperative management. In 2005, Khan et al. published a meta-analysis of 12 randomized controlled trials involving 800 patients. Comparing conservative treatment to open treatment, open repair demonstrated a reduced rerupture rate (3.5% to 12.6%), higher overall complications (34.1% to 2.7%), and higher wound infection (4.0% to 0%). Upon further analysis, the rerupture rate was lower and more comparable to open repair when nonoperative management was stratified into functional rehab (2.4%) versus prolonged immobilization (12.2%). The risk of overall complications and wound infections in the operative group was also lower when stratified into standard open (26.1% and 19.6%, respectively) versus minimally invasive repair (8.3% and 0%, respectively) [1]. In 2010, Willits et al. performed a prospective randomized study comparing surgical versus conservative management. All patients underwent accelerated rehabilitation with early weight-bearing and early range of motion. One hundred and forty-four patients were included in the study. At final follow-up, there was no difference between groups in regard to rerupture rate, strength, range of motion, calf circumference, or functional outcome scores. There were more soft-tissue complications in the operative group [31]. In 2012, a meta-analysis of ten level 1 studies was performed comparing both treatment options. They demonstrated equal rerupture rates if early range of motion was employed and increased risk of overall complications with surgery; however, surgical patients had an earlier return to work (20 days earlier). There was no statistical difference in calf circumference, strength, or functional outcomes [32]. In 2016, Lantto et al. performed a prospective randomized trial comparing operative and nonoperative treatment in regard to clinical outcomes and calf muscle strength recovery. Surgery was an open repair, and both groups underwent identical functional rehabilitation. Sixty patients were included in the study. At 18-month follow-up, there was no difference in the Achilles tendon performance score between the groups. The surgical group had quicker and better recovery of muscle strength at 6 months and 18 months [33]. Recently, in 2019, Wu et al. performed a systematic review and network meta-analysis of 2060 patients included in 29 randomized controlled trials evaluating patients with acute Achilles tendon ruptures treated operatively or nonoperatively. Specifically, they looked at major complication rates, including tendon rerupture, deep infection, and DVT. Overall, they found the major complication rate after acute Achilles tendon injury to be 9.13%. The mean incidence of rerupture was 5%, deep infection was 1.5%, and DVT was 2.67%. The highest risk of major complications was in the nonoperative patients treated with early immobilization. The group with the best chance to minimize major complications were those treated with minimally invasive surgical techniques and accelerated rehab [29].

Return to Play for Higher-Level Athletes

Acute Achilles tendon ruptures often occur during sporting activities with the majority of lower-level athletes returning to their desired preinjury activity level. Unfortunately, the likelihood of return for higher-level athletes is less predictable and often takes longer than the general population. Several studies in the past 10 years have evaluated these types of athletes. Lerch et al. retrospectively evaluated 89 athletes treated nonoperatively for acute Achilles tendon ruptures. All patients were treated with a functional rehab protocol. At a mean follow-up of 34 months, 70% of all patients had returned to their previous sports activity level. Patients grouped into the lower-activity cohort had a 91% return rate, whereas patients in the higher-activity cohort had a 67% return rate [34]. Wise et al. retrospectively evaluated NCAA defensive football players who underwent surgical repair for acute Achilles tendon ruptures in regard to return to play. Fifty-seven athletes were included in the study, and they demonstrated a high rate of return to play (92.5%); however, there was a low rate of these athletes going on to participate in the NFL combine (5.0%) and only 7.5% competed in at least one NFL game. These rates were low when compared to matched controls (20.0% and 21.3%, respectively) [35]. Other studies have demonstrated lower rates of return for professional athletes. Grassi et al. retrospectively evaluated 118 professional soccer players after acute Achilles tendon rupture repairs. Ninety-six percent of athletes returned to unrestricted practice (average 7 months) and competition (average 9 months); however, 18% did not return to their same preinjury level of play. Age >30 years old was a risk factor [36]. In 2017, Trofa et al. performed a retrospective cohort study looking at athletes from four major sports leagues (NBA, NFL, MLB, and NHL) who underwent surgical repair of an acute Achilles rupture. Sixty-two athletes were included in the study, with only 69.4% of patients able to return to play. At 1-year postinjury, those athletes who returned to play demonstrated a significantly lower rate of games played, decreased playing time, and worse statistical performance compared to matched controls. There was no difference between these groups at 2 years postinjury [37]. Similar findings of return-to-play rates have been reported by Parekh et al. (68% among NFL players), Yang et al. (61.3% among NFL players), and Amin (61% among NBA players) [38–40]. A recent systematic review by Johns et al. evaluated Achilles tendon injuries in professional athletes in regard to return-to-play, performance, and career outcomes. Fifteen studies were included in the analysis, resulting in only a 76% return to sport at a mean time of 11 months following the injury. Those athletes who returned to play showed a decrease in performance (player efficiency ratings, power ratings, sport-specific statistics, and position-specific statistics) compared to noninjured controls. They also reported lower return-to-play rates with Achilles injuries compared to anterior cruciate ligament (ACL) injuries, meniscal tears, and ankle fractures [41].

Consensus Statements

In 2010, the American Academy of Orthopaedic Surgeons (AAOS) published its clinical practice guidelines for acute Achilles tendon ruptures. There was a strong consensus in regard to using a proper physical exam for diagnosis (positive Thompson test, decreased plantarflexion strength, palpable gap, increased passive ankle range of motion) and the use of caution with operative management in high-risk patients. There was moderate consensus in regard to early (≤2 weeks) postoperative protected weight-bearing after surgery and the use of a protective device that allows mobilization by 2–4 weeks postoperatively. There was a weak consensus in regard to nonoperative management being a treatment option for all patients, operative treatment being an option for all patients, open/limited open/percutaneous operative techniques being options for treating patients, and the notion that all patients who play sports will return in 3–6 months. Finally, there was no conclusive recommendation in regard to nonoperative patients using functional bracing, operative patients undergoing preoperative immobilization or restricted weight-bearing, the use of allograft or biological adjuncts in operative management, the use of antithrombotic treatment, postoperative physiotherapy use, timing on return to activities of daily living, and timing for nonoperative patients to return to athletic activity [42].

In 2021, the American College of Foot and Ankle Surgeons (ACFAS) released its clinical practice statement in regard to acute Achilles tendon rupture. The census group determined that the following recommendations were "appropriate": taking special consideration and caution for high-risk patients, treating acute partial ruptures nonoperatively, using early weight-bearing and progressive physical therapy regardless of treatment option, and that the use of either posteromedial or posterior midline incisions were appropriate for surgical treatment. The group found the following statements "inappropriate": acute ruptures should always be treated with surgery, advanced imaging should routinely be used, allograft/autograft/xenograft augmentation improves functional outcomes in surgical patients, percutaneous methods have improved functional outcomes compared to traditional open repair, and percutaneous repair results in lower rerupture rate compared to traditional open repair. The census group found the following statements "neither appropriate nor inappropriate": surgical repair should occur within 10 days of injury, percutaneous repair has a lower rate of wound dehiscence and infection, percutaneous repair has increased risk of neurovascular injury, and ischemia in the watershed region of the Achilles tendon is a strong factor in the etiology of the Achilles tendon rupture [43].

Conclusion

The proper treatment of acute midsubstance Achilles tendon ruptures remains a heavily debated topic. Although there are no clear-cut guidelines for optimal outcomes with these patients, there are some trends in the recent literature that foot and ankle surgeons should be aware of when providing management of these injuries.

First, the literature seems to support the use of some form of functional rehabilitation, often consisting of early weight-bearing and early range of motion. Second, if managing these patients conservatively, there may be benefit to early monitoring of the tendon ends with ultrasound and a potential threshold of <5–10 mm needed for successful outcomes. Third, the two most common surgical incision locations, posterior midline and posteromedial, are both often used by surgeons and likely produce similar outcomes in regard to wound healing and infection rates. Fourth, if deciding to perform operative management, more surgeons are trending toward the use of less -invasive and minimally invasive techniques. These techniques have evolved over the years and are often safe in regard to rerupture rates and overall complications. The standard open technique is still a viable option but should be used with caution in patients with increased risks of wound healing complications. Fifth, Achilles tendon injuries are common in athletes, and it is important to counsel your high-level athletes about the lower rate of return to play compared to other common orthopedic injuries. Finally, the debate between operative and nonoperative treatment remains unanswered. Early reports of higher rerupture rates with conservative management have been minimized with the use of functional rehabilitation; however, some believe that the benefit of surgical management may lie within the earlier return to activities/sport, earlier return of muscular function, and improved early performance. Overall, continued research into the various treatment options for acute Achilles tendon ruptures is still needed.

References

1. Khan RJ, Fick D, Keogh A, Crawford J, Brammar T, Parker M. Treatment of acute Achilles tendon ruptures: a meta-analysis of randomized, controlled trials. J Bone Joint Surg Am. 2005;87(10):2202–10. https://doi.org/10.2106/jbjs.d.03049.
2. Lawrence JE, Nasr P, Fountain DM, Berman L, Robinson AH. Functional outcomes of conservatively managed acute ruptures of the Achilles tendon. Bone Joint J. 2017;99(1):87–93. https://doi.org/10.1302/0301-620X.99B1.BJJ-2016-0452.r1.

3. Hufner TM, Brandes DB, Thermann H, Richter M, Knobloch K, Krettek C. Long-term results after functional nonoperative treatment of Achilles tendon rupture. Foot Ankle Int. 2006;27(3):167–71. https://doi.org/10.1177/107110070602700302.

4. Kotnis R, Davis S, Handley R, Willett K, Ostlere S. Dynamic ultrasound as a selection tool for reducing Achilles tendon reruptures. Am J Sports Med. 2006;34(9):1395–400. https://doi.org/10.1177/0363546506288678.

5. Westin O, Helander KN, Silbernagel KG, Moller M, Kalebo P, Karlsson J. Acute ultrasonography investigation to predict reruptures and outcomes in patients with an Achilles tendon rupture. Orthop J Sports Med. 2016;4(10):1–7. https://doi.org/10.1177/2325967116667920.

6. Yassin M, Myatt R, Thomas W, Gupta V, Hoque T, Mahadevan D. Does the size of tendon gap affect patient-reported outcome following Achilles tendon rupture treated with functional rehabilitation. Bone Joint J. 2020;102(11):1535–41. https://doi.org/10.1302/0301-620X.102B11.BJJ-2020-0908.R1.

7. Patel VC, Lozano-Calderon S, McWilliam J. Immediate weightbearing after modified percutaneous Achilles tendon repair. Foot Ankle Int. 2012;33(12):1093–7. https://doi.org/10.3113/fai.2012.1093.

8. Costa ML, MacMillan K, Halliday D, Chester R, Shepstone L, Robinson A, et al. Randomised controlled trials of immediate weight-bearing mobilization for rupture of the tendo Achillis. J Bone Joint Surg Br. 2006;88(1):69–77. https://doi.org/10.1302/0301-620X.88B1.16549.

9. Suchak AA, Bostick GP, Beaupre LA, Durand DC, Jomha N. The influence of early weight-bearing compared to non-weight-bearing after surgical repair of the Achilles tendon. J Bone Joint Surg Am. 2008;90(9):1876–83. https://doi.org/10.2106/JBJS.G.01242.

10. Okoroha KR, Ussef N, Jildeh TF, Khalil LS, Hasan L, Bench C, et al. Comparison of tendon lengthening with traditional versus accelerated rehabilitation after Achilles tendon repair: a prospective randomized controlled trial. Am J Sports Med. 2020;48(7):1720–6. https://doi.org/10.1177/0363546520909389.

11. Maempel JF, Clement ND, Duckworth AD, Keenan OJ, White TO, Biant LC. A randomized controlled trial comparing traditional plaster cast rehabilitation with functional walking boot rehabilitation for acute Achilles tendon ruptures. Am J Sports Med. 2020;48(11):2755–64. https://doi.org/10.1177/0363546520944905.

12. Bruman M, Baumbach SF, Mutschler W, Polzer H. Accelerated rehabilitation following Achilles tendon repair after acute rupture: development of an evidence-based treatment protocol. Injury. 2014;45(11):1782–90. https://doi.org/10.1016/j.injury.2014.06.022.

13. Costa ML, Achten J, Marian IR, Dutton SJ, Lamb SE, Ollivere B, et al. Plaster cast versus functional brace for non-surgical treatment of Achilles tendon rupture (UKSTAR): a multicentre randomised controlled trail and economic evaluation. Lancet. 2020;395(10222):441–8. https://doi.org/10.1016/S0140-6736(19)32942-3.

14. Jamjoom BA. The influence of early weightbearing, controlled motion, and timing of orthosis removal on nonoperative management of Achilles tendon rupture: a systematic review. J Foot Ankle Surg. 2021;5:1067–2516. https://doi.org/10.1053/j.jfas.2020.04.024.

15. Kangas J, Pajala A, Ohtonen P, Leppilahti J. Achilles tendon elongation after rupture repair: a randomized comparison of 2 postoperative regimens. Am J Sports Med. 2007;35(1):59–64. https://doi.org/10.1177/0363546506293255.

16. Barfod KW, Hansen MS, Holmich P, Kristensen MT, Troelsen A. Efficacy of early controlled motion of the ankle compared with immobilization in non-operative treatment of patients with an acute Achilles tendon rupture: an assessor-blinded, randomized controlled trial. Br J Sports Med. 2020;54(12):719–24. https://doi.org/10.1136/bjsports-2019-100709.

17. Barfod KW, Nielsen EG, Olsen BH, Vinicoff PG, Troelsen A, Holmich P. Risk of deep vein thrombosis after acute Achilles tendon rupture: a secondary analysis of a randomized controlled trial comparing early controlled motion of the ankle versus immobilization. Orthop J Sports Med. 2020;8(4):2325967120915909. https://doi.org/10.1177/2325967120915909.

18. Yepes H, Tang M, Geddes C, Glazebrook M, Morris SF, Stanish WD. Digital vascular mapping of the integument about the Achilles tendon. J Bone Joint Surg Am. 2010;92(5):1215–20. https://doi.org/10.2106/JBJS.00743.

19. Highlander P, Greenhagen RM. Wound complications with posterior midline and posterior medial leg incisions: a systematic review. Foot Ankle Spec. 2011;4(6):361–9. https://doi.org/10.1177/1938640011418488.

20. Hippensteel KJ, Johnson J, McCormick J, Klein S. A comparison of wound complications with surgical treatment of Achilles tendon conditions using 2 surgical approaches. FAO. 2019;4(1):1–6. https://doi.org/10.1177/2473011418814004.

21. Bruggeman NB, Turner NS, Dahm DL, Voll AE, Hoskin TL, Jacofsky DJ, et al. Wound complications after open Achilles tendon repair: an analysis of risk factors. Clin Orthop Relat Res. 2004;427:63–6. https://doi.org/10.1097/01.blo.0000144475.05543.e7.

22. Van Maele M, Misselyn D, Metsemakers WJ, Sermon A, Nijs S, Hoekstra H. Is open acute Achilles tendon rupture still justified? A single center experience and critical appraisal of the literature. Injury. 2018;49(10):1947–52. https://doi.org/10.1016/j.injury.2018.08.012.

23. Ma GW, Griffith TG. Percutaneous repair of acute closed ruptured Achilles tendon: a new technique. Clin Orthop Relat Res. 1977;128:247–55. PMID: 340096.

24. Stavenuiter XJ, Lubberts B, Prince RM, Johnson AH, DiGiovanni CW, Guss D. Postoperative complications following repair of acute Achilles tendon rupture. Foot Ankle Int. 2019;40(6):679–86. https://doi.org/10.1177/1071100719831371.

25. Akoh CC, Fletcher A, Sharma A, Parekh S. Clinical outcomes and complications following limited open Achilles repair without an instrumented guide. Foot Ankle Int. 2021;42(3):294–304. https://doi.org/10.1177/1071100720962493.

26. Hsu AR, Jones CP, Cohen BE, Davis WH, Ellington JK, Anderson RB. Clinical outcomes and complications of percutaneous Achilles repair system versus open technique for acute Achilles tendon ruptures. Foot Ankle Int. 2015;36(11):1279–86. https://doi.org/10.1177/1071100715589632.

27. Del Buono A, Volpin A, Maffulli N. Minimally invasive versus open surgery for acute Achilles tendon rupture: a systematic review. Br Med Bull. 2014;109:45–54. https://doi.org/10.1093/bmb/ldt029.

28. Grassi A, Amendola A, Samuelsson K, Svantesson E, Romagnoli M, Bondi A, et al. Minimally invasive versus open repair for acute Achilles tendon rupture: meta-analysis showing reduced complications, with similar outcomes, after minimally invasive surgery. J Bone Joint Surg Am. 2018;100(22):1969–81. https://doi.org/10.2106/JBJS.17.01364.

29. Wu Y, Mu Y, Yin L, Wang Z, Liu W, Wan H. Complications in management of acute Achilles tendon rupture: a systematic review and network meta-analysis of 2060 patients. Am J Sports Med. 2019;47(9):2251–60. https://doi.org/10.1177/0363546518824601.

30. Gatz M, Driessen A, Eschweiler J, Tingart M, Migliorini F. Open versus minimally-invasive surgery for Achilles tendon rupture: a meta-analysis study. Arch Orthop Trauma Surg. 2021;141(3):383–401. https://doi.org/10.1007/s00402-020-03437-z.

31. Willits K, Amendola A, Bryant D, Mohtadi NG, Giffin JR, Folwer P, et al. Operative versus nonoperative treatment of acute Achilles tendon ruptures: a multicenter randomized trial using accelerated functional rehabilitation. J Bone Joint Surg Am. 2010;92(17):2767–75. https://doi.org/10.2106/jbjs.i.01401.

32. Soroceanu A, Sidhwa F, Aarabi S, Kaufman A, Glazebrook M. Surgical versus nonsurgical treatment of acute Achilles tendon rupture: a meta-analysis of randomized trials. J Bone Joint Surg Am. 2012;94(23):2136–43. https://doi.org/10.2106/jbjs.k.00917.

33. Lantto I, Heikkinen J, Flinkkila T, Ohtonen P, Siira P, Laine V, et al. A prospective randomized trial comparing surgical and nonsurgical treatments of acute Achilles tendon ruptures. Am J Sports Med. 2016;44(9):2406–14. https://doi.org/10.1177/0363546516651060.

34. Lerch TD, Schwinghammer A, Schmaranzer F, Anwander H, Ecker TM, Schmid T, et al. Return to sport and patient satisfaction at 5-year follow-up after nonoperative treatment for acute Achilles tendon rupture. Foot Ankle Int. 2020;41(7):784–92. https://doi.org/10.1177/1071100720919029.

35. Wise PM, King JL, Stauch CM, Walley KC, Aynardi MC, Gallo RA. Outcomes of NCAA defensive football players following Achilles tendon repair. Foot Ankle Int. 2020;41(4):398–402. https://doi.org/10.1177/1071100719899072.

36. Grassi A, Rossi G, D'Hooghe P, Aujla R, Mosca M, Samuelsson K, et al. Eight-two per cent male professional football (soccer) players return to play at the previous level two seasons after Achilles tendon rupture treated with surgical repair. Br J Sports Med. 2020;54(8):480–6. https://doi.org/10.1136/bjsports-2019-100556.

37. Trofa DP, Miller JC, Jang ES, Woode DR, Greisberg JK, Vosseller JT. Professional athletes' return to play and performance after operative repair of an Achilles tendon rupture. Am J Sports Med. 2017;45(12):2864–71. https://doi.org/10.1177/0363546517713001.

38. Parekh SG, Wray WH, Brimmo O, Sennett BJ, Wapner KL. Epidemiology and outcomes of Achilles tendon ruptures in the National Football League. Foot Ankle Spec. 2009;2(6):283–6. https://doi.org/10.1177/1938640009351138.

39. Yang J, Hodax JD, Machan JT, Krill MK, Lemme NJ, Durand WM, et al. Factors affecting return to play after primary Achilles tendon tear: a cohort of NFL players. Orthop J Sports Med. 2019;7(3):1–8. https://doi.org/10.1177/2325967119830139.

40. Amin NH, Old AB, Tabb LP, Garg R, Toossi N, Cerynik DL. Performance outcomes after repair of complete Achilles tendon ruptures in national basketball association players. Am J Sports Med. 2013;41(8):1864–8. https://doi.org/10.1177/0363546513490659.

41. Johns W, Walley KC, Seedat R, Thordarson DB, Jackson B, Gonzalez T. Career outlook and performance of professional athletes after Achilles tendon rupture: a systematic review. Foot Ankle Int. 2021;42(4):495–509. https://doi.org/10.1177/1071100720969633.

42. Chiodo CP, Glazebrook M, Bluman EM, Cohen BE, Femino JE, Giza E, et al. American Academy of Orthopaedic Surgeons clinical practice guideline on treatment of Achilles tendon rupture. J Bone Joint Surg Am. 2010;92(14):2466–8. PMID: 20962199.

43. Naldo J, Agnew P, Brucato M, Dayton P, Shane A. ACFAS clinical consensus statement: acute Achilles tendon pathology. J Foot Ankle Surg. 2021;60(1):93–101. https://doi.org/10.1053/j.jfas.2020.02.006.

Nonoperative Treatment of Acute Achilles Tendon Rupture

Mark Glazebrook

Introduction

Rupture of the Achilles tendon (Fig. 5.1) is one of the most common sports-related injuries in the adult population [1]. This is a catastrophic event that most often occurs subcutaneously without skin disruption when forces are placed on the Achilles that exceed its tensile limits [2] or from a penetrating injury. The diagnosis of an acute Achilles tendon rupture is made with careful history, physical examination, and a review of diagnostic imaging if necessary. It is important to understand that the rupture site of the Achilles can occur at various locations along the course of the gastrocnemius-Achilles tendon complex, and the location of the rupture will dictate treatment options.

The operative treatment of an Achilles tendon rupture includes open, minimally invasive, and percutaneous techniques, all involving the placement of sutures, which provide extra protection from elongation and rupture during the early phases of the healing process at the cost of the disruption of blood supply and increased complication rates [3, 4].

The nonoperative treatment of Achilles tendon ruptures with well-supervised functional rehabilitation protocols (Table 5.1) in compliant patients have been shown to provide a similar outcome to operative treatment [3]. The benefits include no further disruption of blood supply at the healing site and decreased rates of surgical complications. The choice of treatment should be made by the patient after consultation with an orthopedic surgeon, who uses current evidence-based medicine techniques to inform the patient of the risks and benefits of both operative and nonoperative treatment options in an unbiased fashion.

Last, regardless of the treatment options chosen, it is important for the patient to have close supervision by an orthopedic surgeon, who can diagnose and treat the complications of both operative and nonoperative treatment.

M. Glazebrook (✉)
Division of Orthopedic Surgery, Department of
Surgery, Dalhousie University, Halifax, NS, Canada

Fig. 5.1 Complete midsubstance rupture of
the Achilles tendon

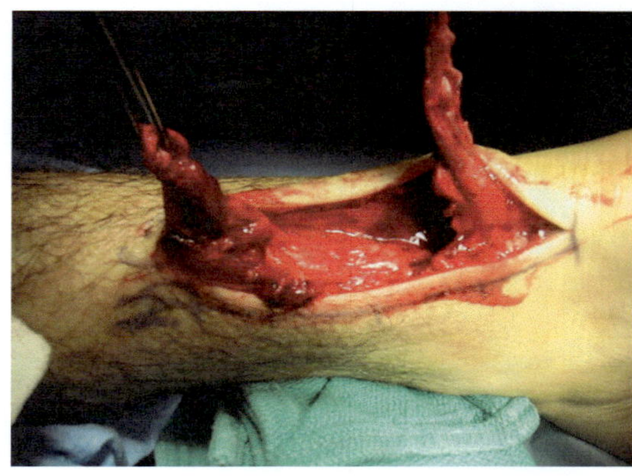

Table 5.1 Glazebrook/Rubinger Achilles protocol for nonoperative treatment (GAPNOT)

Time period	Protocol
0–2 weeks	• Plaster cast with ankle plantarflexed to approx. 20 degrees; non-weight-bearing with crutches.
2–4 weeks	• *Achilles-specific* (or other) walking boot with 40-degree plantarflexed heel lifts. • Protected weight-bearing with crutches: 　　– Week 2–3: 25%. 　　– Week 3–4: 50%. 　　– Week 4–5: 75%. 　　– Week 5–6: 100%. • Active plantar- and dorsiflexion range of motion exercises to neutral, inversion/eversion in slight plantarflexion. • Modalities to control swelling (US, IFC with ice, acupuncture, light/laser therapy). • EMS to calf musculature with seated heel raises when tolerated. • Patients being seen two to three times per week depending on availability and the degree of pain and swelling in the foot and ankle. • Knee/hip exercises with no ankle involvement, e.g., leg lifts from sitting, prone, or side-lying. • Non-weight-bearing fitness/cardio work, e.g., biking with one leg (with boot walker on), deep water running (usually not started till 3–4-week point). • Hydrotherapy if available (within motion and weight-bearing limitations). • Emphasize the need of the patient to use pain as a guideline. If in pain, back off activities and weight-bearing.
4–6 weeks	• Continue weight-bearing as tolerated. • Continue the 2–4-week protocol. • Progress EMS to calf with lying calf raises on shuttle with no resistance as tolerated around weeks 5–6. **Please ensure that the ankle does not go past neutral while doing exercises**. • Continue with physiotherapy two to three times per week. • Emphasize patient doing non-weight-bearing cardio activities as tolerated with the boot walker on.
6–8 weeks	• Continue physiotherapy two times a week. • Continue with modalities for swelling as needed. • Continue with EMS on the calf with strengthening exercises. **Do not go past the neutral ankle position**. • Remove heel lifts in stages dependent on Achilles length. Remove one lift daily as tolerated. Always leave one to two lifts to represent a regular shoe lift, depending on the boot design. • Weight-bearing as tolerated, usually 100% weight-bearing in boot walker now. • Graduated resistance exercises (open and closed kinetic chain as well as functional activities)—start with resisted tubing exercises. • **With weighted-resisted exercises, do not go past the neutral ankle position**. • Gait retraining now with 100% weight-bearing. • Fitness/cardio to include weight-bearing as tolerated, e.g., biking. • Hydrotherapy.

Table 5.1 (continued)

Time period	Protocol
8–12 weeks	**Ensure the patient understands that the tendon is still very vulnerable and that patients need to be diligent with activities of ADL and exercises. Any sudden loading of the Achilles (e.g., trip, step up stairs, etc.) may result in a rerupture.** • Wean off boot (usually over a 2–5-day process—varies per patient), at night as well. • Wear an Achilles compression ankle brace to provide extra stability and swelling control once the boot walker is removed. • Return to crutches/cane as necessary and gradually wean off. Have the patient always wear shoes, limiting time in bare/sock feet. • Continue to progress range of motion, strength, and proprioception exercises. • Add exercises such as stationary bicycle, elliptical, and walking on the treadmill as the patient tolerates. • Add wobble board activities—progress from seated to supported standing to standing as tolerated. • Add calf stretches in standing (gently). **Do not allow the ankle to go past the neutral position**. • Add double heel raises and progress to single heel raises when tolerated. **Do not allow the ankle to go past the neutral position.** • Continue physiotherapy one to two times per week depending on how independent the patient is at performing exercises at home and their access to the appropriate home excercise equipment.
12–16 weeks	• Continue to progress range of motion, strength, and proprioception exercises. • Retrain strength, power, and endurance. Ensure the patient understands that the tendon is still very vulnerable and that patients need to be diligent with activities of ADL and exercises. Avoid lunges, squats, etc. as these places excessive stretch on the tendon.
16+ weeks	• Increase dynamic weight-bearing exercise, including sports-specific retaining, i.e., skipping, jogging, or weight training.
6–9 months	• Return to normal sporting activities that do not involve contact or sprinting, cutting jumping, etc. if the patient has regained 80% strength.
12 months	• Return to sports that involve running/jumping as directed by the medical team and tolerated if the patient has regained 100% strength.

Diagnosis of Achilles Tendon Rupture

The diagnosis of an acute Achilles tendon rupture is made with careful history, physical examination, and a review of diagnostic imaging. When taking the history, it is important to establish the circumstances of the event that caused the injury. Specifically, it is important to know if the rupture was a subcutaneous rupture, meaning the tendon failed without a penetrating injury to the skin. Laceration injuries, such as that could occur with a hockey skate blade, will sharply divide the tendon and surrounding structures, resulting in recoil of the tendon ends. Plantarflexion of the foot may not reoppose the tendon ends, preventing nonoperative treatment. With a subcutaneous rupture, the magnitude of the force may be variable and related to a preexisting disease. A large force that is typical of a noncontact rupture may result from an eccentric contraction with the tendon elongated because of the foot placed in a dorsiflexed position. Tendon rupture may also result from a large traumatic force such as a fall from a height. Last, tendon rupture may result from a relatively low force if there is preexisting tendon disease [5, 6]. Regardless of the magnitude of the force required to cause a subcutaneous rupture, the end result is usually a tendon that is severely traumatized with a resultant trauma zone where the tendon ends are disrupted, contused, and frayed, like that seen when a rope fails. This failure of the Achilles tendon leads patients to often describe a sudden snap, acute severe pain localized to the rupture site, and often difficulty with weight-bearing activities. Last, if you are not the initial treating physician, it is very important to understand the timing of the patient's first treatment. Patients who present for treatment delayed without immobilization in the plantarflexed position and weight-bearing may not be appropriate for nonoperative treatment.

The physical examination is best done with the patient in the prone position and the feet hanging over the end of the bed. The key physical exam features that will confirm an acute Achilles tendon rupture include a palpable gap (Fig. 5.2), a lack of plantarflexion response with calf squeeze (Thompson test), localized pain, swelling, and ecchymosis. Tests are repeated with the knee in flexion and extension. Finally, it is important to identify the location of the rupture. Midsubstance Achilles tendon ruptures that are most common may be treated with or without surgery. When the injury occurs at the gastrocnemius or myotendinous junction, operative treatment is rarely indicated. However, when the injury is in the most distal part of the tendon or at the Achilles tendon insertion on the calcaneus with or without a bone avulsion fragment, surgical treatment should be considered.

Diagnostic imaging should be used as needed to confirm Achilles tendon rupture if clinical history and physical exam are not definitive or the location of the rupture is in question. A simple a lateral plain X-ray will exclude a bony avulsion (Fig. 5.3), which will likely dictate a need for operative treatment. An ultrasound is not essen-

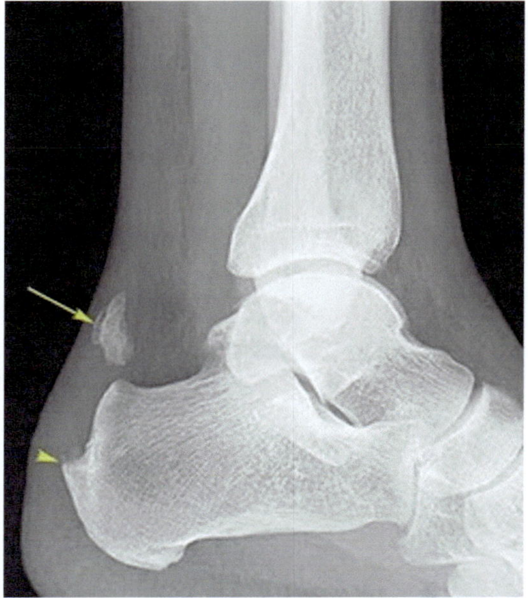

Fig. 5.3 Lateral X-ray showing an avulsed bone fragment with distal Achilles tendon rupture

tial but may be helpful to confirm the diagnosis. Magnetic resonance imaging (MRI) has a high sensitivity for identifying a complete versus partial rupture. However, caution should be exercised with the interpretation of the MRI signal. Radiologists tend to report a "Gap size." It is more likely that the gap reported is a zone of trauma where the traumatized frayed ends of the ruptured Achilles tendon produce a different MRI signal than a normal tendon. Further, the current best available evidence from a randomized controlled study [4] ignored the presence or absence of the gap when employing nonoperative treatment and showed similar results to operative treatment irrespective of a potential "Gap."

Nonoperative Treatment of Achilles Tendon Ruptures

Patients with a confirmed diagnosis of acute subcutaneous rupture of the Achilles tendon are appropriate for nonoperative treatment if they do not have an avulsion of the Achilles tendon of the calcaneus (Fig. 5.3). Further, it is very important that the diagnosis occurs early and ideally within

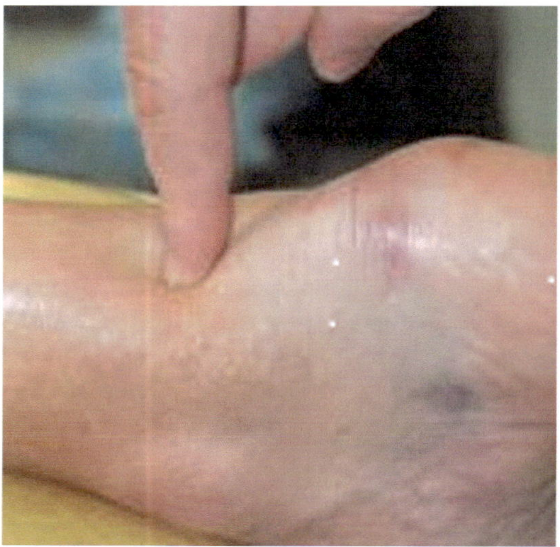

Fig. 5.2 Palpable gap defect of complete midsubstance Achilles tendon rupture

2 days of injury. This will allow the start of nonoperative treatment with a 2-week period of non-weight-bearing with the foot in a plantarflexed position and minimal weight-bearing activities during that period. It is important that they meet the below criteria. If not, they should be considered for surgical repair.

Nonoperative treatment methods include a few different techniques. A functional rehabilitation protocol can include early weight-bearing, early controlled range of motion (ROM), or both [7]. The degree to which a patient is weight-bearing and the amount of time before controlled ROM exercises begin is variable between protocols, but there is evidence in the literature that suggests it is indeed an important component in the success of nonoperatively treated Achilles tendon ruptures. Nilsson-Helander [7] found that using functional braces results in more favorable outcomes than casting, as demonstrated by a lower rerupture rate. Suchak et al. [8] investigated early weight-bearing and its consequences on health-related quality of life and found that it increased the quality of life in the early stages of rehabilitation. Lastly, a study conducted by Olsson et al. [9] that demonstrated early controlled ROM and early loading of the tendon resulted in favorable clinical outcomes.

Compliance by the patient and physiotherapist with the accelerated rehabilitation protocol is of utmost importance as deviation can result in tendon elongation, leading to residual weakness. It has been found that clinical outcomes correlate with the degree of tendon lengthening and that early, well-supervised mobilization can reduce the degree of tendon elongation [10]. The currently available evidence in the literature shows that when the accelerated rehabilitation protocol is administered correctly, there is no significant difference in the clinically important outcomes for patients who receive operative or nonoperative treatments. However, if the nonoperative treatment functional rehabilitation protocol cannot be supervised and administered correctly, then strong consideration should be given to operative treatment [3].

The best-studied accelerated rehabilitation protocol for the nonoperative treatment of mid-substance Achilles rupture was described by Willets et al. [4] in a high-quality level 1 randomized control trial. In this chapter, we describe the Glazebrook/Rubinger Achilles protocol for nonoperative treatment (GAPNOT, Table 5.1), which is a standardized accelerated rehabilitation protocol modified from the previous study of Willets et al. [2].

GAPNOT begins with an early diagnosis and appropriate patient selection to allow the initiation of nonoperative treatment with immobilization in a plantarflexed position and non-weight-bearing for 2 weeks. At some point during this 2-week period, the patient should be given the choice of treatment after consultation with an orthopedic surgeon, who uses current evidence-based medicine techniques [11] to inform the patient, in an unbiased fashion, of the risks and benefits of both operative and nonoperative treatment options.

Orthopedic surgeon follow-up supervision should continue at 6, 12, 26, and 52 weeks after the rupture. During these visits, healing is assessed with history and physical examination to check for resolving pain, swelling, ecchymosis, gradual return to activity specified by the GAPNOT protocol, and filling of the palpable defect. The physician should also examine the rupture sight to ensure the restoration of the continuity of the tendon and assess the patient's Achilles tendon length using careful passive dorsiflexion with the knee in an extended position as compared to the contralateral side. Patients should be counseled about avoiding a fall or stumble as well as activities that may force the ankle beyond the 90-degree dorsiflexion position.

After 2 weeks of immobilization, patients who choose to undergo nonoperative treatment for their Achilles tendon rupture are placed in the Achilles-specific cast boot with approximately 40-degree heel lifts to start progressive weight-bearing and the GAPNOT protocol initiated under the supervision of a physiotherapist. The progressive return to weight-bearing should be done by adding 25% body weight per week over a 4-week period. During this time, patients commenced pain-free, gradual active plantar- and dorsiflexion exercises below 90 degrees of ankle dorsiflexion, and conventional physiotherapy modalities are used for the control of pain and swelling as needed. Electrical muscle stimulation with active heel raises in the sitting position may also be initiated at about the 3-week mark, ensuring the ankle does not go past 90 degrees of ankle dorsiflexion. It is important that passive ranging of the ankle into dorsiflexion beyond 90 degrees is avoided during the 2–8-week stage. During this stage, communication with the physician is optimal to deal with complications such as reruptures, tendon elongation, noncompliance of the patient, and blood clots. It is important that all exercises and weight-bearing are pain free, and patients should reduce activity if they notice any pain, swelling, or tension on the injured side.

Between 6 and 8 weeks, the heel lifts are gradually reduced in height while fully weight-bearing, followed by a further week to wean from the Achilles-specific boot. Patients often used the assistance of a cane while weaning from the boot walker. An Achilles-specific compression garment is recommended to patients when weaning from the boot walker but is not mandatory. While weaning from the boot walker, it is imperative to do this gradually with a "step to" gait initially so as not to lengthen the Achilles tendon. Patients are recommended to always wear shoes, even indoors, and avoid shoes with low heel rise. The patient can lengthen their stride gradually as the tendon lengthens naturally. They are still instructed to do stairs one at a time, protecting the Achilles tendon.

Between 8 and 12 weeks, the patient can initiate active plantarflexion strengthening exercises but avoid activities that would dorsiflex the ankle past neutral. Thereafter strength, power, and endurance are worked on. It is imperative that patients are educated to avoid activities that place the foot beyond 90 degrees of ankle dorsiflexion. They are allowed normal activities of daily living to set the appropriate length of Achilles tendon. Physical therapy should still avoid stretching to achieve a normal range of motion at this stage.

During this period (10–16 weeks), complications of a rerupture and elongation of the tendon may be more common due to patients regaining a more normal activity pattern. Education and careful monitoring of the activities the patient is doing is essential to help prevent rerupture elongation. Patients often stop attending physical therapy during this period as they feel they are "better" when they can walk normally again. Patient compliance with the program is essential for the best outcomes.

From 6 months, a gradual return to sporting activities was encouraged, but patients were advised to avoid contact sports and high-intensity activities such as sprinting, cutting, and jumping. From 9 to 12 months, a full return to sporting activity is allowed.

Complications

Complications with nonoperative treatment of Achilles are significantly lower than with operative treatment; however, certain complications have been identified to occur with nonoperative treatments, including rerupture, elongation, decreased strength, and blood clots. Most of these complications are more common if patients are noncompliant with the protocol. This can be minimized with good patient education, close supervision, and good communication between the physical therapist and physician.

Complete rerupture is an uncommon but devastating complication of both operative and nonoperative treatment, with rates being reported in the literature between 3 and 4% [4]. Patients who are identified with complete reruptures should be assessed by a surgeon for consideration of operative treatment; while repeat nonoperative treatment is an option, it has not been studied. Patients should be educated on this.

Partial rerupture is an uncommon complication of both operative and nonoperative treatment. When patients are identified with partial reruptures, they should be immediately immobilized in a plantarflexed position and made non-weight-bearing and assessed by a surgeon for possible consideration of operative treatment. If operative treatment is deemed unnecessary, the protocol should be adjusted with consensus between the physical therapist and the physician as to which time point in the GAPNOT protocol the patient needs to revert to.

Elongation is likely more common with non-operative treatment if the protocol is not administered properly or patients are noncompliant. While this may occur at any time point, it is more likely to occur during the 6–16-week mark as patients have removed the heel wedges and started walking, gaining confidence. Elongation can be identified on follow-up visits by poor progression of strengthening and a careful examination of the patient's extent of passive dorsiflexion with the knee in an extended position compared to the contralateral side. If elongation is identified, the protocol should be adjusted with a consensus between the physical therapist and the physician as to which time point in the GAPNOT protocol the patient may need to revert to. If elongation is extreme, the patient should be advised of risks and benefits of surgical shortening of the tendon versus continued nonoperative treatment [12] as necessary.

Deep vein thrombosis and pulmonary embolism are rare occurrences but are serious potential complications with immobilization and casting. This should be considered with calf pain, swelling, and shortness of breath, and emergency treatment should be sought immediately. The best method to mitigate this complication should begin with patient education during lower leg immobilization and consideration for an anticoagulant should also be consider while the leg is immobilized.

With proper Achilles tendon length, calf atrophy and poor strength are minor complications in the long term when patients do not complete the physical therapy protocol. This often results because patients can resume all normal activities of daily living and sporting activities and do not understand the need for doing isolated and specific calf-strengthening exercises. When this is identified, patients are educated on the importance of isolated Achilles strengthening exercises on the affected side.

Summary

Historically, when functional rehabilitation was NOT employed for the nonoperative treatment of an acute midsubstance rupture of the Achilles tendon, the benefits of surgical treatment have been cited as increased strength, decreased rerupture, and a faster return to high-level activity. However, several high level 1 studies [3, 13] have demonstrated that nonoperative treatment with functional rehabilitation provides equivalent outcomes to surgical treatment. As a result, there has been an increased incidence of patients avoiding the risks of surgery and choosing nonoperative treatment.

It is essential that patients and surgeons alike understand that nonoperative treatment does not mean no treatment. In fact, nonoperative treatment protocols, such as the GAPNOT protocol described here, must be closely supervised by an experienced physiotherapist and physician with open communication to allow optimal results and avoid complications. If this cannot be done, patients should be educated on the historical benefits of surgery in the absence of functional rehabilitation.

Treatment failure and resultant complications with nonoperative treatment are almost always due to noncompliance, overzealous activity, or neglect by the physiotherapist or physician. As such, patient selection and education are important, and following the GAPNOT protocol is essential. Further, close supervision and good communication by both the physical therapist and the physician are mandatory to avoid, identify, and treat the complications of nonoperative treatment.

Acknowledgment Thanks are due to Daniela Rubinger, BScPT, MCPA, who has made contributions to this manuscript and, more importantly, to the hundreds of patients treated for Achilles tendon ruptures.

References

1. Hess GW. Achilles tendon rupture: a review of etiology, population, anatomy, risk factors, and injury prevention. Foot Ankle Spec. 2010;3(1):29–32.
2. Kastelic J, Palley I, Baer E. A structural mechanical model for tendon crimping. J Biomech. 1980;13(10):887–93.
3. Soroceanu A, et al. Surgical versus nonsurgical treatment of acute Achilles tendon rupture: a meta-analysis of randomized trials. J Bone Joint Surg Am. 2012;94(23):2136–43.
4. Willits K, et al. Operative versus nonoperative treatment of acute Achilles tendon ruptures: a multicenter

randomized trial using accelerated functional rehabilitation. J Bone Joint Surg Am. 2010;92(17):2767–75.

5. Kannus P, Jozsa L. Histopathological changes preceding spontaneous rupture of a tendon. A controlled study of 891 patients. J Bone Joint Surg Am. 1991;73(10):1507–25.

6. Puddu G, Ippolito E, Postacchini F. A classification of Achilles tendon disease. Am J Sports Med. 1976;4(4):145–50.

7. Nilsson-Helander K, et al. Acute achilles tendon rupture: a randomized, controlled study comparing surgical and nonsurgical treatments using validated outcome measures. Am J Sports Med. 2010;38(11):2186–93.

8. Suchak AA, et al. The influence of early weight-bearing compared with non-weight-bearing after surgical repair of the Achilles tendon. J Bone Joint Surg Am. 2008;90(9):1876–83.

9. Olsson N, et al. Stable surgical repair with accelerated rehabilitation versus nonsurgical treatment for acute Achilles tendon ruptures: a randomized controlled study. Am J Sports Med. 2013;41(12):2867–76.

10. Brumann M, et al. Accelerated rehabilitation following Achilles tendon repair after acute rupture - development of an evidence-based treatment protocol. Injury. 2014;45(11):1782–90.

11. Glazebrook MA, Glazebrook HM. Scientific evidence-based foot and ankle care. In: Haskell AA, editor. Coughlin and Mann's surgery of the foot. Amsterdam: Elsevier; 2022.

12. Stathakis A, Wadden C, Glazebrook M. Asymmetric Z-tendon shortening to maximize excision of abnormal tendon tissue: a technique tip to treat elongated tendons with pathology. Tech Foot Ankle Surg. 2019;18(1):43–7.

13. Wilkins R, Bisson LJ. Operative versus nonoperative management of acute Achilles tendon ruptures: a quantitative systematic review of randomized controlled trials. Am J Sports Med. 2012;40(9):2154–60.

Part II

Acute Injuries of the Achilles Tendon

Ruptures of the Medial Gastrocnemius Tendon ("Tennis Leg")

Amanda N. Fletcher and Samuel B. Adams

Introduction and Historical Perspective

Tennis leg refers to a partial or complete tear of the medial head of the gastrocnemius. The term "lawn tennis leg" was coined by R.W. Powell in 1883, where he attributed the injury to an isolated rapture of the plantaris sustained in a tennis player [1]. He described a 41-year-old healthy man who had sudden, sharp pain when reaching for the ball while playing tennis. The patient experienced acute onset pain, tenderness, and swelling but was able to return to sports after 4 weeks of rest. In 1958, Arner and Lindholm refuted the theory of this presentation being attributed to a plantaris tendon tear by surgically exploring five patients with tennis legs [2]. They noted a transverse rupture of the medial gastrocnemius at the musculotendinous junction with intact plantaris in all five patients.

While the plantaris was implicated in this injury for many years, it has been established that injury to the medial head of the gastrocnemius is much more common and now defines the term "tennis leg" [3]. Given the evolving knowledge of the pathogenesis, authors use the term tennis leg to refer to an acute muscle injury involving the superficial calf: plantaris, soleus, the medial head of the gastrocnemius, gastrocnemius-soleus aponeurosis, or a combination of injuries. The term also encompasses a spectrum of injury, severity from muscle strain to complete rupture.

Anatomy

The gastrocnemius muscle has a medial and lateral head that originate posteriorly from the medial and lateral femoral condyles, respectively. The two heads unite into a broad aponeurosis, which eventually joints with the deep tendon of the soleus to form the Achilles tendon, inserting on the middle 1/3 of the posterosuperior calcaneus. The gastrocnemius is innervated by the tibial nerve, and each head receives its blood supply from a sural branch of the popliteal artery. The gastrocnemius is vulnerable to injury because it spans three joints (knee, tibiotalar, and subtalar) and is subjected to excessive stretch. Ruptures of the medial gastrocnemius most commonly occur at the musculotendinous junction, specifically where the medial head of the gastrocnemius inserts into the soleus aponeurosis. The musculotendinous junction is the weakest point in the muscle-tendon unit under passive strain [4]. A normal tendon does not typically tear in response to excess strain, but rather, it is from within muscle fibers close to the tendon that the failure occurs.

A. N. Fletcher (✉) · S. B. Adams
Department of Orthopaedic Surgery, Duke University Medical Center, Durham, NC, USA
e-mail: amanda.fletcher@duke.edu; samuel.adams@duke.edu

Epidemiology and Mechanism of Injury

Tennis leg has most commonly been described in middle-aged patients with a male predominance. In a series of 720 patients with a strain of the posterior calf musculature, the age ranged from adolescents (<15 years old) to elderly (>60 years old), and the greatest incidence occurred in middle-aged patients around 45 years of age [5]. Despite the historical eponym, injuries to the medial head of the gastrocnemius muscle are not isolated to tennis players. In this same large series, injuries most commonly involved football (18%), squash (16.5%), and tennis (16.2%) [5]. While sports involving running and jumping are commonly involved, these injuries may also occur with more routine activities, such as walking upstairs or stepping off of a curb. Given the middle-age predominance and often "weekend warrior" presentation, the pathogenesis has been suggested to involve a degenerative process analogous to a rupture of the long head of the biceps, rotator cuff of the shoulder, or the Achilles tendon [6].

The mechanism of injury typically involves concomitant knee extension and ankle dorsiflexion. In this position, the gastrocnemius muscle is stretched to its maximum length, increasing the tension on the muscle. A powerful contraction of the gastrocnemius muscle with concomitant overstretching of the muscle leads to excessive tensile force and the disruption of the musculotendinous junction. This may occur during the extension of the knee and forced dorsiflexion of the ankle. resulting in a tightened heel cord distally and sudden overstretching of the gastrocnemius muscle belly proximally. However, concomitant knee extension with active ankle plantarflexion can also result in injury as the gastrocnemius attempts to contract in an already lengthened state.

History and Physical Exam

The typical presentation of a tennis leg is characterized by a sudden onset of pain in the midportion of the calf. Patients may present reporting an audible "popping" or "snapping" and the sensation of pulling or tearing in their calf muscle. The injury event often leads to an acute onset of pain and swelling in the calf with painful ambulation. Patients may even report a prodromal soreness in their calf prior to the injury. Froimson questioned his patients specifically about this, and nearly half recalled prodromal calf discomfort [7].

Clinical findings can include calf swelling, tenderness, and ecchymosis over the middle third of the medial calf. Maximal tenderness is typically over the musculotendinous junction of the medial gastrocnemius. Occasionally, there is a palpable mid-calf defect in the setting of a complete tendon rupture. Patients will frequently hold the foot in plantarflexion, which avoids tensioning the gastrocnemius. The pain is exacerbated by passive dorsiflexion or active plantarflexion of the ankle. Some patients have decreased plantarflexion power and are unable to sustain toe standing or toe walking given the associated pain and/or weakness. While plantarflexion strength is diminished and there is decreased muscle tone in the medial head of the gastrocnemius, a negative Thompson test is noted [8]. Swelling is variable depending on the degree of injury. Rarely, the swelling is so extensive that it causes an acute compartment syndrome [9–12]. Thus, it is crucial to examine the patient's compartments and to be aware of the signs and symptoms of compartment syndrome.

Differential Diagnosis and Concomitant Pathologies

The differential diagnosis for a patient presenting with a painful and swollen calf should include tennis leg, a ruptured popliteal cyst (Baker's cyst), Achilles tendon rupture, deep venous thrombosis (DVT), cellulitis, thrombophlebitis, pyomyositis, abscess, hematoma, arteriovenous malformation, tumor, and compartment syndrome. Additionally, it is important to recognize that tennis leg can present with concomitant compartment syndrome or DVT. Acute compartment syndrome has been reported in case reports of tennis leg, however, iatrogenic compartment syndrome may also occur after tennis leg is misdiagnosed as DVT and anticoagulation is started [9–11, 13]. In a study of sonographic evaluation and the diagnosis of tennis leg, 35 consecutive patients with acute traumatic injury of the calf underwent an ultrasound examination. Of these patients, five were found to have a gastrocnemius vein thrombosis in addition to tennis leg, and one patient was misdiagnosed and actually had a Baker's cyst [14]. In another clinical ultrasound study of 141 patients referred with the diagnosis of tennis leg, Delgado et al. reported a DVT in isolation in 14 patients (9.9%) [3]. An additional seven patients (5.0%) had DVT in association with another finding, suggesting concomitant muscle injury. This highlights the common occurrence of DVT mimicking or complicating tennis leg, and thus, a complete and intentional workup is necessary to ensure patient safety and proper management.

Imaging

The history and clinical examination are often sufficient to diagnose tennis leg; however, an ultrasound or magnetic resonance imaging (MRI) should be utilized to confirm the diagnosis and exclude other potential pathologies. Ultrasound is considered the gold standard for diagnosing tennis leg [14]. Ultrasound is portable, noninvasive, and inexpensive and can be utilized for both diagnosis and follow-up. However, ultrasound does require a provider trained to perform and interpret musculoskeletal ultrasound imaging.

In an uninjured patient, ultrasound examination demonstrates a uniform, organized, homogeneous, and linear appearance of the medial gastrocnemius muscle. There is a natural taper of the distal medial gastrocnemius muscle superficial to the soleus muscle. The hypoechoic and hyperechoic lines end in the muscle aponeurosis, and the distal tendon appears hypoechogenic and parallel [15]. The most consistent sonographic finding of tennis leg is the disruption or discontinuity of the normally linear appearance of the medial gastrocnemius muscle [16] (Fig. 6.1). In a series of 33 patients with tennis leg, Flecca et al. reported that an ultrasound evaluation of all patients showed a disruption or discontinuity of the normal muscular structure and a fluid collection interposed between the disrupted medial head of the gastrocnemius muscle and the underlying aponeurosis of the soleus muscle evidenced by anechoic to hypoechoic areas [14]. They reported that this fluid collection or hematoma occurs in 80% of patients, presumably due to muscle disruption and hemorrhage. Bianchi et al. retrospectively reviewed sonographic images of 65 patients with clinically suspected tennis legs and described the typical sonographic features and sonographic progression of the diagnosis [15]. Mild injuries were evidenced by distal muscle fibers and septa that did not reach the aponeurosis, whereas more severe injuries presented with hematoma.

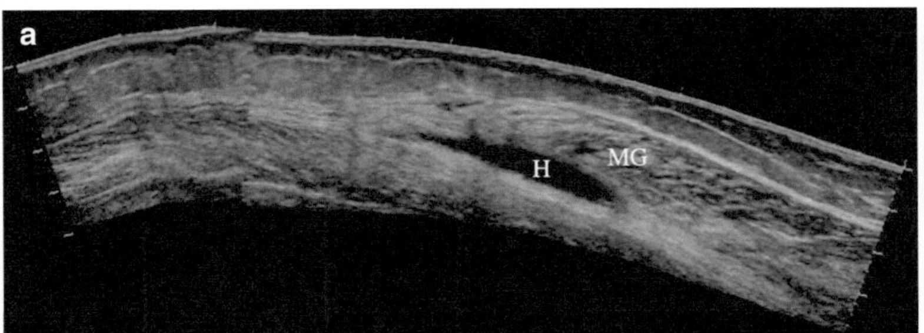
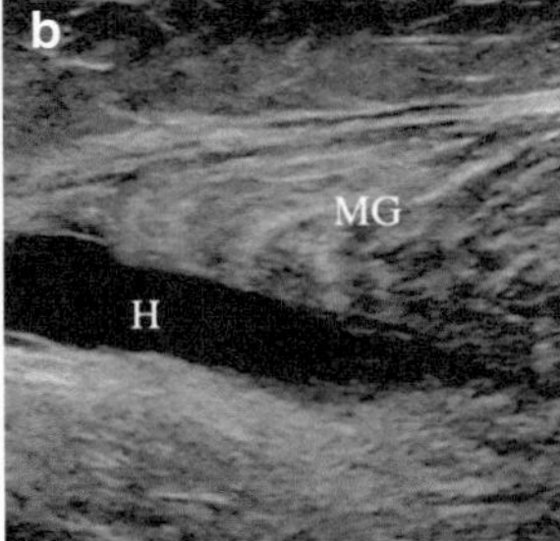

Fig. 6.1 (a) Long-axis extended field and (b) long-axis magnification ultrasound images demonstrating a complete rupture of the medial head of the gastrocnemius (MG) and underlying hematoma (H). There is disruption of the normal, parallel, hyper- and hypoechogenic lines within the tendon and muscle of the medial head of the gastrocnemius

Based on the completeness of the disruption of the normal appearance, partial and complete lesions can be differentiated on ultrasound. Complete ruptures were reported in 21.5% of cases by Bianhci et al. and up to 27.3% of cases by Flecca et al. [14, 15]. Additionally, Flecca et al. noted that the degree of fluid collection in patients with complete rupture (6–16 mm; mean: 9.7 mm) was significantly greater than those seen in patients with partial rupture (4–8 mm; mean: 6.8 mm) [14]. In Delgado et al.'s report of the sonographic findings in 141 patients with the clinical diagnosis of tennis leg, partial rupture of the medial head of the gastrocnemius was noted in 66.7% of patients, and a fluid collection between the aponeuroses of the gastrocnemius and the soleus without evidence of muscle rupture was found in 21.3% of patients [3]. Plantaris tendon rupture occurred in only 1.4% of patients, and partial rupture of the soleus was seen in 0.7% of patients. Additionally, given that 10% of patients in their cohort had an isolated and unsuspected DVT, despite the classic clinical presentation of tennis leg, it is essential to include Doppler during sonography to rule out thrombosis. Comparison views to the contralateral extremity may also be useful in the setting of mild injuries.

MRI may also be utilized to diagnose tennis leg; however, the high cost and limited availability in ambulatory settings limit use. Multiple different presentations of tennis leg have been reported on MRI [17] (Fig. 6.2). Muscle injury presents as hyperintensity of the medial head of the gastrocnemius or even concomitant involvement of the soleus or plantaris. T1-weighted images may show a disruption of the normal architecture of the musculotendinous junction, while T2-weighted images show increased signals in the injured muscle due to edema. Intramuscular hematoma within the medial head of the gastrocnemius or peri-muscular hematoma has also been described. Hematoma is visible as a homogenous or heterogenous mass with a high-intensity signal on T1- and T2-weighted scans.

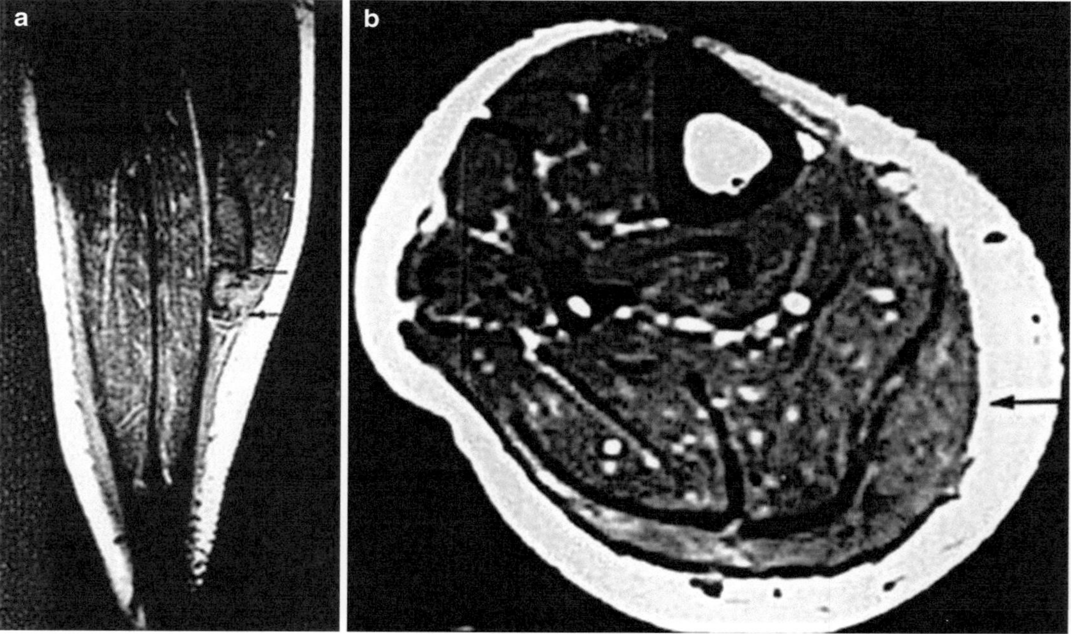

Fig. 6.2 (**a**) T1-weighted coronal magnetic resonance images (MRI) demonstrating a partial rupture of the medial head of the gastrocnemius and subsequent hematoma (arrows). (**b**) T1-weighted axial images demonstrating altered signal in the medial head of the gastrocnemius (arrow). Reproduced with permission from Yu, J., Garrett, W.E. (2008). Ruptures of the Medial Gastrocnemius Muscle ("Tennis Leg"). In: Nunley, J. (eds) The Achilles Tendon. Springer, New York, NY. https://doi.org/10.1007/978-0-387-79205-7_4

Depending on the severity of injury, muscle retraction may also be present and appear as a mass-like structure in the mid-calf. MRI is usually unnecessary but can be helpful in differentiating between tennis leg and other pathologies in equivocal cases.

Treatment

Nonoperative Management

The literature regarding the management of tennis legs is limited to case reports and small retrospective case series without prospective or randomized controlled evidence. However, the majority of tennis leg injuries are successfully managed with conservative management and surgery reserved for rare refractory cases. Acute treatment is aimed at limiting hemorrhage and pain with activity modification, ice, compression, elevation, nonsteroidal anti-inflammatories, a heel lift, and early physical therapy.

Nonsteroidal anti-inflammatory medications have been reported to help decrease recovery time in tennis legs [5]. Kwak et al. performed a case-control study to examine the effect of compression on patient recovery in 30 patients with diagnosed tennis legs [18]. All patients were treated with rest, ice, leg elevation, and nonsteroidal anti-inflammatory medication, and the compression cohort was also treated with an elastic band and neoprene cast sleeves for 2 to 4 weeks. They reported sonographic decreases in hemorrhage amount, more rapid union of the medial head of the gastrocnemius with the soleus muscle, and earlier ambulation. Applying a heel wedge/lift or an ankle-foot orthosis in slight plantarflexion helps alleviate discomfort by reducing the strain on the injured gastrocnemius. The body also compensates for the lift by holding the knee slightly flexed, further relaxing the gastrocnemius muscle belly.

Rest is recommended in the acute inflammation period occurring 1 to 5 days postinjury. While crutches may initially be required, patients should progress their weight-bearing as tolerated. A rehabilitation protocol should be initiated immediately following injury. Prescribing a home exercise program versus formal physical therapy is at the discretion of the surgeon, taking into account injury severity, disability, and patient motivation and compliance. It is recommended that passive stretching is initiated immediately following the injury. With the knee fully extended, the posterior calf musculature can be passively stretched to tolerance. Isometric ankle dorsiflexion and plantarflexion can also begin at this time. At 2 to 4 weeks, patients can progress to resisted exercise [19]. This involves gradually increasing resistance against the movement of the ankle progressing from resistance bands to calf raises with body weight. The majority of patients are able to resume activity and sport at 6 weeks [20].

Surgical Management

Surgical treatment for tennis leg is rare and reserved for patients with symptoms refractory to nonoperative measures. Surgical treatment with delayed repair of the medial head of the gastrocnemius following rupture has been scarcely described [20, 21]. Cheng et al. propose the consideration of surgery for complete ruptures and for patients with prolonged pain (4 to 6 months months) with evidence of contracture [21]. Large intramuscular hematomas may impair clinical progress and may also be an indication of surgical referral. Additionally, they suggest surgical repair in young patients who are actively involved in sports to ensure strength for continued sports activity.

Cheng et al. reported their repair technique and a two-patient case series: one case of long-standing symptoms and one of recent rupture of the musculotendinous junction [21]. They utilized a single longitudinal incision centered over the middle of the defect. After evacuation of the hematoma, the retracted proximal muscle fibers are dissected and reattached to the distal end using absorbable and nonabsorbable sutures with the foot held in plantarflexion. They advocate excising scar tissue in chronic injuries so that sutures engage healthy, contractile muscle tissue to achieve proper reattachment. Their postoperative protocol included immobilization for three weeks in a long leg cast with the knee flexed 60° and the ankle plantar flexed 20°–30°, followed by an additional 3 weeks in a short leg cast with continued ankle plantarflexion. After removal of the cast, the patient begins range of motion exercises with progressive weight-bearing.

Similarly, Jennings and Peterson reported operative repair in an adult male who experienced calf cramping and pain during activity owing to a neglected rupture of the medial head of the gastrocnemius [20]. They utilized a single longitudinal incision overlying the retracted medial head, and the sural nerve was immediately identified and protected. The retracted medial head was mobilized, and a short tendinous portion that developed from the lamination of the distal fascial insertion was retained with the proximal muscle. The superficial tendinous lamination of the triceps surae was then elevated as a "trap door" about 3 cm distally. The medial head of the gastrocnemius was then advanced distally and secured into this triceps surae "trap door" using a No. 2 Orthocord suture (DePuy Mitek, Raynham, MA). Postoperatively, a short leg cast was placed with the foot in the resting equinus. At 2 weeks postoperatively, the patient was transitioned to a removable boot with three heel lifts for weight-bearing. Active knee extension and ankle range of motion were encouraged, and the heel lifts were gradually reduced. Good functional outcome with symptom resolution was achieved in their patient.

Prognosis

Among athletes, outcomes generally are reported to be excellent with a return to full activity within 4 to 6 weeks [22]. In older, deconditioned patients or those with coexisting musculoskeletal or painful conditions, recovery may be prolonged and patients should be counseled appropriately. In the largest series studying tennis legs including 720 patients, Millar et al. reported successful conservative management in the majority of patients with recurrence of only 0.7% of patients [5]. They advocated for a regimen of passive stretch-

ing, exercises for the antagonists and later the agonists, and quadriceps exercises. Additionally, prevention of the injury is best obtained by regular stretching and strength development routines. Shields et al. compared the isokinetic performance of the injured leg with that of the normal leg for 1 to 3 years following conservative treatment with a heel lift, calf sleeve, and physical therapy. They reported no significant loss in plantarflexion strength in the injured extremity after healing, and all patients returned to their previous level of athletic activity [23].

Failure to heal the injury with ongoing pain or cramping has been reported in rare cases. More serious, long-term functional deficits can occur when the ruptured muscle forms a fibrotic band and causes joint contracture. Prolonged immobilization following a tennis leg injury with a lack of stretching exercises can result in extensive fibrotic band formation and severe contracture involving both the knee and ankle joints. Ryu et al. reported concomitant contracture of the knee and ankle joints after a neglected gastrocnemius muscle rupture with 4 weeks of complete immobilization [24]. Upon surgical intervention, the authors identified a long fibrotic band, continuous from the distal musculotendinous junction to the proximal tendinous insertion of the medial head of gastrocnemius, resulting in a concomitant knee flexion contracture and ankle equinus deformity. Similarly, Takigami et al. reported a case of pes equinus deformity due to gastrocnemius contracture resulting from trauma to the muscle [25]. In their case, the cord-like fibrosis was about 6 cm long, and the resulting ankle equinus was resolved through an excision of the scar tissue. Given these iatrogenic complications, it is imperative to initiate early range of motion and stretching exercises immediately following injury.

References

1. Powell RM. Lawn tennis leg. Lancet. 1883;2:44.
2. Arner O, Lindholm A. What is tennis leg? Acta Chir Scand. 1958;116:73–7.
3. Delgado GJ, Chung CB, Lektrakul N, et al. Tennis leg: clinical US study of 141 patients and anatomic

investigation of four cadavers with MR imaging and US. Radiology. 2002;224(1):112–9.

4. Garrett WE Jr, Nikolaou PK, Ribbeck BM, Glisson RR, Seaber AV. The effect of muscle architecture on the biomechanical failure properties of skeletal muscle under passive extension. Am J Sports Med. 1988;16(1):7–12.

5. Millar AP. Strains of the posterior calf musculature ("tennis leg"). Am J Sports Med. 1979;7(3):172–4.

6. McClure JG. Gastrocnemius musculotendinous rupture: a condition confused with thrombophlebitis. South Med J. 1984;77(9):1143–5.

7. Froimson A. Tennis leg. JAMA. 1969;209:415–6.

8. Dürig M, Schuppisser JP, Gauer EF, Müller W. Spontaneous rupture of the gastrocnemius muscle. Injury. 1977;9(2):143–5.

9. Chagou A, Benameur H, Zine A, Bouabid S, Boussougua M, Jaafar A. Compartment syndrome complicating tennis leg: about a case. Pan Afr Med J. 2020;37:310.

10. Jarolem KL, Wolinsky PR, Savenor A, Ben-Yishay A. Tennis leg leading to acute compartment syndrome. Orthopedics. 1994;17(8):721–3.

11. Tao L, Jun H, Muliang D, Deye S, Jiangdong N. Acute compartment syndrome after gastrocnemius rupture (tennis leg) in a nonathlete without trauma. J Foot Ankle Surg. 2016;55(2):303–5.

12. Straehley D, Jones WW. Acute compartment syndrome (anterior, lateral, and superficial posterior) following tear of the medial head of the gastrocnemius muscle. A case report. Am J Sports Med. 1986;14(1):96–9.

13. Anouchi YS, Parker RD, Seitz WH Jr. Posterior compartment syndrome of the calf resulting from misdiagnosis of a rupture of the medial head of the gastrocnemius. J Trauma. 1987;27(6):678–80.

14. Flecca D, Tomei A, Ravazzolo N, Martinelli M, Giovagnorio F. US evaluation and diagnosis of rup-ture of the medial head of the gastrocnemius (tennis leg). J Ultrasound. 2007;10(4):194–8.

15. Bianchi S, Martinoli C, Abdelwahab IF, Derchi LE, Damiani S. Sonographic evaluation of tears of the gastrocnemius medial head ("tennis leg"). J Ultrasound Med. 1998;17(3):157–62.

16. Monseau AJ, Balcik BJ, Denne N, Sharon MJ, Minardi JJ. Point-of-care ultrasound diagnosis of tennis leg. Clin Pract Cases Emerg Med. 2019;3(1):36–9.

17. Menz MJ, Lucas GL. Magnetic resonance imaging of a rupture of the medial head of the gastrocnemius muscle. A case report. J Bone Joint Surg Am. 1991;73(8):1260–2.

18. Kwak HS, Lee KB, Han YM. Ruptures of the medial head of the gastrocnemius ("tennis leg"): clinical outcome and compression effect. Clin Imaging. 2006;30(1):48–53.

19. Domeracki SJ, Landman Z, Blanc PD, Guntur S. Off the courts: occupational "tennis leg". Workplace Health Saf. 2019;67(1):5–8.

20. Jennings A, Peterson R. Delayed reconstruction of medial head of gastrocnemius rupture: a surgical option. Foot Ankle Int. 2013;34(6):904–7.

21. Cheng Y, Yang HL, Sun ZY, Ni L, Zhang HT. Surgical treatment of gastrocnemius muscle ruptures. Orthop Surg. 2012;4(4):253–7.

22. Campbell JT. Posterior calf injury. Foot Ankle Clin. 2009;14(4):761–71.

23. Shields CL Jr, Redix L, Brewster CE. Acute tears of the medial head of the gastrocnemius. Foot Ankle. 1985;5(4):186–90.

24. Ryu DJ, Kim JM, Kim BS. Concomitant contracture of the knee and ankle joint after gastrocnemius muscle rupture: a case report. J Foot Ankle Surg. 2017;56(1):87–91.

25. Takigami J, Hashimoto Y, Yamasaki S, Hara Y, Nishikino S, Nakamura H. Gastrocnemius contracture caused by traumatic injury without fracture: a case report. Foot Ankle Int. 2011;32(12):1152–4.

Percutaneous and Minimally Invasive Surgery for Acute Achilles Tendon Tears

Raul M. Espinoza, Felipe Chaparro, Cristian Ortiz, Giovanni Carcuro, and Manuel J. Pellegrini

Introduction

The Achilles tendon is the strongest in the human body and is critical for foot plantarflexion. A rupture of this tendon has a significant impact on a patient's function, especially in the young population. Typically, these ruptures occur spontaneously and affect men between 30 and 39 years of age. Suboptimal treatment can produce weakness, an altered gait, and a detrimental effect on sports performance and on activities of daily living.

The goal of treatment is to restore tendon length and strength as close as possible to a pre-injury situation, allowing patients to return to their previous functions and activities without associated complications [1].

The optimal treatment for this pathology is still a matter of debate, particularly with publications demonstrating that conservative treatment with early functional rehabilitation has achieved comparable outcomes to those obtained with surgical treatment. Twaddle and Poon [2] published a randomized prospective study comparing the

R. M. Espinoza
Foot and Ankle Center, Clínica Universidad de Los Andes, Santiago, Chile

Department of Orthopaedic Surgery, Hospital Regional de Talca, Clínica Lircay, Talca, Chile

F. Chaparro
Foot and Ankle Center, Clínica Universidad de Los Andes, Santiago, Chile

Foot and Ankle Center, Department of Orthopaedic Surgery, Clínica Universidad de Los Andes, Hospital San Jose, Santiago, Chile
e-mail: fchaparro@clinicauandes.cl

C. Ortiz
Foot and Ankle Center, Clínica Universidad de Los Andes, Santiago, Chile

Foot and Ankle Center, Department of Orthopaedic Surgery, Clínica Universidad de Los Andes, Santiago, Chile
e-mail: caortiz@clinicauandes.cl

G. Carcuro
Foot and Ankle Center, Clínica Universidad de Los Andes, Santiago, Chile

Department of Orthopaedic Surgery, Clínica Universidad de Los Andes, Santiago, Chile
e-mail: gcarcuro@clinicauandes.cl

M. J. Pellegrini (✉)
Foot and Ankle Center, Clínica Universidad de Los Andes, Santiago, Chile

Department of Orthopaedic Surgery, Hospital Clinico Universidad de Chile, Clínica Universidad de Los Andes, Santiago, Chile
e-mail: mpellegrini@clinicauandes.cl

treatment of acute Achilles tendon ruptures associated with an early motion protocol. They found no significant differences between patients with and without surgery. The rerupture rate was low and comparable in both groups, which led to the conclusion that early controlled motion is the essential step in a patient's treatment and not the surgical status.

Although successful, conservative treatment has an inherent risk of tendon elongation, prolonged rehabilitation, delayed return to sports and activities of daily living, and muscular weakness [3–8]. Because of the reasons mentioned above, we prefer surgical treatment to treat this injury, unless contraindicated.

Open surgical treatment was the standard of care for treating acute Achilles tendon ruptures. The most popular is the Krackow suture technique [9], approaching the ruptured ends of the tendon with a stable and resistant configuration. High-quality tissue volume will securely allow the tendon to heal and reduce the risk of rerupture. One major disadvantage of this approach is the high risk of wound complications. Khan and colleagues [10] published a meta-analysis of randomized controlled trials for the treatment of acute Achilles tendon ruptures. They concluded that open surgical treatment was associated with a significantly higher risk of complications than conservative treatment. Movin et al. [11] found that the complication rates of conservative treatment ranged from 0% to 10%, whereas surgical complication rates were as low as 4.7% but as high as 34%. These complications included infection, wound-healing problems, sural nerve injuries, and scar issues [10, 12, 13]. However, the rerupture rate associated with conservative treatment ranged from 8.4% to 17.7%, whereas this rate was reduced to 1.4–3.5% in surgical treatment. Therefore, detractors of surgical treatment often cite these higher complication rates to be associated with open surgery—those who favor surgical repair quote the higher rerupture rate associated with nonoperative treatment to justify their approach. In this scenario, surgeons introduced minimally invasive techniques to reduce complications associated with open surgery.

Anatomical Considerations in Minimally Invasive Surgery

Several anatomical considerations for a safe approach to the minimally invasive treatment of the Achilles' tendon exist, the main of which is the sural nerve [14]. Webb et al. [15] published an anatomical description of the sural nerve, located superficial to the crural fascia and the paratenon. At 10 cm proximal from the tendon's footprint, the nerve travels in a lateral to medial direction. Hence, the techniques developed must consider this trajectory and anatomical situation to avoid transitory or permanent nerve damage.

Moreover, it is of paramount importance to have in mind the vascular supply of the Achilles tendon. The posterior tibial artery irrigates the proximal and distal portions of the tendon, while the peroneal artery vascularizes the middle segment [16]. The highest probability of tendon rupture is located at 4–7 cm from the insertion site, given the insufficient vascular supply to this tendon area. Despite not having a genuine synovial sheath, the Achilles tendon has a richly vascularized paratenon. Therefore, careful soft tissue handling and minimizing dissection will allow for better and faster healing of the tendon [17]. Carr and Norris [18] describe anterior vessels into the mesotenon, providing additional irrigation. Although the repair of the paratenon is essential, we feel that avoiding further injury to the tendon via a minimally invasive approach overcomes this advantage.

Lastly, the skin over the Achilles tendon has scarce irrigation, which implies a higher probability of presenting complications such as delayed wound healing and infection. Conveniently, the skin between the medial malleolus and the medial border of the Achilles tendon has better vascularization and is frequently selected for the surgical approach [16].

Evolution of the Minimally Invasive Surgery

Historically, conservative treatment with cast immobilization was the treatment of choice when selecting the nonsurgical management of this pathology. Nevertheless, the development of ankle stiffness, muscle atrophy, and loss of proprioception raised concern about the effectiveness of this treatment modality. Early functional rehabilitation seeks to reduce these complications, as suggested by some studies in which similar results are reported compared to surgical management [12]. Young et al. demonstrated similar rerupture rates after excluding patients presenting for treatment after 72 h from injury.

Mullaney et al. published that conservative management fails after an improper position of the tendon stumps with the corresponding tendon elongation, which leads to the decrease the triceps plantarflexion power. The musculotendinous junction cannot shorten optimally to produce average plantarflexion power [19]. Because of these concerns, surgical management is our treatment choice, relying on a complete approximation of tendon stumps, restoring the length and tension of the gastrocnemius-soleus complex. In the literature, surgical management demonstrates increased plantarflexion strength [3], faster rehabilitation, four earlier return to work [12, 13, 20], and a higher rate of return to sport [20]. All studies demonstrated lower rerupture rates in surgical treatment compared with nonsurgical treatment. Willits et al. [3] showed in a randomized trial that at 1-year and 2-year velocity testing, the surgical group demonstrated a higher plantarflexion strength ratio than the nonsurgical group.

Surgical management generally is divided into open, percutaneous, and minimally invasive repair. This treatment modality has associated complications like delayed wound healing or wound border necrosis, superficial or deep infection, scar issues, sural nerve injury, rerupture, and deep venous thrombosis. In open surgery, they could have a rate as high as 34% of the patients [11].

In seeking to reduce these high complication rates, surgeons developed percutaneous repair techniques. The concept is to approximate the ruptured tendon without exposing the rupture site.

Ma and Griffith [21] were the first to introduce a percutaneous method for Achilles tendon ruptures with local anesthesia and without a tourniquet. Their technique requires three small stab incisions on the medial and lateral aspects of the Achilles tendon to pass nonabsorbable sutures through the tendon using a Bunnell stitch proximally and a box-type configuration distally. The surgeon ties the sutures on the medial aspect of the rupture site, outside of the paratenon. Their investigation reported 18 patients with two minor complications and an ankle power of 89% of the contralateral lower extremity after 2 years of follow-up. The authors concluded that their technique was a better option than the open technique or conservative treatment by restoring tendon length and strength while minimizing complications.

Nevertheless, Klein et al. [22] described that the incidence of sural nerve damage with this technique was 13%. Rozis et al. [23] report a prospective study with 82 patients randomized into an open surgery group or percutaneous surgery group using the Ma and Griffith technique. Complications included sural nerve injuries and infections, with 7.3% and 0% for the percutaneous group and 0% and 7% for the open surgery group. There were no reruptures. While the percutaneous techniques resolved part of the problem by reducing the wound complication matter, they increased the injuries to the sural nerve.

Hockenbury and Johns [24], in a cadaveric study, compared five specimens repaired with the Ma and Griffith technique and five specimens repaired with an open technique. Three out of five specimens had sural nerve entrapment in the percutaneous group. Moreover, they proved that open repairs tolerate twice the degree of ankle dorsiflexion before failure than those repaired using Ma and Griffith's technique.

Delponte et al. [25] developed a modified percutaneous technique using two harpoon-like devices (Tenolig (R), FH Orthopedics (Chicago, IL)). In this technique, the surgeon performs two small incisions approximately 5 cm proximal to the ruptured tendon. The harpoon is preloaded with sutures that have metallic barbs securing the proximal stump to pull it distally. Once the appropriate length and tension are restored, the sutures are locked to a metallic disk using crimps, which remain superficial to the skin for 6 weeks. After promising preliminary results with this technique, a posteriorly published series reported a high rate of complications [1]. Gorschewsky et al. [26] modified the harpoon technique using a fibrin sealant through a small incision at the rupture site. Sixty-four patients were treated with this method with favorable results, reporting no cases of no sural nerve damage, and all patients returned to sports after nearly 5 months.

Webb and Bannister [15] described a new technique to avoid sural nerve damage, creating three midline stab incisions over the posterior aspect of the tendon. With a no. 1 nylon suture loaded on a 90-mm cutting needle, the tendon ends are approximated using two box stitches. They report on 27 patients treated with this technique after a 3-year follow-up period. There was only one case of a mild wound problem and complex regional pain syndrome but no rerupture or sural nerve entrapment cases. Wagnon and Akayi [27] published a retrospective series of 57 patients treated with the Webb-Bannister technique, comparing their results to those from an open repair. They found similar functional results but fewer complications with the minimal incision technique.

Majewski et al. [14] retrospectively studied 84 patients treated at two different hospitals. Surgeons in both centers used a similar percutaneous technique, but they added an ancillary incision to expose and protect the sural nerve before suture placement in one hospital. This addition led to 0% of nerve injury in comparison to 18% in the other group.

Minimally invasive techniques use the advantage of a minimal open incision and percutaneous placement of the sutures, minimizing complications from both treatment methods and ensuring a better approximation of the tendon ends. By placing sutures underneath the paratenon, this technique has lowered nerve injury rates in comparison with the open and percutaneous techniques.

Del Buono et al. [28] reported a systematic review of 12 studies comparing open and minimally invasive repairs in 781 patients; 375 were open and 406 with a minimally invasive repair. They state that minimally invasive repairs have a better postoperative range of motion, present lower complication rates, are less expensive, and are less demanding than open repairs. With the advances in surgical instrumentations and the perfection of the technique, minimally invasive Achilles tendon repair has provided sufficient data to justify its use for repairs.

Amlang et al. [29] developed a technique where through a small incision at 3 cm proximal to the rupture site, two specially designed instruments (Dresden instruments) are inserted to catch the distal stump of the tendon, in between the paratenon and the crural fascia. Two sutures are inserted percutaneously through this instrument at the distal stump 1. Afterward, the Dresden instruments are pulled out to recover the sutures through the proximal incision and tie them under optimal tension to the proximal stump. In 62 repairs in 61 patients, they reported two reruptures, no cases of sural nerve injury, and 92% of reasonable and excellent outcomes with an average of 96 AOFAS score.

Henriquez et al. [30] compared 17 patients treated with Dresden repair and 15 with open repair and observed similar values of plantarflexor strength, range of motion, calf and ankle perimeter, and single heel raising test between the groups. Meantime, return to work was longer for patients who had open versus percutaneous repair (5.6 months versus 2.8 months). No patients had nerve injuries.

Keller et al. [31] also demonstrated favorable outcomes with 100 percutaneous repairs with the Dresden technique, with a 98% rate of patient satisfaction and only two reruptures. Also, Elton and Bluman [32] reported a similar technique using curved ring forceps instead.

Kakiuchi [33] developed a suture guide made with looped Kirschner wires and inserted it under the paratenon from the rupture site of the tendon with a minimal incision. Then percutaneous placement of the sutures in the tendon stumps through the Kirschner guide allowed the authors to bring the sutures inside the paratenon, rescue them at the rupture site, and then, under direct vision of the tendon stumps, tie them to ensure the correct position of the tendon stumps. This maneuver avoids the entrapment of the sural nerve. Results in 12 patients showed better functional scores and higher return to sports than open surgery at a mean of 5.1 years of follow-up.

Kakiuchi's technique is the precursor of the Achillon device (Integra LifeSciences, Plainsboro, New Jersey) published by Assal et al. [34], designed to standardize the technique to repair the Achilles tendon. This device is a guiding instrument with an inner and outer corresponding arm. Through a 2-cm longitudinal incision at the rupture site, the Achillon is inserted deep into the Achilles tendon's paratenon. First, three sutures are delivered into the proximal stump through the instrument. The device is then removed, pulling out six suture strands from the incision. The procedure is repeated for the distal tendon stump. When the proper tension is set, the sutures are tied, creating three box configuration sutures. They reported their results in 82 patients with a mean AOFAS score of 96 points at 26 months of follow-up and no differences in plantarflexion strength with the uninjured side. There were no wound complications, no infections, and no nerve injuries. Three reruptures were documented in noncompliant patients.

Calder and Saxsby [35], in a prospective study on 46 patients using the Achillon device, reported a mean AOFAS of 98 and no reruptures at 12 months of follow-up. One patient had a superficial wound infection, and two had transitory paresthesias in the sural nerve territory that resolved within 3 months.

Kolodziej et al. [36], in a randomized trial, enrolled 47 patients with a follow-up time of 24 months. There were no reruptures or nerve injuries and no difference in functional and clinical outcomes with open repair.

A meta-analysis published in 2018 showed fewer wound complications and no differences in rerupture rate, sural nerve injury, return to sports, or AOFAS score with the Achillon device compared with open repair [37]. However, there were some deficiencies in this device. The jig is not very stout, is a single-use device increasing the cost, does not eliminate the risk of needle damage to the sural nerve, and has a nonanatomic straight design. All three sutures pass through the tendon in the same transverse plane, predisposing to early failure through suture cutout, and there is no option of locking the suture construct [1].

In 2010, the percutaneous Achilles repair system (PARS) (Arthrex, Naples, Florida) made improvements to the deficiencies of the Achillon device. The PARS jig is metallic and nondisposable, and it is stout and less prone to bending, decreasing the risk of the needles missing the inner arms. Its design is more anatomic than Achillon, with an anterior contour, which effortlessly glides around the tendon while applying counterpressure. This device allows inserting up to seven different sutures at once in various positions with an option of making all sutures transverse or up to two locked suture configurations.

Hsu et al. [38] reviewed 270 consecutive cases of operatively treated acute Achilles tendon ruptures, 101 with PARS, and 169 with open repair. A more significant number of patients treated with PARS (98%) could return to baseline physical activities by 5 months compared with the open group (82%). There were no significant differences in the rates of sural neuritis, wound, superficial, deep infection, or reoperation. There was no deep vein thrombosis (DVT) or reruptures in either group. Demetracopoulos et al. [39] studied and compared the strength of the construct of three nonlocking sutures, like the Achillon technique, with a construct with locking and nonlocking sutures used, like the PARS technique. They found greater stability in a construct with both locking and nonlocking sutures with a load to failure of 385.0 N compared with 299.6 N in the nonlocking-only construct.

The Achilles Midsubstance SpeedBridge repair (Arthrex, Inc., Naples, FL, USA) is a knotless technique that has recently been developed. The PARS device is used proximally to catch the tendon stump, and distally bone anchors are used to fix the sutures to the calcaneal bone [40]. The latter reduces failure risk at the knots and suture cutout from the distal part of the tendon, which has previously been reported with the traditional PARS technique [41]. Another potential advantage is the absence of knots that could irritate the soft tissue envelope at the rupture site [40].

Clanton et al. reported a biomechanical study with four different techniques and introduced SutureTape (Arthrex, Inc) as the suture chosen for Achilles Midsubstance SpeedBridge repair [41]. Similar elongation to the open repair was observed after cyclic loading.

Pellegrini et al. [42] described a modification of this technique, introducing the jig between the crural fascia and the paratenon. By translating the incision, 3 cm proximal, the rupture site hematoma remains intact, maintaining the biological conditions to improve repair. They called this technique PARS-Dresden, and it is the authors' treatment of choice for Achilles tendon ruptures.

Techniques of Minimal Invasive Surgery

Indications/Contraindications

Surgical management of Achilles midsubstance ruptures is indicated in young active patients who desire to maintain optimal function and return to their previous activity level as soon as possible. Patients presenting with ruptures within 3 weeks from injury are operated on using this technique.

Contraindications for surgical management include nonambulatory patients, poorly controlled medical conditions, and inability or unwillingness to participate in early rehabilitation. Smoking and diabetes are relative contraindications for the procedure and must be evaluated on a case-to-case basis [42].

The Dresden Technique [29]

- General or regional anesthesia can be used, although regional is preferred when feasible.
- This technique is performed with the patient in a prone position with no thigh tourniquet. However, if desired, the tourniquet should be placed on the thigh, not the calf, to avoid limiting the excursion of the gastrocnemius-soleus complex.

- Drape both legs to adjust the gastrocnemius-soleus complex's tension compared to the contralateral normal side.
- The rupture site and the skin incision are marked.
- A 3-cm longitudinal, dorsomedial incision is made at 3 cm from the rupture site (Fig. 7.1).
- The crural fascia is prepared and opened, revealing the paratenon. The paratenon is not opened (Fig. 7.2).
- The first Dresden instrument is introduced into the layer between the crural fascia and the paratenon (Fig. 7.3).
- The instrument aperture is positioned 1 cm proximal to the insertion of the Achilles tendon at the calcaneus.

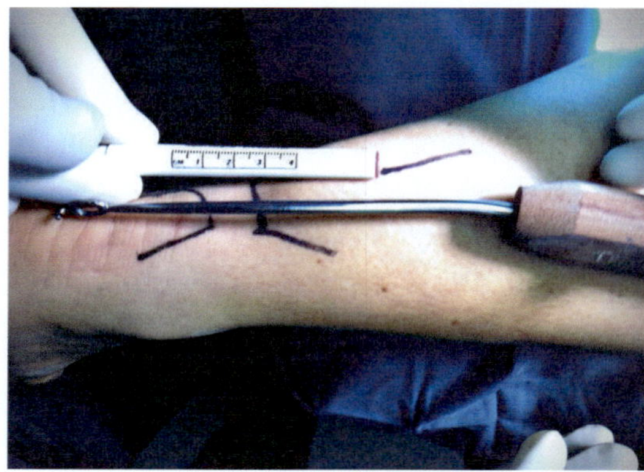

Fig. 7.1 After outlining the rupture site and the skin incision, we perform a 3-cm longitudinal, dorsomedial incision approximately 3 cm proximal to the rupture site

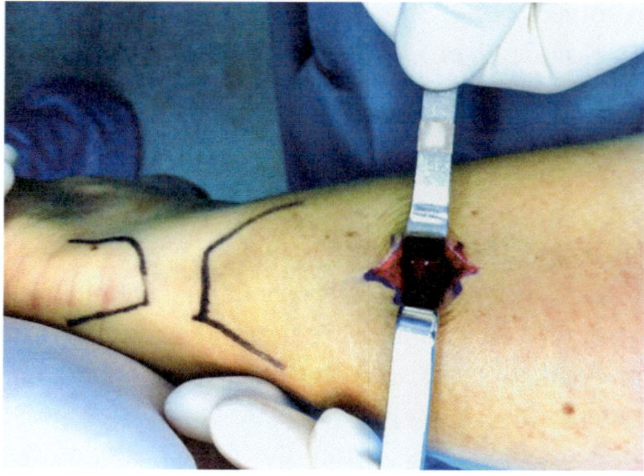

Fig. 7.2 The crural fascia is opened and the paratenon exposed. Dissection is performed carefully not to open the paratenon

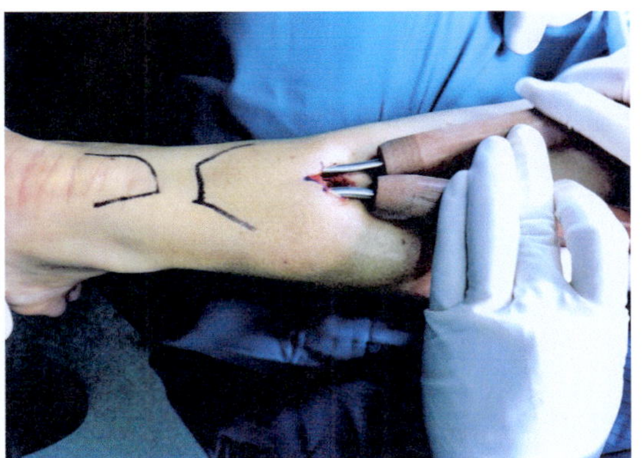

Fig. 7.3 The Dresden instruments are introduced into the layer between the crural fascia and the paratenon (subfascial epi/paratenon plane), one medial and the other lateral to the Achilles tendon. This step is crucial to avoid injury to the sural nerve

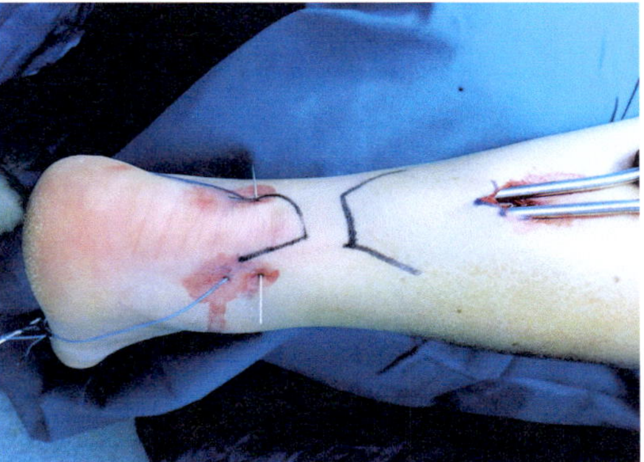

Fig. 7.4 Two sutures are introduced at the distal stump, separated by 1 cm and starting at 1 cm from the tendon's footprint. A straight needle is used to catch both instruments' aperture sites and pass the suture through the tendon. The same step is repeated after retrieving the Dresden devices 1 cm proximal to introduce the second suture

- Using a straight needle with a 2.0 FiberWire (Arthrex, Inc., Naples, FL, USA), pierce through the skin through the aperture of the instrument and the Achilles tendon.
- The second instrument is introduced on the contralateral side of the tendon as far as the needle. The needle is pulled back into the tendon. The second instrument is pushed until the opening of the instrument is at the level of the needle. The needle is now passed through the aperture of the second instrument, and the thread is pulled through.
- After that, a second suture is placed at 1 cm proximally using the method described (Fig. 7.4).
- The suture ends on one side and held securely, and the instrument is pulled out of the contralateral side. The suture ends, which have already been pulled out, are then fixed, and the second instrument is removed (Fig. 7.5).
- Pull the sutures firmly until there is maximum plantarflexion of the foot to check if the sutures are firmly in place. The pullout strength of each suture is revised separately.
- The suture's proximal anchorage is ensured by a suture using a robust and free needle with 3/8 curvature from lateral or medial toward central. The distance of both sutures should be approximately 5 mm. The assistant holds the

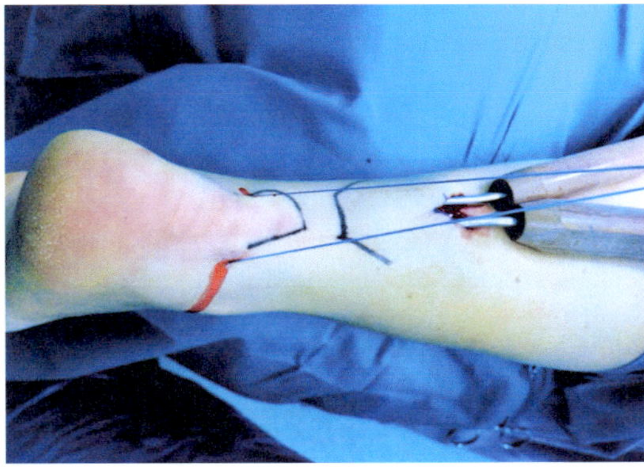

Fig. 7.5 The instrument is retrieved at the proximal incision. The sutures are provided with axial traction to ensure their firm attachment to the distal stump. After separate traction of each suture, full ankle plantarflexion should be observed

foot in maximum plantarflexion, and a knot is tied and firmly tightened. The knot is held under tension (Fig. 7.6).

- The assistant lets go of the foot, and the plantarflexion angle is measured with the knee bent at 90° (Matles test). The initial tension is then adjusted to the same on each side, and knotting is completed.
- The second suture is fixed approximately 1–2 cm proximal to the first knot in the same

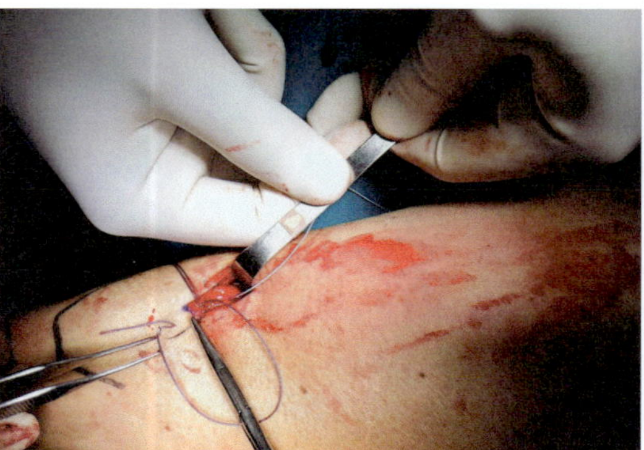

Fig. 7.6 The suture's proximal anchorage is ensured from lateral or medial toward central. The assistant holds the foot in maximum plantar flexion, and the knots are firmly tightened

way, whereby primary stability can be increased by additional looping.

- The knots are "buried" by tying up both sutures and inserting them directly next to the knots.
- Wound closure is performed in a layered fashion.
- In cases of distal Achilles tendon rupture, the instruments are advanced to the calcaneus. The sutures are anchored in a transcalcaneal position through the instrument's opening via a 2.5-mm drill hole using a drill sleeve.

The PARS Technique [1, 40, 42]

- General or regional anesthesia can be used, although regional is preferred when feasible.
- This technique is performed with the patient in a prone position with no thigh tourniquet. However, if desired, the tourniquet should be placed on the thigh, not the calf, to avoid limiting the excursion of the gastrocnemius-soleus complex.
- Drape both legs to adjust the gastrocnemius-soleus complex's tension compared to the contralateral normal side.
- Proximal and distal Achilles stumps are delimited in the skin, and a 3-cm transverse incision is marked at 1 cm proximal to the tendon gap (Fig. 7.7).

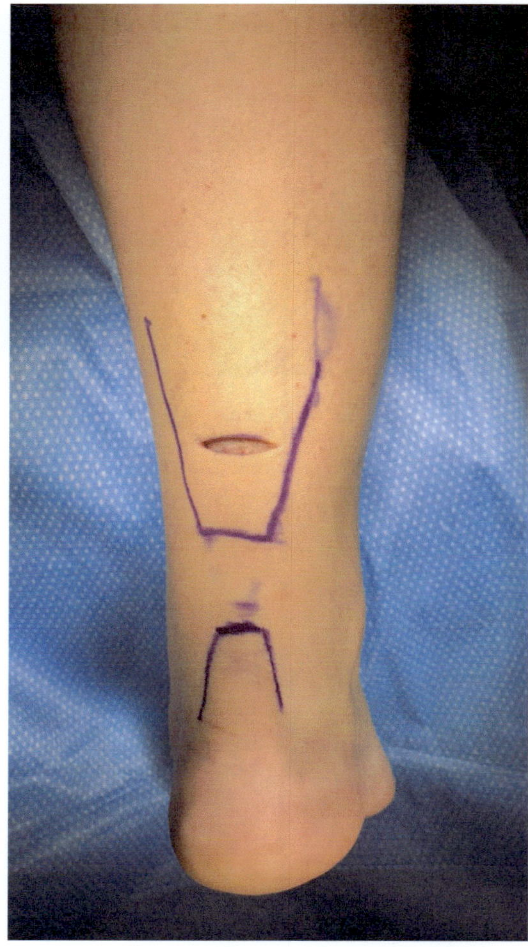

Fig. 7.7 Proximal and distal Achilles stumps are delimited in the skin, and a 3-cm transverse incision is made 3 cm proximal to the tendon gap

- The incision is carried out into the deep fascia, opening the paratenon.
- Carefully, blunt dissection is performed at the medial and lateral borders of the proximal stump to identify the tendon width correctly. Afterward, the inner arms of the PARS jig are inserted into the wound and accommodated to the tendon width by adjusting the wheel at the jig's base (Fig. 7.8).
- The surgeon must firmly press the jig toward the Achilles tendon to ensure that the instrument will capture enough tissue. The outer arms of the PARS jig have seven holes, which are chronologically numbered from 1 to 7.

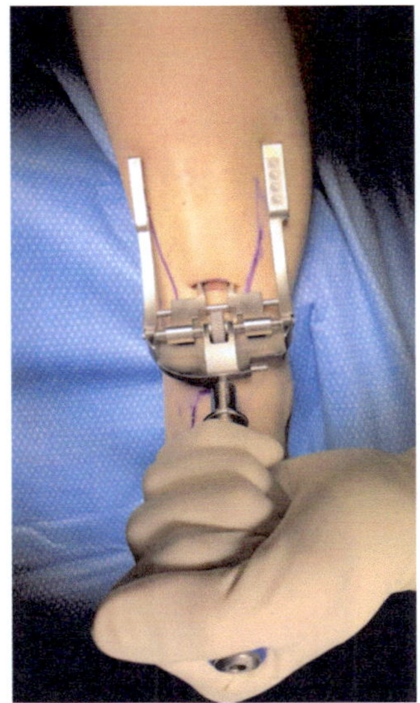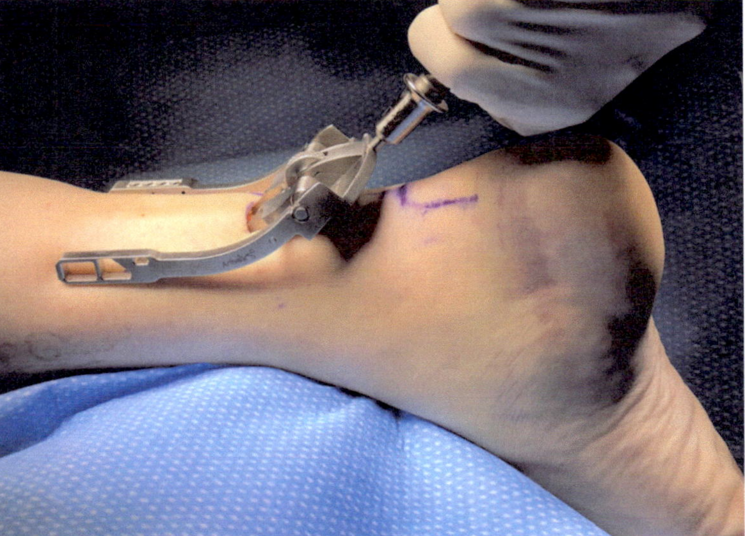

Fig. 7.8 The inner arms of the PARS jig are inserted into the wound and accommodated to the tendon width

- A needle is passed through hole number 1 and left in place during the rest of the procedure, stabilizing the jig and facilitating Achilles tendon capture.
- Then the PARS needle with the nitinol loop is passed through hole number 2. A blue #2 SutureTape is pulled through the leg, leaving tails on both sides of equal length.
- Again, the PARS needle is passed through holes 3 and 4. White and green #2 SutureTape with loops are pulled through the leg, leaving tails on both sides of equal length. The surgeon needs to be sure that one looped end is left on each side of the leg to lock one suture of the construct (blue SutureTape at number 2) during the operation.
- The PARS needle is passed through hole number 5, and the white and black #2 SutureTape are pulled through the leg, leaving tails on both sides of equal lengths.
- Finally, the white #2 SutureTape is pulled through the leg using the needle that was left in place at hole number 1 (Fig. 7.9).
- The jig is pulled down for removal, and sutures are recovered at the wound to be organized the way they have initially been placed through the PARS jig (Fig. 7.10).

- The #2 blue SutureTape is passed under the numbers 3 and 4 looped SutureTape and backed through the loop of the white and green looped suture at each side.
- By pulling on the nonlooped side (one at a time) of numbers 3 and 4 white and green looped sutures, #2 SutureTape is passed through the Achilles tendon into the other side. This step locks the blue SutureTape in place, leaving a construct with two transverse sutures and one locked at each side of the tendon (Fig. 7.10).
- Pull the white and black/white suture individually to ensure the suture does not pull through the tendon. If either suture pulls out, the jig is reinserted, and the suture passing needle is passed with its designated suture.
- The jig is reinserted into the distal stump, and the same order for suture passing is conducted, as detailed for the proximal stump.
- Once all sutures are passed, there should be three sutures with excellent tension proximally and distally on each side.
- The sutures are tied down with the foot held in a plantarflexed position by an assistant. The black/white sutures are tied on one side, followed by shuttling the knot more proximally

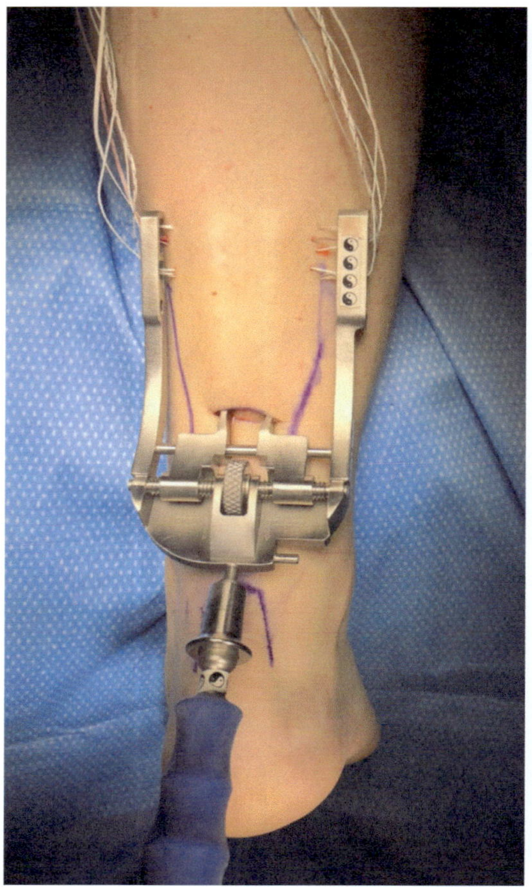

Fig. 7.9 A needle with a nitinol loop is passed through the Jig's holes in an ordered fashion

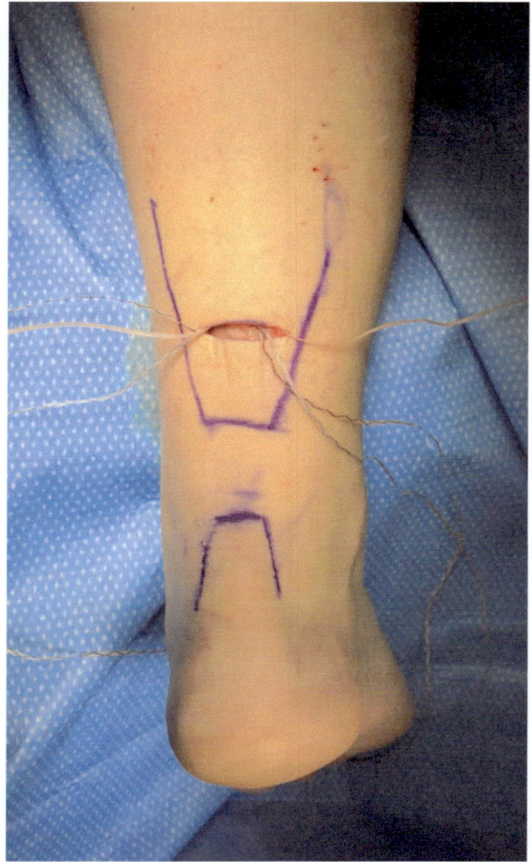

Fig. 7.10 The jig is pulled down for removal, and sutures are recovered at the wound to be organized in the way they were placed initially through the PARS jig

by pulling on the contralateral free suture. The other side of the black/white suture is tied next.

- The blue locking sutures are tied on both sides.
- The white suture is tied on one side, followed by shuttling the knot more proximally by pulling on the contralateral free suture. The other side of the white suture is tied next.
- The repair is tested by the restoration of the Thompson test and with moderate dorsiflexion pressure on the foot. If the repair fails with gentle pressure or there is no plantarflexion with calf squeeze, the quality of the repair should be reevaluated and revised if needed.
- Wounds are closed in a layered manner, and a sterile dressing is applied.

The PARS-Dresden Technique [42]

- General or regional anesthesia can be used, although regional is preferred when feasible.
- This technique is performed with the patient in a prone position with no thigh tourniquet; however, if desired, the tourniquet should be placed on the thigh, not the calf, to avoid limiting the excursion of the gastrocnemius-soleus complex.
- Drape both legs to adjust the gastrocnemius-soleus complex's tension compared to the contralateral normal side.
- Proximal and distal Achilles stumps are delimited in the skin, and a 3-cm transverse incision

is marked at 3 cm proximal to the tendon gap (Fig. 7.7).

- The incision is carried out into the deep fascia without opening the paratenon.
- This structure can be easily identified as a thin layer surrounding the Achilles tendon after blunt dissection of the deep fascia.
- The development of the subfascial epi/paratenon plane is of paramount importance to avoid the entrapment of the sural nerve as the nerve course is superficial to the deep fascia layer.
- Carefully, blunt dissection is performed at the medial and lateral borders of the proximal stump to identify the tendon width correctly. Afterward, the inner arms of the PARS jig are inserted into the wound and accommodated to the tendon width by adjusting the wheel at the jig's base.
- The surgeon must firmly press the jig toward the Achilles tendon to ensure that the instrument will capture enough tissue. The outer arms of the PARS jig have seven holes, which are chronologically numbered from 1 to 7 (Fig. 7.8).
- The PARS technique is used in the proximal tendon stump (Figs. 7.9 and 7.10).
- Two stab incisions are made 2 cm apart over the calcaneus near the Achilles insertion.
- The 3.4 drill bit is used to prepare the hole for a 4.75-mm Swivelock (Arthrex) anchor fixation. Drilling direction should aim 45° proximal and 30° to the midline to achieve an optimal purchase (Fig. 7.11).
- Each hole must be tapered until every thread of the tap disappears into the bone, avoiding potential anchor breakage during fixation. The PARS needles are left in the prepared holes as a guide for tunnel direction in anticipation of final fixation.
- Banana SutureLasso (Arthrex) is introduced through the medial stab incision and drove through the distal medial half of the Achilles tendon into the proximal Achilles stump (Fig. 7.12).
- Sutures are loaded into the Nitinol lasso and retrieved at the incision. The same steps are

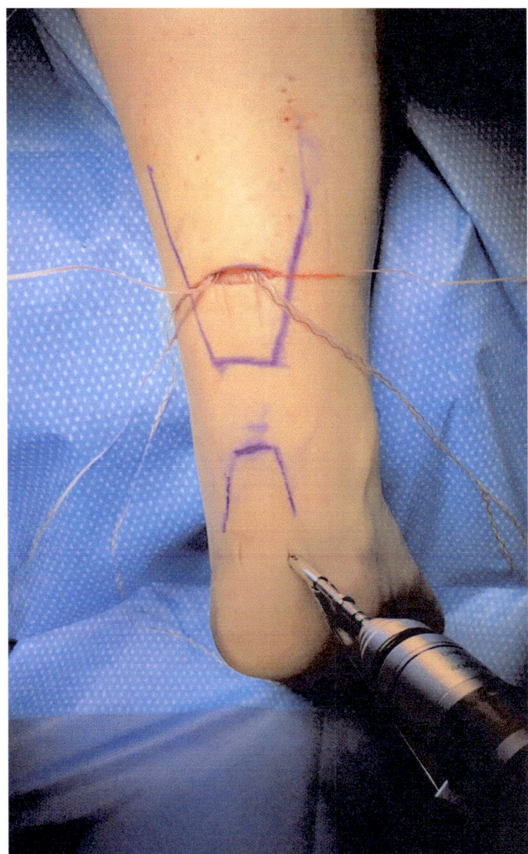

Fig. 7.11 Two stab incisions are made 2 cm apart near the Achilles insertion, and the 3.4 drill bit is used to prepare the hole into the calcaneus for a 4.75-mm Swivelock (Arthrex) anchor fixation. Drilling direction should aim perpendicular to the bone and 30° to the midline

realized to deliver the lateral sutures into the lateral stab incision.

- Ensure that maximal tension has been applied to the sutures and that medial sutures are fixed into the medial tunnel using a 4.75-mm Swivelock with the foot in slight hyper-plantarflexion (Fig. 7.13).
- After that, the lateral sutures are fixed in a similar manner using another 4.75-mm Swivelock. Wounds are closed in a layered way, and a sterile dressing is applied. No immobilization is used after surgery (Fig. 7.14).

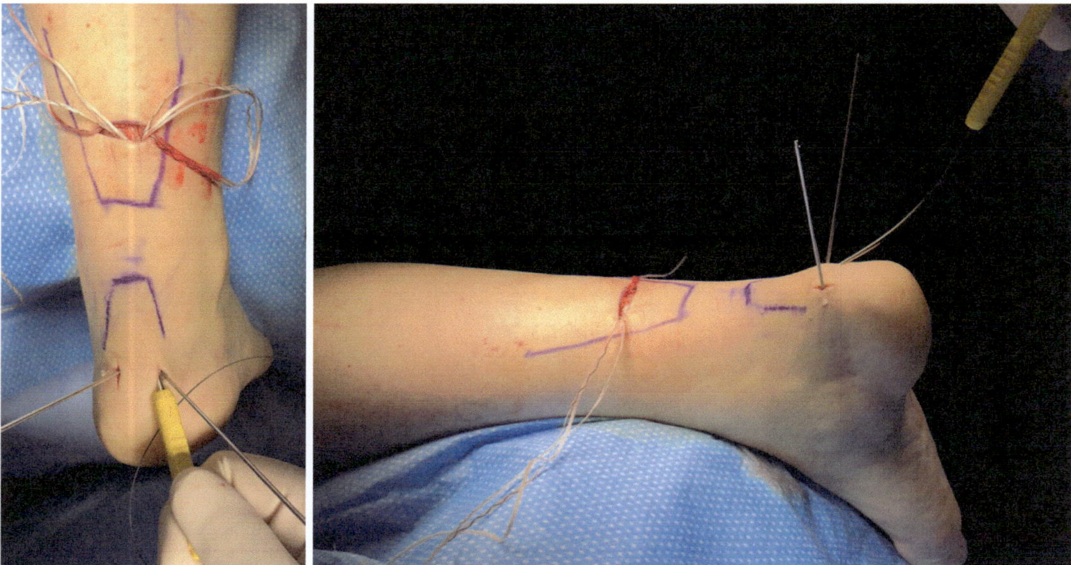

Fig. 7.12 A Banana SutureLasso (Arthrex) is introduced through the medial stab incision and driven through the distal medial half of the Achilles tendon into the proximal Achilles stump

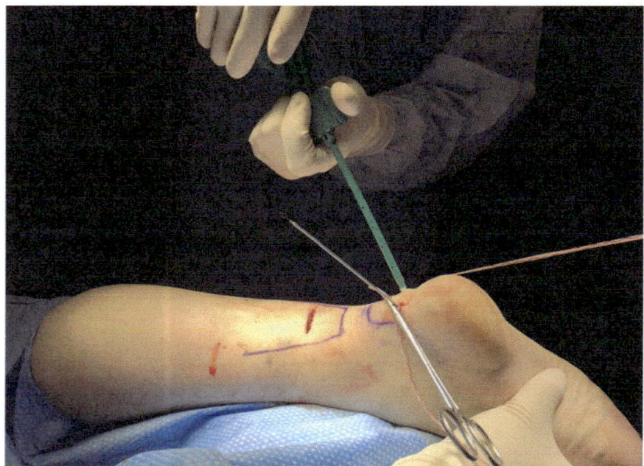

Fig. 7.13 The sutures rescued to the distal incisions are fixed into the tunnels using a 4.75-mm Swivelock with the foot in slight hyper-plantarflexion

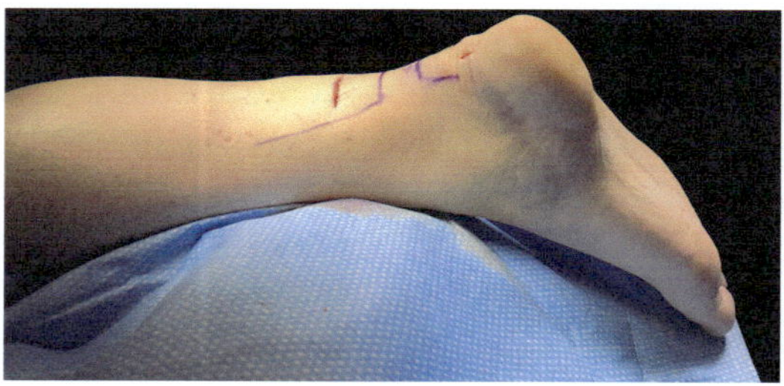

Fig. 7.14 Final view after the procedure

Postoperative Rehabilitation Protocol [42]

Patients are operated on and discharged the same day or stay overnight. No immobilization of any kind is used on these patients. All patients are authorized to weight bear on two crutches as tolerated. Early weight-bearing should be reconsidered if a soft bone is detected during anchor placing.

We do not follow up on patients using ultrasound at any time during the recovery period unless there is clinical suspicion of rerupture, deep infection, or unexplained pain source. Thromboprophylaxis is initiated on day 1 using dabigatran for 30 days.

Dressings are changed during the first postoperative visit at 7 days, and physiotherapy is started at this time.

We follow a stepwise rehabilitation protocol as follows:

- Week 1: Gentle mobilization and active dorsiflexion are encouraged. No passive dorsiflexion is authorized.

- Week 2: Sutures are removed, and compression socks are recommended. Progressive plantarflexion exercises are started at this time.
- Week 3: Crutches are progressively removed as tolerated, and plantarflexion exercises continue. Cardiovascular exercises are initiated.
- Week 4: Initiate biking and passive dorsiflexion. Patients may stop using crutches if tolerated. Exercises progress in intensity as tolerated but avoid impact activities—proprioceptive and gait training.
- Week 8: Patients can progress to swimming or continue biking until week 12. Continue to progress with a range of motion, strength, and proprioception.
- Week 12: This involves eccentric strengthening, progressive impact, loading, speed work, and plyometric training. Patients can progress to sports-specific activity as tolerated.
- Weeks 20 to 24: Patients can return to unrestricted sports if they can perform 20 single heel rises and have completed sports-specific protocols.

Conclusions

Minimally invasive repair of acute Achilles tendon ruptures has proven to be a safe and reliable treatment modality. In comparison with open repairs, patients resume their function level and activities with a low complication rate. Smokers and poorly controlled diabetics are overall poor surgical candidates. However, we believe that a minimally invasive technique is considered for patients with high comorbidities requiring surgery.

We have witnessed how these techniques have evolved over the years. General concepts in an optimal strategy include minimal dissection, avoidance of fixation in the distal stump, preservation of the tendon's rupture hematoma, and early mobilization. For the reasons mentioned above, we believe that the PARS-Dresden technique offers the best combination of these ideas.

References

1. Patel MS, Kadakia AR. Minimally invasive treatments of acute Achilles tendon ruptures. Foot Ankle Clin. 2019;24:399–424.
2. Twaddle BC, Poon P. Early motion for Achilles tendon ruptures: is surgery important? A randomized, prospective study. Am J Sports Med. 2007;35:2033–8.
3. Willits K, et al. Operative versus nonoperative treatment of acute Achilles tendon ruptures: a multicenter randomized trial using accelerated functional rehabilitation. J Bone Joint Surg Am. 2010;92:2767–75.
4. Nilsson-Helander K, et al. Acute achilles tendon rupture: a randomized, controlled study comparing surgical and nonsurgical treatments using validated outcome measures. Am J Sports Med. 2010;38:2186–93.
5. Morrey BF. Operative versus nonoperative treatment of acute achilles tendon ruptures: a multicenter randomized trial using accelerated functional rehabilitation. Yearbook Orthop. 2011;2011:228–30.
6. Liu Y et al. Early functional rehabilitation versus traditional immobilization for repair of acute Achilles tendon ruptures: a meta-analysis based on randomized controlled trials. 2020, https://doi.org/10.37766/inplasy2020.8.0100.
7. Olsson N, et al. Stable surgical repair with accelerated rehabilitation versus nonsurgical treatment for acute Achilles tendon ruptures: a randomized controlled study. Am J Sports Med. 2013;41:2867–76.
8. Heikkinen J, et al. Soleus atrophy is common after the nonsurgical treatment of acute Achilles tendon ruptures: a randomized clinical trial comparing surgical and nonsurgical functional treatments. Am J Sports Med. 2017;45:1395–404.
9. Krackow KA, Thomas SC, Jones LC. Ligament-tendon fixation: analysis of a new stitch and comparison with standard techniques. Orthopedics. 1988;11:909–17.
10. Khan RJK, et al. Treatment of acute achilles tendon ruptures. A meta-analysis of randomized, controlled trials. J Bone Joint Surg Am. 2005;87:2202–10.
11. Movin T, Ryberg A, McBride DJ, Maffulli N. Acute rupture of the Achilles tendon. Foot Ankle Clin. 2005;10:331–56.
12. Soroceanu A, Sidhwa F, Aarabi S, Kaufman A, Glazebrook M. Surgical versus nonsurgical treatment of acute Achilles tendon rupture: a meta-analysis of randomized trials. J Bone Joint Surg Am. 2012;94:2136–43.
13. Wilkins R, Bisson LJ. Operative versus nonoperative management of acute Achilles tendon ruptures: a quantitative systematic review of randomized controlled trials. Am J Sports Med. 2012;40:2154–60.
14. Majewski M, Rohrbach M, Czaja S, Ochsner P. Avoiding sural nerve injuries during percutaneous Achilles tendon repair. Am J Sports Med. 2006;34:793–8.

15. Webb JM, Bannister GC. Percutaneous repair of the ruptured tendo Achillis. J Bone Joint Surg Br. 1999;81:877–80.
16. Chen TM, et al. The arterial anatomy of the Achilles tendon: anatomical study and clinical implications. Clin Anat. 2009;22:377–85.
17. Amlang MH, Christiani P, Heinz P, Zwipp H. Die perkutane Naht der Achillessehne mit dem Dresdner instrument the percutaneous suture of the Achilles tendon with the Dresden instrument. Oper Orthop Traumatol. 2006;18:287–99.
18. Carr AJ, Norris SH. The blood supply of the calcaneal tendon. J Bone Joint Surg Br. 1989;71:100–1.
19. Mullaney MJ, McHugh MP, Tyler TF, Nicholas SJ, Lee SJ. Weakness in end-range plantar flexion after Achilles tendon repair. Am J Sports Med. 2006;34:1120–5.
20. Cetti R, Christensen SE, Ejsted R, Jensen NM, Jorgensen U. Operative versus nonoperative treatment of Achilles tendon rupture. A prospective randomized study and review of the literature. Am J Sports Med. 1993;21:791–9.
21. Ma GW, Griffith TG. Percutaneous repair of acute closed ruptured achilles tendon: a new technique. Clin Orthop Relat Res. 1977:247–55.
22. Klein W, Lang DM, Saleh M. The use of the Ma-Griffith technique for percutaneous repair of fresh ruptured tendo Achillis. Chir Organi Mov. 1991;76:223–8.
23. Rozis M, et al. Outcome of percutaneous fixation of acute Achilles tendon ruptures. Foot Ankle Int. 2018;39:689–93.
24. Hockenbury RT, Johns JC. A biomechanical in vitro comparison of open versus percutaneous repair of tendon Achilles. Foot Ankle. 1990;11:67–72.
25. Davies MS, Solan M. Minimal incision techniques for acute Achilles repair. Foot Ankle Clin. 2009;14:685–97.
26. Gorschewsky O, Pitzl M, Pütz A, Klakow A, Neumann W. Percutaneous repair of acute Achilles tendon rupture. Foot Ankle Int. 2004;25:219–24.
27. Wagnon R, Akayi M. The Webb-Bannister percutaneous technique for acute Achilles' tendon ruptures: a functional and MRI assessment. J Foot Ankle Surg. 2005;44:437–44.
28. Buono AD, Del Buono A, Volpin A, Maffulli N. Minimally invasive versus open surgery for acute Achilles tendon rupture: a systematic review. Br Med Bull. 2014;109:45–54.
29. Amlang MH, Christiani P, Heinz P, Zwipp H. Die perkutane Naht der Achillessehne mit dem Dresdner Instrument. Oper Orthop Traumatol. 2006;18:287–99.
30. Henríquez H, Muñoz R, Carcuro G, Bastías C. Is percutaneous repair better than open repair in acute Achilles tendon rupture? Clin Orthop Relat Res. 2012;470:998–1003.
31. Keller A, Ortiz C, Wagner E, Wagner P, Mococain P. Mini-open tenorrhaphy of acute Achilles tendon ruptures. Am J Sports Med. 2014;42:731–6.
32. Elton JP, Bluman EM. Limited open Achilles tendon repair with modified ring forceps: technique tip. Foot Ankle Int. 2010;31:914–5.
33. Kakiuchi M. A combined open and percutaneous technique for repair of tendo Achillis. Comparison with open repair. J Bone Joint Surg Br. 1995;77-B:60–3.
34. Assal M, et al. Limited open repair of Achilles tendon ruptures. J Bone Joint Surg Am. 2002;84:161–70.
35. Calder JDF. Early, active rehabilitation following mini-open repair of Achilles tendon rupture: a prospective study. Br J Sports Med. 2005;39:857–9.
36. Kołodziej Ł, Bohatyrewicz A, Kromuszczyńska J, Jezierski J, Biedroń M. Efficacy and complications of open and minimally invasive surgery in acute Achilles tendon rupture: a prospective randomised clinical study—preliminary report. Int Orthop. 2013;37:625–9.
37. Alcelik I, et al. Achillon versus open surgery in acute Achilles tendon repair. Foot Ankle Surg. 2018;24:427–34.
38. Hsu AR, et al. Clinical outcomes and complications of percutaneous Achilles repair system versus open technique for acute Achilles tendon ruptures. Foot Ankle Int. 2015;36:1279–86.
39. Demetracopoulos CA, Gilbert SL, Young E, Baxter JR, Deland JT. Limited-open Achilles tendon repair using locking sutures versus nonlocking sutures. Foot Ankle Int. 2014;35:612–8.
40. McWilliam JR, Mackay G. The internal brace for Midsubstance Achilles ruptures. Foot Ankle Int. 2016;37:794–800.
41. Clanton TO, et al. A biomechanical comparison of an open repair and 3 minimally invasive percutaneous Achilles tendon repair techniques during a simulated, progressive rehabilitation protocol. Am J Sports Med. 2015;43:1957–64.
42. Pellegrini MJ, Butteri A, Chaparro F, Carcuro G, Ortiz C. New option for Achilles tendon ruptures, combining the best of all: the PARS-Dresden. Tech Foot Ankle Surg. 2019;18:50.

Minimally Invasive Treatment of Achilles Tendon Tears

Fernando Aran [iD], Karl M. Schweitzer Jr, and James K. DeOrio

Introduction

In an effort to reduce wound complications, improve patient outcomes, and achieve earlier return to sport, orthopedic surgeons have been trying to perfect minimally invasive techniques for acute Achilles tendon repairs. This started with the Ma and Griffith technique first published in 1977 [1]. As a truly percutaneous technique, there was a much lower wound complication rate, but sural nerve injuries were a real concern. Cretnik et al. reported a 0.7% wound complication rate vs 13% in their open group in 2005 [2], but sural nerve injuries were reported as high as 13% [3]. In order to avoid sural nerve injuries, a number of modifications were made. One of the earliest modifications done by Cretnik et al. was to do the repair on an awake patient with local anesthetic. If the patient had severe pain with the passage of one of the sutures, it was removed and replaced. They reported their incidence of sural nerve injury at 4.5% with this technique [2]. This technique was not widely adopted.

Subsequently, the idea of capturing the suture within the paratenon with a loom-like device was developed. This was first done with a custom device by Assal et al. This device was then patented and sold as the Achillon Achilles repair system. The technique calls for a 2 cm vertical incision centered medial to the tendon at the level of the rupture. The incision is then carried deep, and the paratenon is opened. The Achillon device is a plastic loom that is inserted along the residual tendon that allows the passage of three sutures in a transverse fashion both proximally and distally to the tear. The corresponding proximal and distal sutures are tied together through the incision. Their initial report was for 87 patients who underwent this technique and was published in 2002. They reported no wound issues, no sural nerve complications, and three reruptures with an average 26 month follow-up, which equated to a 3.7% rerupture rate [4]. A systematic review later revealed that the complication rates were as follows: 3.2% rerupture, 2% wound complications, 1.2% sural nerve injuries, 1.2% suture reactions or irritations, and 0.8% infections [5]. The Achillon system was disposable and therefore costly. In addition, surgeons were concerned that you could not create a locking suture construct that could strengthen the repair [6]. Biomechanical testing of Achilles tendon repairs had demonstrated that locking suture constructs were superior in load-to-failure testing [7].

F. Aran · K. M. SchweitzerJr · J. K. DeOrio (✉)
Department of Orthopaedic Surgery, Duke University
Medical Center, Durham, NC, USA
e-mail: Fernando.Aran@duke.edu;
Karl.Schweitzer@duke.edu;
James.DeOrio@duke.edu

PARS Technique

The Percutaneous Achilles Repair System (PARS) was then created as an additional minimally invasive technique. The original PARS technique used a 2 cm transverse incision, and a metal loom was placed first proximally to pass and capture sutures at the proximal residual tendon. This technique called for five independent suture passes with a locking technique of the crossing sutures to pass the second suture, which resulted ultimately in three sutures being tied: two unlocked and one locked. This was repeated proximally and distally. The sutures were tied sequentially: first, nearest to the rupture and progress to the middle suture, then to the farthest from the tear to avoid the bunching of the tendon. The first large retrospective cohort by Hsu et al., published in 2015, compared open repair vs the PARS technique. In total, there were 270 patients; 101 underwent PARS repair. Ninety-eight percent were able to return to baseline activities compared to 82% in the open group. Complications in this cohort for the PARS were 3% superficial wound dehiscence treated with local wound care and 2% reoperation for foreign body reaction to FiberWire suture. In the open group, for comparison, there was 3% sural neuritis, 4.1% superficial wound dehiscence treated with local wound care, 1.8% superficial infection treated with oral antibiotics, and 1.8% reoperation for deep infection. In total, there was a difference of 5% complication rate in the PARS group vs 10.6% in the open group [6]. The PARS system gained wide adoption after this paper and has become the preferred system for minimally invasive Achilles tendon repair for many surgeons.

Current MIS Achilles Tendon Techniques and Further Evolution

From the time of the first percutaneous Achilles technique to the modern day, the incidence of Achilles ruptures has increased significantly due to the increase in participation in sport in the adult population. The incidence in 1979 was 2.1 per 100,000 and increased to 21.5 per 100,000 in 2011 [8]. Most studies have demonstrated a decrease in wound complications, quicker return to sport, and reduced sural nerve complications with modern minimally invasive surgery (MIS) techniques.

At our institution, we have adopted many of the original PARS technique suggestions, but we have also made a few modifications. Below, we will present our suggested technique, along with photographic and illustrative support.

It is advisable that the patient who suffers an Achilles tendon rupture is identified in an expeditious manner. If the decision is made to proceed with surgery, it should ideally be done within a 2-week period to ensure that the tendon is still mobile and can be manipulated with the percutaneous technique. In Hsu et al.'s study, there was an average of 6 days from injury to surgery ± 3 days on average [6]. This requires an efficient clinic or referral system to capture these patients within the short window of opportunity to use this system.

Technique

We place a thigh tourniquet on our patients and lay them prone on the operating room table. The leg is prepped and draped in a sterile fashion, and the tourniquet is inflated. The Achilles tendon is palpated, and the rupture site is identified. A 2–3 cm incision is placed vertically, midline over the rupture. The paratenon is incised, and the proximal residual tendon is identified and then held with one Alice clamp (Fig. 8.1) Sometimes it is necessary to free up the tendon from the surrounding paratenon to gain excursion; this becomes more important the farther away you are from injury. To do so, a ½ inch key elevator is used to free up the tendon while keeping the tendon under tension with the Alice clamps.

Next, the PARS Achilles jig is inserted under the paratenon, while the tendon continues to be held in tension by the Alice clamps. The jig is opened or closed until it matches the width of the tendon and then inserted until it reaches the full depth of the jig. The first PARS needle is placed

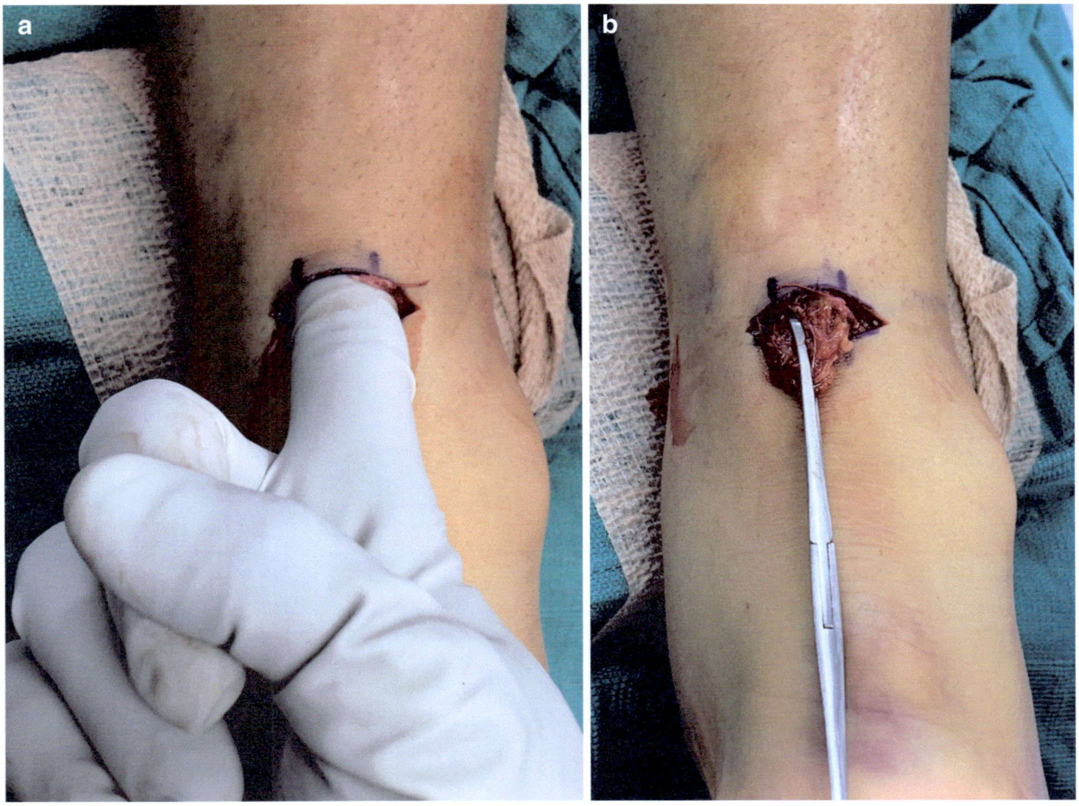

Fig. 8.1 (**a**) Identifying the proximal residual Achilles tendon. (**b**) Holding the proximal tendon with an Alice clamp

through the hole numbered #1 and is left in place. This will maintain the tendon length and position while the other needles and their corresponding sutures are passed (Fig. 8.2). You follow with holes 2–5 in a similar manner, passing the sutures from one side to the other. Sutures 3 and 4 are crossing and will be used to form the locking construct with suture number 2. It is important that the loops for sutures 3 and 4 end up on opposite sides. Once all five sutures are passed, the technique is to wrap suture 2 around 3 and 4 and then pass each side into its corresponding loop before pulling it through. This creates the locking mechanism for the suture construct (Fig. 8.3). There are two additional suture passing holes in the jig that may be used for additional fixation. Holes 6 and 7 allow you to lock suture number 5 and are recommended to be used in high-level

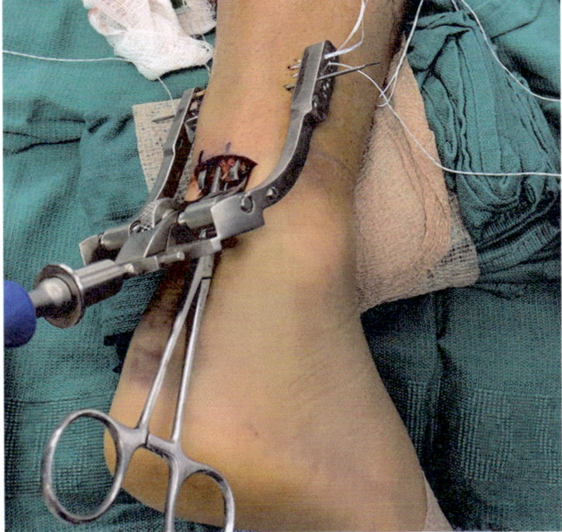

Fig. 8.2 Passing sutures in a sequential fashion through a jig

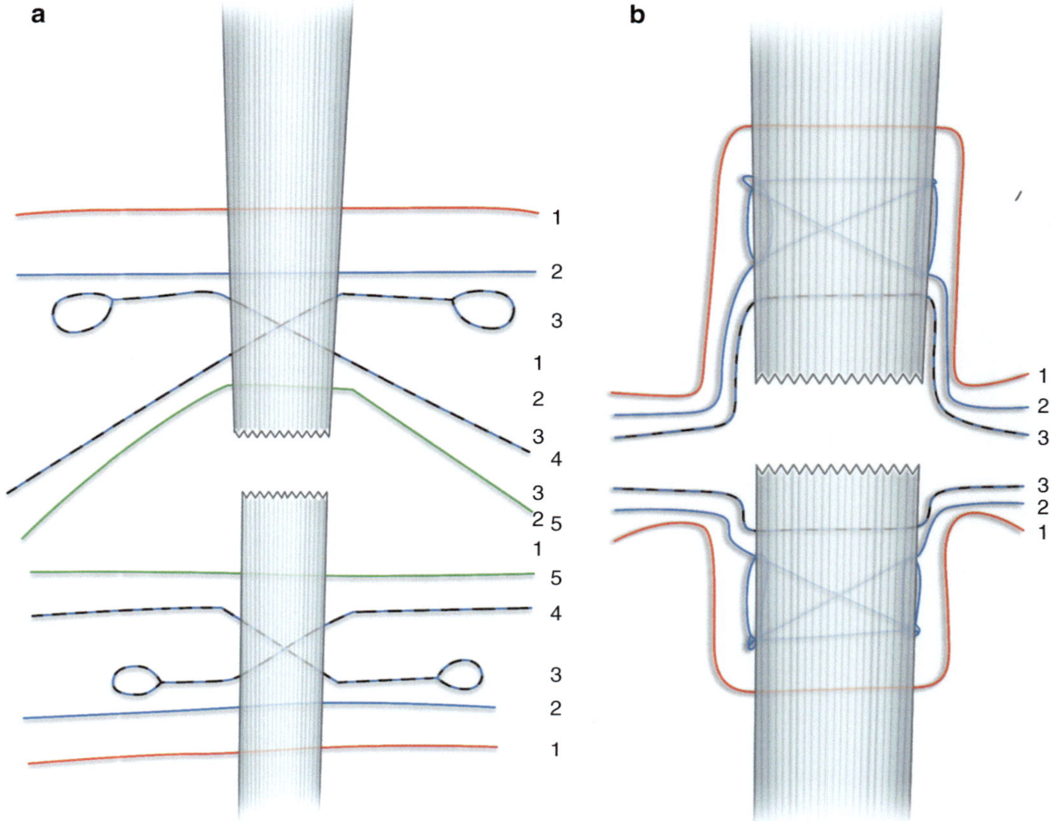

Fig. 8.3 (**a**) Illustration of suture passage through a PARS jig. (**b**) Suture relationship once the locking technique is performed

athletes. The technique is then repeated on the distal residual tendon still connected to the calcaneus.

With this technique, you will have three sutures on each side of the tendon, both proximally and distally, for a total of 12 sutures, which are exiting your incision (Fig. 8.4). These can then be tied in a sequential fashion from closest to the rupture to the farthest. The foot is maximally plantar flexed. You tie the corresponding sutures proximally and distally. One of the original design surgeons recommends tying the non-locked sutures first and then the locked sutures last. In this manner, it is believed that you pull the tendon ends closer together. The paratenon is then closed with 3-0 Vicryl, the subcutaneous tissues are closed with 3-0 Vicryl, and the skin closed with 3-0 nylon. In the original outcome

paper, there were some reoperations due to foreign body reactions to the FiberWire suture. In modified techniques, the FiberWire has been replaced with suture tape, which has higher pullout strength and smaller knot stacks (Figs. 8.5 and 8.6].

Additionally, another modification to the technique has been added which may prove useful [9]. This is used when the Achilles tendon rupture happens in the setting of a chronic Achilles tendonitis or there is an inadequate tendon stump on the calcaneus. Here, the tissue for repair may be suboptimal and have low pullout strength. The modification used by our senior author uses a bone tunnel in the calcaneus and passes the suture from the proximal stump through this bone tunnel for fixation. There has been a similar commercial solution that uses two suture anchors for

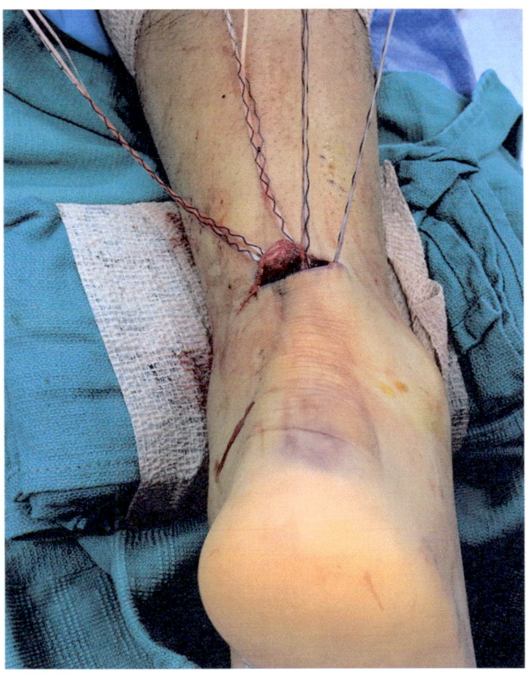

Fig. 8.4 Proximal and distal sutures exiting at incision

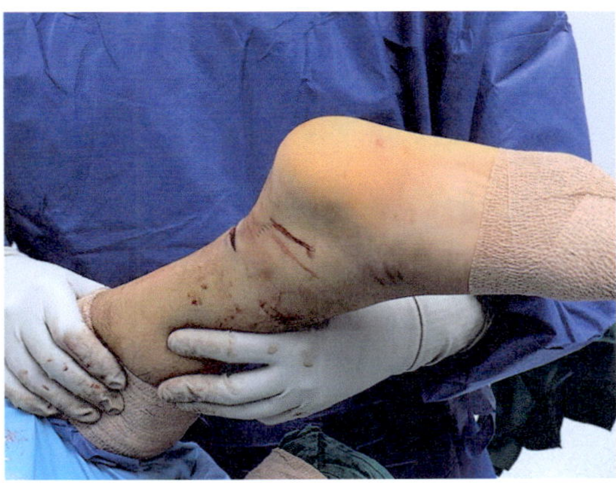

Fig. 8.5 Completed repair in resting plantar flexion before the skin is closed

the distal fixation. The six proximal strands of the suture are passed distally and fixed through a knotless technique to anchors in the calcaneus.

A similar technique has been described with a proximal incision instead of a mid-rupture incision by the Wagner brothers and the use of bony anchors [10].

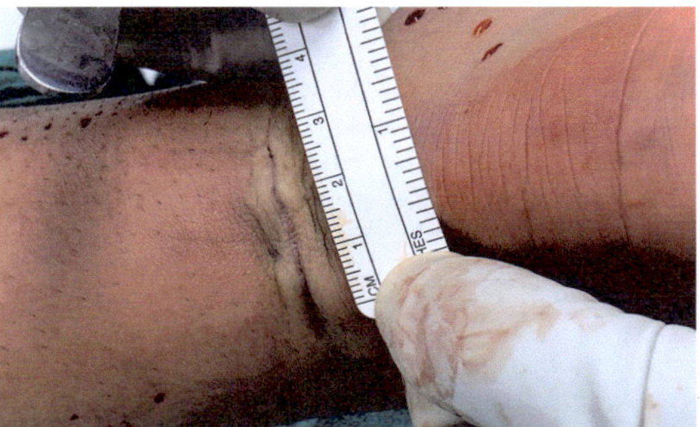

Fig. 8.6 Closed subcutaneous layer and paratenon; incision length is typically 3 cm

In summary, MIS techniques for acute Achilles tendon repairs and advancements in the technique have led to lower sural nerve issues while maintaining the advantage of lower wound complications. Furthermore, the results have been excellent, and the rerupture rate was the lowest of any technique available.

References

1. Ma GW, Griffith TG. Percutaneous repair of acute closed ruptured achilles tendon: a new technique. Clin Orthop Relat Res. 1977;128:247–55.
2. Cretnik A, Kosanovic M, Smrkolj V. Percutaneous versus open repair of the ruptured Achilles tendon: a comparative study. Am J Sports Med. 2005;33(9):1369–79. https://doi.org/10.1177/0363546504271501. Epub 2005 Apr 12
3. Klein W, Lang DM, Saleh M. The use of the Ma-Griffith technique for percutaneous repair of fresh ruptured tendo Achillis. Chir Organi Mov. 1991;76:223–8.
4. Assal M, Jung M, Stern R, Rippstein P, Delmi M, Hoffmeyer P. Limited open repair of Achilles tendon ruptures: a technique with a new instrument and findings of a prospective multicenter study. J Bone Joint Surg Am. 2002;84(2):161–70.
5. Bartel AF, Elliott AD, Roukis TS. Incidence of complications after Achillon® mini-open suture system for repair of acute midsubstance achilles tendon ruptures: a systematic review. J Foot Ankle Surg. 2014;53(6):744–6. https://doi.org/10.1053/j.jfas.2014.07.009. Epub 2014 Sep 8
6. Hsu AR, Jones CP, Cohen BE, Davis WH, Ellington JK, Anderson RB. Clinical outcomes and complications of percutaneous Achilles repair system versus open technique for acute Achilles tendon ruptures.

Foot Ankle Int. 2015;36(11):1279–86. https://doi.org/10.1177/1071100715589632. Epub 2015 Jun 8

7. Demetracopoulos CA, Gilbert SL, Young E, Baxter JR, Deland JT. Limited-open Achilles tendon repair using locking sutures versus nonlocking sutures: an in vitro model. Foot Ankle Int. 2014;35(6):612–8. https://doi.org/10.1177/1071100714524550.

8. Lantto I, Heikkinen J, Flinkkilä T, Ohtonen P, Leppilahti J. Epidemiology of Achilles tendon ruptures: increasing incidence over a 33-year period.

Scand J Med Sci Sports. 2015;25(1):e133-8. https://doi.org/10.1111/sms.12253. Epub 2014 May 23

9. Clanton T, Stake IK, Bartush K, Jamieson MD. Minimally invasive Achilles repair techniques. Orthop Clin North Am. 2020;51(3):391–402. https://doi.org/10.1016/j.ocl.2020.02.005. PMID: 32498958

10. Wagner E, Wagner P. Mini-open Achilles tendon rupture repair. JBJS Essent Surg Tech. 2019;9(4):e46.1-2. https://doi.org/10.2106/JBJS.ST.18.00139. PMID: 32051783; PMCID: PMC6974314

Traditional Open Repair of Achilles Tendon Tears

9

Claude T. Moorman III and Maria K. A. Kaseta

Acute ruptures of the Achilles tendon are common injuries associated with trauma, male gender, obesity, and a history of injected corticosteroids [1]. Although there is a significant increase in the incidence of Achilles tendon injuries over the last 2 decades [2], there is no consensus regarding the optimal management (operative vs. nonoperative) of acute ruptures of the Achilles tendon [3–7]. This chapter describes the operative technique favored by the senior author as well as a physical therapy protocol that has resulted in excellent outcomes.

A number of studies have shown that surgical repair results in less morbidity and improved function. For example, surgically repaired tendons are at lower risk of rerupture [4, 7, 8], and patients who elect surgery achieve normal push-off power [9, 10]. One randomized prospective study compared operative versus nonoperative treatment of acute ruptures of the Achilles tendon in 111 patients and demonstrated better results (resuming sports activities, fewer subjective complaints) in the operative group at 1-year follow-up, although there were fewer minor complications in the nonoperative group [11]. Other advantages of surgical repair include decreased ankle stiffness and calf atrophy, fewer tendocutaneous adhesions, and a lower risk of thrombophlebitis [12, 13].

Open operative treatment of acute ruptures of the Achilles tendon is probably the method of choice for athletes and patients who wish to continue with high-demand physical activity [4, 9]. Two recent meta-analyses of randomized controlled trials showed that operative management has a reduced risk of rerupture compared with conservative measures but was associated with an increased risk of complications, including wound infections, delayed wound healing, adhesions, and disturbed sensations [4, 7].

Case Study

While playing golf, a 35-year-old man ran up a hill, felt a sudden onset of pain behind his right ankle, and heard a popping sound. He turned around as he thought he had been struck with an errant golf ball. He came to the clinic 6 days later with right lower extremity pain (2 on a 10-point visual analog scale). His aching pain was continuous, was worse in the morning, and aggravated when standing. He had been treating his pain with ice and non-weight-bearing (by sitting and lying down).

On physical examination, the patient was healthy except for non-weight-bearing on the right side. The leg length examination revealed that his limbs were equal. His right ankle range of motion was 30 degrees of dorsiflexion, 0

C. T. Moorman III
Department of Orthopaedic Surgery, Edward
N. Hanley Jr, MD Professor & Chair, Atrium Health
Musculoskeletal Institute, Charlotte, NC, USA
e-mail: T.Moorman@orthocarolina.com

M. K. A. Kaseta (✉)
Orthopaedic Surgeon, Konstantopouleion General
Hospital of N. Ionia, Athens, Greece

S. B. Adams (ed.), *The Achilles Tendon*, https://doi.org/10.1007/978-3-031-45594-0_9

degrees of plantarflexion, 15 degrees of inversion, and 30 degrees of eversion. The Thompson test was positive, and a mild ankle effusion was noted. His knee and hindfoot were in neutral alignment. He had a palpable defect in his Achilles tendon 3 cm proximal to the calcaneal insertion with tenderness at this site. His plantarflexion strength was 3/5. No additional motor or sensory deficits were noted. His peripheral pulses were normal with no edema. His personal and family histories were unremarkable. The clinical diagnosis was that he had a right Achilles tendon rupture.

The operation was performed 2 days after his initial clinical examination. Preoperative regional anesthesia was induced in the anesthesia holding area. The patient was taken to the operating room and placed in a prone position. The lower extremity was scrubbed using Hibiclens and alcohol, prepped using DuraPrep, and then draped using sterile drapes and towels. The extremity was exsanguinated using an Esmarch, and the tourniquet was inflated to 300 mm Hg. The tourniquet time for the procedure was 45 min.

An incision was made along the lateral portion of the midline. Dissection was carried down to identify the sural nerve that was retracted carefully. The peritenon was then identified and incised longitudinally over the torn portion. Both ends of the tear were then delivered to the wound site. Tajima sutures with No. 2 Orthocord sutures were placed into position using tapered needles. Two Tajima stitches were placed proximally, and two were placed distally. The foot was held in a 90-degree neutral position, and the sutures were tied down securely. Next, interrupted 0 Vicryl sutures were used to repair the tendon edges over the scaffolding, and then the paratenon was closed with 2-0 Vicryl over the site. The subcutaneous tissue was closed using 2-0 Vicryl. A running 3-0 Prolene subcuticular stitch was used for the skin. A bulky dry sterile dressing and a posterior splint were applied.

There was minimal blood loss, no drains, and no complications.

After the procedure, the patient was placed in a posterior splint and was non-weight-bearing for 10 days.

At 10 days, the splint was removed, and he was placed in a Cam walker with the ankle in a neutral position for weight-bearing. During this period, the patient began 30 cycles of rebound active dorsiflexion, three times per day, to provide gentle stress to the healing collagen to encourage healing along the lines of stress.

At 6 weeks, the patient was given the option of using an ankle-foot orthosis in his regular shoe but could return to the boot as needed. Thus, the injury was protected with non-weight-bearing and a boot or an ankle-foot orthosis for 3 months after the operation.

At 3 months, weight-bearing as tolerated was permitted in the absence of any immobilization. He was permitted to begin progression back to his sport but not allowed full participation until 6 months. The patient was evaluated clinically and subjectively. He went back to his athletic activities after 6 months and on the last follow-up had a normal tendon contour, full range of motion, and full strength with a resumption of all activities.

In an attempt to improve the overall outcome of patients with Achilles tendon rupture and to reduce complications, a number of different surgical techniques have been described, including open [14, 15], percutaneous [16, 17], and combined procedures [18]. Open surgical methods are of two types: those involving direct tendon repair with different suture techniques (e.g., Kessler, Bunnel, Tajima, Krakow, triple bundle) [19] and those involving reconstruction using grafts (e.g., gastrocnemius fascia, plantaris tendon, fascia lata, peroneus brevis, flexor digitorum longus (FDL), flexor hallucis longus (FHL)) [9], or synthetic materials (e.g., carbon fiber, Dacron grafts) [20, 21].

The choice of surgical procedure requires consideration of a number of factors, including mechanism of injury; the time from the initial injury [3, 5, 10, 15, 19, 22]; the presence of connective tissue diseases (which usually requires augmentation) [10]; local factors (e.g., ischemia, atrophy of gastrocnemius-soleus muscle, scars, infections) [5, 10]; and demographics such as age, gender, and athletic activity of the patient [10]. According to Wapner [10], primary end-to-end repair can be done up to 3 months postoperatively. In general, however, the longer the time from the initial injury, the less likely a primary end-to-end repair can be performed successfully with acceptable physician and patient outcomes.

Several authors define chronic ruptures of the Achilles tendon as injuries left untreated for more than 4 weeks [3]. The gap between ruptured ends, assessed preoperatively with magnetic resonance imaging (MRI) and intraoperatively after excision of the impaired tissue, is the determining factor for the type of surgical repair. In a neglected Achilles tendon rupture, the subsequent contraction of the tendon and the formation of fibrous scar tissue make even relatively small gaps less likely to achieve a successful end-to-end repair [5, 22]. An end-to-end anastomosis is usually possible in 1- to 2-cm defects [5, 22]. For 2- to 5-cm defects, either V-Y myotendinous lengthening, graft augmentation, or both are surgical options [5, 22] For defects larger than 5 cm, a graft reconstruction method should be employed [5]. An FHL transfer seems to be a reliable and effective way to deal with large, chronic defects [5, 6, 10].

If surgical repair is chosen, it is recommended to wait for 4–7 days to allow for the reduction of swelling and to lessen the degree of fraying and friability of the tendon that could occur if the repair is performed immediately postinjury [4, 23, 24]. We prefer to perform the repair within 2 weeks of the injury to minimize gapping and to facilitate tissue handling. As always, the optimal management plan should include not only the selection of the surgical technique but also the patient's health status, expectations, and goals.

Primary Repair Using the Tajima Suture Technique

We favor the (four-strand) Tajima suture technique, which is widely used by hand surgeons for flexor tendon repair and is an excellent soft-tissue-holding suture [25, 26]. The patient is positioned prone with the feet lying just over the end of the table. Using a thigh tourniquet is optional but advisable. The contralateral extremity is draped, so it can be used for intraoperative comparison of resting dynamic tension of the repaired tendon [5, 9].

A linear posterolateral incision, approximately 10 cm long, is made about 1 cm lateral to the tendon (Fig. 9.1). The incision ends proximal to where the shoe counter strikes the heel. It has to be off-center to prevent later irritation by shoes, which can happen if the incision is directly over the tendon midline [19]. Care should be taken to maintain full thickness and to avoid undermining the skin flaps. The sural nerve is usually found directly under the incision and must be carefully protected. The incision is deepened sharply into the deep fascia. Finally, the deep fascia and the peritendinous tissues are incised longitudinally to expose the rupture. The incision should be made through all three layers (deep fascia, mesotenon, thin layer closest to the tendon) directly to the middle of the tendon itself [23]. Gently retract the skin throughout the procedure using only skin hooks or handheld retractors [23].

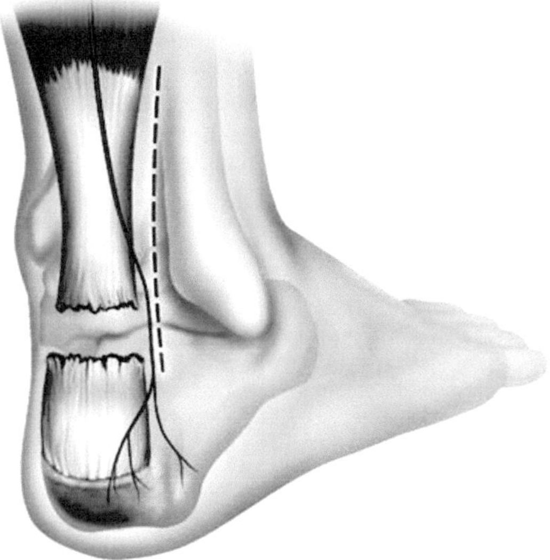

Fig. 9.1 The posterolateral approach to the ankle. The sural nerve lies underneath the incision plane, so it must be carefully identified and protected

The hematoma is evacuated, and the quality and extent of damage are assessed. Any obvious redundant, detached, or devitalized tissue should be sharply excised [3, 19, 23]. Posteriorly, the tendon is invariably separated, while anteriorly, it is possible to find some fibers intact but attenuated [23].

Two sutures are used on each side of the rupture and are tied in the middle (Fig. 9.2). A long, tapered needle is used with nonabsorbable No. 5 polyester suture material. The needle is passed through one of the ruptured ends of the tendon and then out of the tendon 5 cm proximal to or distal from the injured end. This suture then is passed across and exits the tendon. Next, the suture is passed back down within the tendon and out of the injured surface. The process is repeated for the opposite side of the tendon. The knots are tied within the tendon to unite the injured ends. This process is repeated, only this time the suture exits the tendon 2.5 cm from the cut surfaces (Fig. 9.2).

One of the most important aspects of surgical repair is the correct tensioning of the tendon. The ankle is held in a neutral position as sutures are tied. Each strand is pulled to obtain a sense of the correct tension and compared to the opposite limb [5]. Often, the tendon fibers will not be in continuity. The proximal and distal ends of the tendon are "milked" together along the tensioned sutures to the point of contact for a scaffold of healing. Simple 0-braided absorbable sutures are used to further approximate the repair (Fig. 9.3).

The peritenon is a major source of blood supply to the tendon as well as the border between the tendon and the subcutaneous layer preventing adhesions. This layer is closed carefully using a 2-0 absorbable suture (Fig. 9.4) [5]. The subcuta-

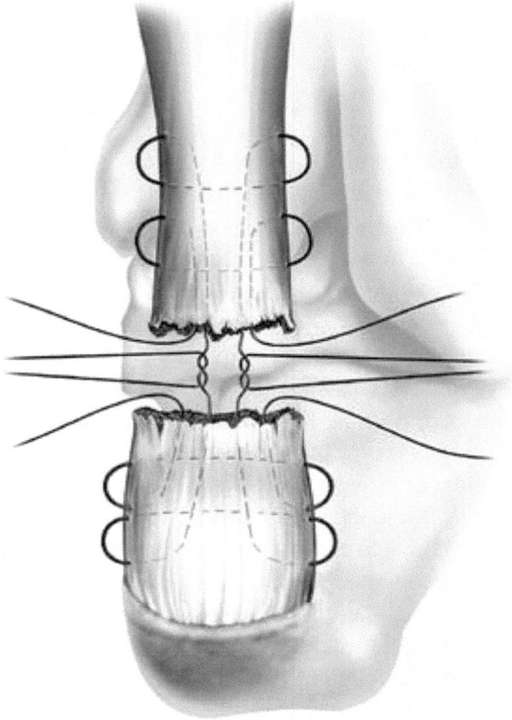

Fig. 9.2 The Tajima suture with four strands. Note that one set of sutures exits the tissue at 5 cm, and a parallel set of sutures exits the tissue at 2.5 cm

neous layer is closed with interrupted 2-0 braided absorbable sutures. The skin is closed with a running 3-0 monofilament nonabsorbable pullout suture. Swelling of the repaired tendon may complicate wound closure, and a fasciotomy of the posterior aspect of the leg has been proposed to resolve this issue [5]. The neurovascular status of the limb must be assessed. A posterior ankle splint set in a neutral position is applied, and the operated limb is elevated on a frame. The sutures are removed about 2 weeks postsurgery.

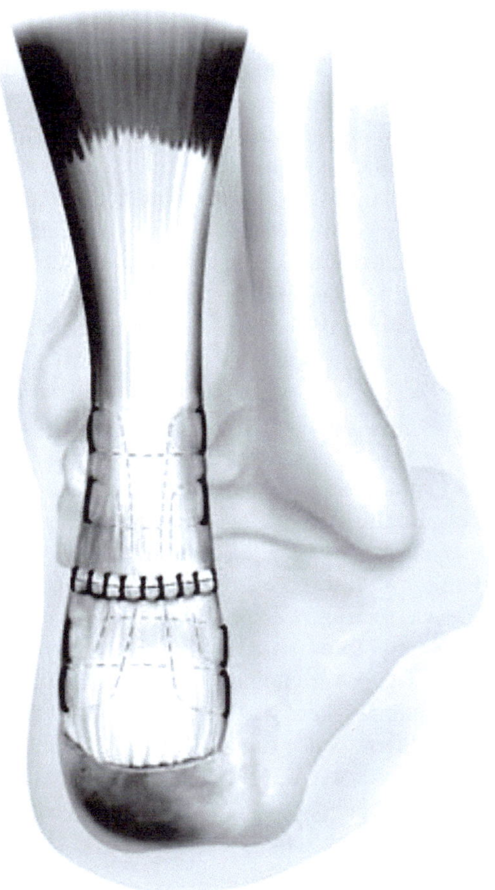

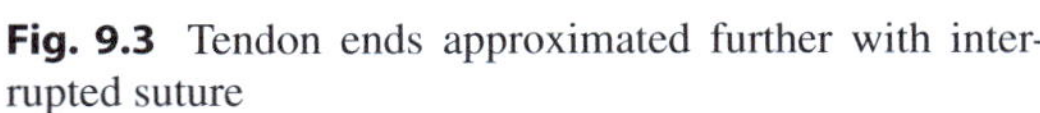

Fig. 9.3 Tendon ends approximated further with interrupted suture

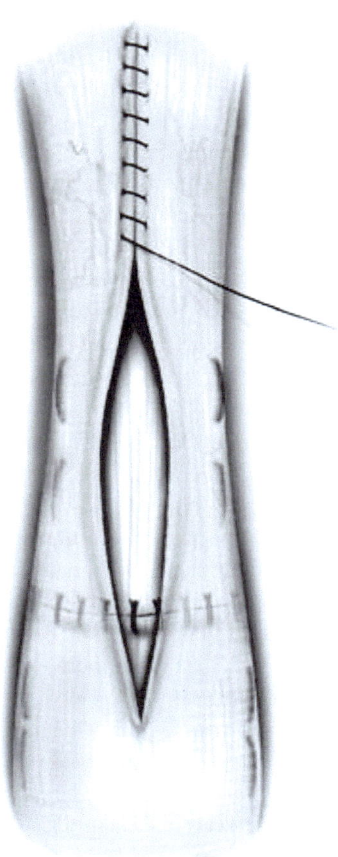

Fig. 9.4 Retinacular layer closure

Rehabilitation

Physical therapy is an essential component to improve the patient's postinjury recovery of activity and satisfaction [27, 28]. An early start to rehabilitation is recommended as there is a significant decrease in complication rates in patients treated with surgery and early mobilization versus those treated with surgery and immobilization [4, 7]. Prolonged immobilization is associated with an increased incidence of calf atrophy, articular cartilage weakening and degeneration, osteoporosis, skin necrosis, adhesions, deep venous thrombosis, and even pulmonary embolism [3, 22]. A meta-analysis confirms that there are more excellent subjective responses, fewer scar adhesions, and fewer transient sural nerve deficits in patients who began an early rehabilitation protocol (when there was no difference in rerupture rate and percentage of superficial and deep infections among them) [29].

The posterior splint is removed within 10–14 days, during which weight-bearing is forbidden. When the splint is removed, a walking boot (neutral position) is applied and patients start progressively weight-bearing as they feel comfortable. Patients are encouraged to perform mobilization of the involved ankle three times per day by performing 30 cycles of active dorsiflexion-recoil passive plantarflexion with the knee flexed 90 degrees (Fig. 9.5a, b). No active plantarflexion is permitted (Fig. 9.5c). Active dorsiflexion is used to provide gentle traction to the repair to promote collagen healing along the lines of stress [13]. Recoil plantarflexion (not active) allows a return to the neutral position. After 6 weeks, the patient can switch to an ankle-foot orthosis or remain in a boot (usually 50% each). At 3 months, the patient is weight-bearing without immobilization. Generally, 6 months is required for a full return to sports.

Over the past 5 years, the senior author has performed this surgical technique on more than 100 acute Achilles tendon ruptures. Despite the proximity of this approach to the sural nerve, no sural nerve palsies occurred. Complications were few as only four patients had delayed wound healing. There were no infections or other major complications. There was only one rerupture in a weight lifter, who, against medical advice, decided to return to full activity 3 months postoperatively. All but one patient returned to their full levels of previous activity.

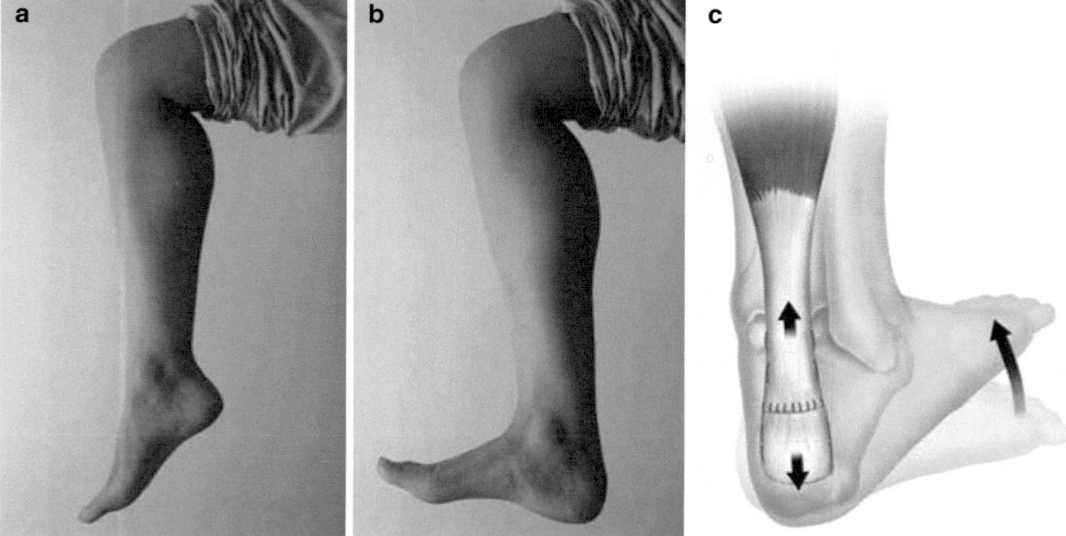

Fig. 9.5 (**a, b**) Active dorsiflexion-recoil passive plantarflexion with the knee flexed 90 degrees; 30 cycles three times per day. (**c**) No active plantarflexion

Other Surgical Options

Watson et al. [30] tested three suture methods (the Kessler, the Bunnell, and the Krackow locking loop) as to the initial strength of Achilles tendon repair. The locking loop suture method was significantly stronger than either of the other two configurations. The latter two did not differ significantly from each other.

Jaakkola and colleagues [31] compared the tensile strength of ruptured Achilles tendons repaired using either the triple-bundle technique or the Krakow locking loop technique. They showed a significantly stronger repair with the triple-bundle technique. Jaakkola et al. [32] evaluated the triple-bundle technique for acute Achilles tendon rupture repair, followed by early postoperative ankle range of motion versus nonoperative treatment with delayed ankle range of motion in 73 patients. They found that operative treatment reduced immobilization and weight-bearing time. Yet at a follow-up of 3.5 years or greater, there was no statistical difference in American Orthopaedic Foot and Ankle Society (AOFAS) hindfoot scores, strength, or patient satisfaction between the two groups. There were more complications in the nonoperative group with three reruptures (7.7%) versus only one deep wound dehiscence in the operative group (3%).

Mandelbaum and coworkers [12] used a Krackow suture technique [33] and early postoperative mobilization in 32 patients, achieving excellent results and no reruptures. All patients returned to preinjury activity levels at an average of 4 months after repair. By 12 months, there were no significant differences in ankle motion, isokinetic strength, or endurance compared with the uninvolved side.

Maffulli et al. [34] used a single modified Kessler suture in two groups. The first group followed an early weight-bearing ankle mobilization protocol, while the second group followed a more traditional postoperative protocol. Both groups had a similar fraction of excellent results and no reruptures, but the first group had faster recovery and return to work, with less use of rehabilitation recourses. Gastroc-soleus muscle strength deficit and muscle atrophy, however, were not prevented.

Finally, Speck and Klaue [13] used a Kessler-type suture and simple apposition sutures combined with an accelerated rehabilitation protocol in 20 patients with excellent results and no reruptures. All patients reached their preinjury levels of sports activities with no significant difference in ankle mobility or isokinetic strength.

Potential Complications

There are several possible complications of Achilles tendon injuries. One large review reported that the complication rate in operatively treated patients was 20%, but most complications were minor [35]. Skin complications include keloid formation, wound necrosis, and skin and soft tissue defects, any of which could require free tissue transfers [9, 36]. Adhesions of the tendon to the overlying skin are considered minor complications and usually require little, if any, treatment. In a few cases, surgical lysis and early mobilization are recommended [23].

After an open repair, the tendon can thicken by up to three to four times its natural size [34]; however, this usually resolves within 18 months.

Ankle stiffness is a result of failure to achieve sufficient tendon length during the procedure and subsequent prolonged immobilization. Excessive tendon length is also unacceptable because push-off strength would be inadequate [5]. If normal strength has not completely been restored after 6 months, the patient must continue rehabilitation because improvement is expected to continue [9]. Oral or intravenous antibiotics treat infections, but surgical debridement may also be necessary [23].

Reruptures can usually be controlled by closely following the postoperative rehabilitation protocol [7]. In the unfortunate case of a rerupture, the patient should be managed as though he or she has an acute rupture. It might be a good idea to reconstruct the tendon with an FHL transfer because rerupture has not been reported with that technique [10]. Sural nerve damage and sural neuroma usually occur after a lateral approach; however, we still prefer a lateral approach because with careful incision and identification of the nerve, this complication easily can be avoided. Our experience with this approach is that the incidence of wound-healing problems is very small [37]. It is important to leave the surrounding tissue as a protective layer after the identification of the nerve. In the case of sural neuroma formation, it has been proposed to transect the nerve more proximally where the subcutaneous tissue is intact [10].

Achilles tendon rupture is a condition that responds well to surgical repair. The technique described is a relatively simple, robust repair with relatively few minor wound complications. The immediate positioning of the ankle postoperatively in the neutral position with an early mobilization rehabilitation protocol is important for a successful outcome.

References

1. Seeger JD, West WA, Fife D, et al. Achilles tendon rupture and its association with fluoroquinolone antibiotics and other potential risk factors in a managed care population. Pharmacoepidemiol Drug Saf. 2006;15(11):784–92.
2. Maffulli N, Waterston SW, Squair J, et al. Changing incidence of Achilles tendon rupture in Scotland: a 15-year study. Clin J Sport Med. 1999;9(3):157–60.
3. Tafuri SA, Daly N. Achilles tendon trauma. In: Banks AS, et al., editors. McGlamry's comprehensive textbook of foot and ankle surgery. 3rd ed. Philadelphia: Lippincott Williams & Wilkins; 2006. p. 1706–23.
4. Wong J, Barrass V, Maffulli N. Quantitative review of operative and nonoperative management of Achilles tendon ruptures. Am J Sports Med. 2002;30(4):565–75.
5. Myerson MS. Achilles tendon ruptures. AAOS Instr Course Lect. 1999;48:219–30.
6. Wapner KL. Achilles tendon ruptures and posterior heel pain. In: Kelikian AS, editor. Operative treatment of the foot and ankle. Stamford, Connecticut: APPLETON & LANGE; 1999. p. 369–87.
7. Khan RJ, Fick D, Keogh A, et al. Treatment of acute Achilles tendon ruptures. A meta-analysis of randomized, controlled trials. J Bone Joint Surg Am. 2005;87(10):2202–10.
8. Bhandari M, Guyatt GH, Siddiqui F, et al. Treatment of acute Achilles tendon ruptures: a systematic overview and metaanalysis. Clin Orthop Relat Res. 2002;400:190–200.
9. Coughlin MJ. Disorders of tendons. In: Coughlin MJ, Mann RA, editors. Surgery of the foot and ankle. 7th ed; 1999. p. 786–861.
10. Wapner KL. Chronic Achilles tendon rupture. In: Nunley JA, Pfeffer GB, Sanders RW, Trepman E, editors. Advanced reconstruction foot and ankle. Rosemont: American Academy of Orthopedic Surgery; 2004. p. 163&8.
11. Cetti R, Christensen SE, Ejsted R, et al. Operative versus nonoperative treatment of Achilles tendon rupture. A prospective randomized study and review of the literature. Am J Sports Med. 1993;21(6):791–9.
12. Mandelbaum BR, Myerson MS, Forster R. Achilles tendon ruptures. A new method of repair, early range of motion, and functional rehabilitation. Am J Sports Med. 1995;23(4):392–5.
13. Speck M, Klaue K. Early full weightbearing and functional treatment after surgical repair of acute Achilles tendon rupture. Am J Sports Med. 1998;26(6):789–93.
14. Assal M, Jung M, Stern R, et al. Limited open repair of Achilles tendon ruptures: a technique with a new instrument and findings of a prospective multicenter study. J Bone Joint Surg Am. 2002;84–A(2):161–70.
15. Lennox DW, Wang GJ, McCue FC, et al. The operative treatment of Achilles tendon injuries. Clin Orthop Relat Res. 1980;148:152–5.
16. Ma GW, Griffith TG. Percutaneous repair of acute closed ruptured Achilles tendon: a new technique. Clin Orthop Relat Res. 1977;128:247–55.
17. Zandbergen RA, de Boer SF, Swierstra BA, et al. Surgical treatment of Achilles tendon rupture: examination of strength of 3 types of suture techniques in a cadaver model. Acta Orthop. 2005;76(3):408–11.
18. Kakiuchi M. A combined open and percutaneous technique for repair of tendo Achillis. Comparison with open repair. J Bone Joint Surg (Br). 1995;77(1):60–3.
19. Azar FM, Pickering RM. Traumatic disorders. In: Canale T, editor. Campbell's operative orthopaedics. 9th ed. St Louis, Missouri: Mosby-Year Book, Inc.; 1998. p. 1405–49.
20. Levy M, Velkes S, Goldstein J, et al. A method of repair for Achilles tendon ruptures without cast immobilization. Preliminary report. Clin Orthop Relat Res. 1984;187:199–204.
21. Jenkins DH, Forster IW, McKibbin B, et al. Induction of tendon and ligament formation by carbon implants. J Bone Joint Surg (Br). 1977;59–B(1):53–7.
22. Canete AC, Deiparine HP. Treatment of chronic Achilles tendon rupture with triple bundle suturing technique and early rehabilitation: early results. Tech Orthop. 2006;21(2):134–42.
23. Schuberth JM. Achilles tendon trauma. In: Scurran BL, editor. Foot and ankle trauma. 2nd ed. New York, NY: Churchill Livingstone Inc.; 1996. p. 205–31.
24. Miller MD, Howard RF, Plancher KD. Achilles tendon repair. In: Lampert R, editor. Surgical atlas of sports medicine. Printed in Hong Kong. Saunders: An imprint of Elsevier Science (USA); 2003. p. 183–6.
25. Urbaniak JR. Repair of the flexor pollicis longus. Hand Clin. 1985;1(1):69–76.

26. Tran HN, Cannon DL, Lieber RL, et al. In vitro cyclic tensile testing of combined peripheral and core flexor tenorrhaphy suture techniques. J Hand Surg [Am]. 2002;27(3):518–24.

27. Rajasekar K, Gholve P, Faraj AA, et al. A subjective outcome analysis of tendo-Achilles rupture. J Foot Ankle Surg. 2005;44(1):32–6.

28. Dugan DH, Hobler CK. Progressive management of open surgical repair of Achilles tendon rupture. J Athl Train. 1994;29(4):349–51.

29. Suchak AA, Spooner C, Reid DC, et al. Postoperative rehabilitation protocols for Achilles tendon ruptures: a meta-analysis. Clin Orthop Relat Res. 2006;445:216–21.

30. Watson TW, Jurist KA, Yang KH, et al. The strength of Achilles tendon repair: an in vitro study of the biomechanical behavior in human cadaver tendons. Foot Ankle Int. 1995;16(4):191–5.

31. Jaakkola JI, Hutton WC, Beskin JL, et al. Achilles tendon rupture repair: biomechanical comparison of the triple bundle technique versus the Krakow locking loop technique. Foot Ankle Int. 2000;21(1):14–7.

32. Jaakkola JI, Beskin JL, Griffith LH, et al. Early ankle motion after triple bundle technique repair vs. casting for acute Achilles tendon rupture. Foot Ankle Int. 2001;22(12):979–84.

33. Krackow KA, Thomas SC, Jones LC. A new stitch for ligament-tendon fixation. Brief note. J Bone Joint Surg Am. 1986;68(5):764–6.

34. Maffulli N, Tallon C, Wong J, et al. Early weight-bearing and ankle mobilization after open repair of acute midsubstance tears of the Achilles tendon. Am J Sports Med. 2003;31(5):692–700.

35. Wills CA, Washburn S, Caiozzo V, et al. Achilles tendon rupture. A review of the literature comparing surgical versus nonsurgical treatment. Clin Orthop Relat Res. 1986;207:156–63.

36. Stanec S, Stanec Z, Delimar D, et al. A composite forearm free flap for the secondary repair of the ruptured Achilles tendon. Plast Reconstr Surg. 1999;104(5):1409–12.

37. Calliada F, Orlandi S, Pellegrini F. Clinico-statistical review of 74 cases of subcutaneous rupture of the Achilles tendon. Chir Ital. 1979;31(5):1018–25.

Management of Achilles Tendon Tears in Athletes

Naji S. Madi, Aman Chopra, and Selene G. Parekh

Introduction

The Achilles tendon is the strongest tendon in the body. Multiple benefits have been linked to the evolutionary development of this tendon, and these include being an energy saver for running twice as fast, being a shock absorber during gait, and allowing humans to jump [1].

Achilles tendon tears are among the most detrimental injuries for athletes, with the potential to be a career-ending injury for professional athletes [2]. It is believed that a tear happens due to an eccentric overload of the tendon, usually during sports; a violent dorsiflexion of a plantarflexed ankle; or an abrupt forced plantarflexion. However, some evidence suggests predisposing factors that include degenerative changes, nonuniform vascularity, and genetic influence [1]. In a histopathologic study of spontaneous tendon rupture, it was shown that a healthy tendon state was not seen in any ruptured tendon [3]. Achilles tendon ruptures in professional athletes usually undergo an operative repair, followed by an extensive rehabilitation protocol, with at least 36% of athletes reportedly never returning to play [4].

Anatomy

This is the largest tendon in the human body. It is formed by the two heads of the gastrocnemius that cross the knee and then fuse in a single muscle belly in the posterior superficial compartment of the lower leg. The soleus muscle lies closer to the bone, deeper to the gastrocnemius muscle. The triceps surae forms by the fusion of these two muscles, and it inserts as the Achilles tendon on the posterior surface of the calcaneal tuberosity. The contribution of each muscle to the tendon is variable. The Achilles tendon has an average length of 15 cm (11–26 cm). The middle part of the tendon has the poorest blood supply from the peroneal artery, while the posterior tibial artery supplies the proximal and distal parts of the tendon [5].

Epidemiology

In the general population, Achilles tendon tears most commonly occur in a middle-aged man who participates in occasional athletic activities, also known as the "weekend warrior." Different sorts of sports activities have been shown to be associated with tears. In the United States, basketball,

N. S. Madi (✉)
Department of Orthopaedic Surgery,
West Virginia University, Morgantown, WV, USA

A. Chopra
School of Medicine, Georgetown University,
Washington, D.C., USA
e-mail: ac2090@georgetown.edu

S. G. Parekh
Department of Orthopaedic Surgery,
West Virginia University, Morgantown, WV, USA

Rothman Orthopaedic Institute,
Morgantown, WV, USA

tennis, and football are Augusta sports with tears, while in Europe and Canada, soccer and volleyball were the most involved activities. Eighty percent of ruptures occur in males. Females are usually older than males at the time of injury [6]. The incidence of contralateral Achilles tendon tear remains significantly higher than that in the general population (6% versus 18/100.000) [7].

Thirty percent of Achilles tendon tears are not related to sports activities, and other factors have been reported to increase this risk, such as quinolone use [8], prior steroid injections around the Achilles tendon [9], anabolic steroid use, and blood type O [10]. In active-duty military personnel, African Americans were at a higher risk of tendon rupture, including the Achilles tendon [11].

In reviewing Achilles tendon ruptures in the National Football League (NFL), Parekh et al. found an incidence of ruptures per game of 0.93%, with the average age at the time of injury being 29 years (older than the average age of NFL players). The players had been in the league for an average of 6 years before the injury was sustained. Defensive tackle players had the highest number of Achilles tendon ruptures, with almost half of the injuries occurring in skilled positions (quarterbacks, running backs, wide receivers, cornerbacks) [3]. When analyzing the impact of the field surface, Krill et al. found that over 70% of Achilles ruptures occurred within the first half of the NFL regular season, with no difference in injury rates when playing on either artificial turf or grass from 2009 to 2017 [12].

In a review of Achilles tendon ruptures that occurred in selected seasons in the National Basketball Association (NBA), the players had an average age of 28 years at the time of injury, and they played for an average of 6.8 seasons before the Achilles rupture occurred. The ruptures were most common to occur during early-season game play, followed by preseason and late season. The rupture was significantly more common in forward than guard players. Video analysis identified the "takeoff" with the ankle dorsiflexed, knee in early flexion, and hip in extension to be the most common mechanism of injury [13].

In Major League Baseball (MLB) [14], Achilles tendon tears were less common as compared to other sports, but the incidence seems to be increasing in recent years. The most common Achilles tendon ruptures (69%) occurred during the preseason or regular season, followed by the offseason and the playoffs. Injuries were more common on the nonpower (front) side than the power (rear) side. Injuries to the power side had more detrimental effects on the player's performance (less plate appearances, fewer triples, decreased speed score).

Diagnosis

Clinical Findings

The typical presentation includes acute pain, sudden instability, and a popping sound or sensation in the back of the leg. According to the American Academy of Orthopaedic Surgeons, at least two of the following tests should be positive to establish the diagnosis: clinical Thompson test (calf squeeze test), decreased ankle plantarflexion strength, presence of a palpable gap, and Matles test (increased passive ankle dorsiflexion with gentle manipulation) [15]. Difficulty with weight-bearing and limping are commonly seen. False-negative Thompson test can occur due to intact foot flexors [16]. Diagnosis can be delayed in patients with a high body mass index (BMI), ruptures that are not sustained during sports, and an age greater than 55 years.

Imaging

The acute Achilles tendon tear is primarily a clinical diagnosis. However, radiographs should be obtained to rule out a Haglund deformity, insertional calcifications, or a calcaneus avulsion fracture. An ultrasound or magnetic resonance imaging (MRI) has been used to confirm the diagnosis. The ultrasound is more cost-effective and shows an area of hypoechogenic signal over the tear. The MRI shows a disruption of the signal over the ruptured tendon [17].

Operative Management

The most appropriate treatment for Achilles tendon rupture remains unclear, but the consensus for athletes is surgery. Athletes younger than 30 years old might represent a more challenging group with a higher incidence of rerupture after surgical repair as compared to those older than 30 [18]. In general, operative repair showed lower rerupture rates (3.1% vs 13%), higher plantarflexion strength (87% vs 78%), better return to athletic activities, improved ankle range of motion, and fewer complaints [19].

Variable methods have been described to repair an acute Achilles tendon tear. It includes open, mini-open, and percutaneous techniques [20]. The senior author (S.G.P) prefers a surgical technique that is a limited open repair without an instrumented guide [21] (Fig. 10.1). The patient is placed in a prone position, and a nonsterile thigh tourniquet is used. A 3-cm longitudinal incision is made midline over the Achilles tear and through the peritenon (Fig. 10.2). The proximal stump is identified and grasped with an Alice clamp (Fig. 10.3). Three No. 2 Orthocord sutures

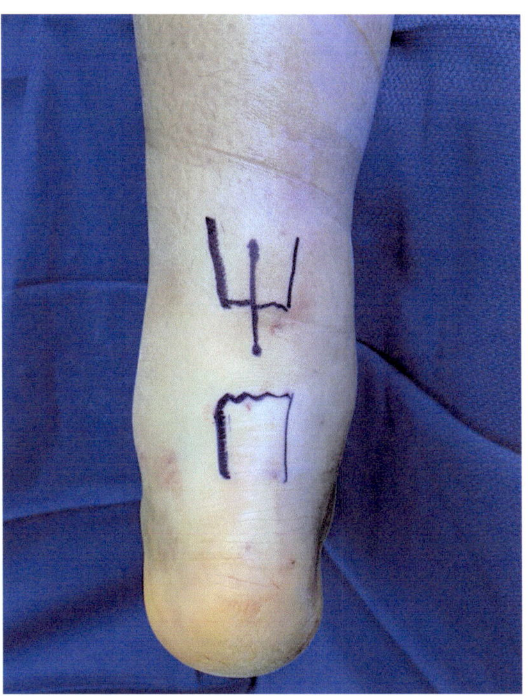

Fig. 10.2 The gap at the rupture site is palpable, and the two ends of the Achilles tendon and the skin incision are marked (Akoh CC, Fletcher A, Sharma A, Parekh SG. Clinical Outcomes and Complications Following Limited Open Achilles Repair Without an Instrumented Guide. Foot & Ankle International)

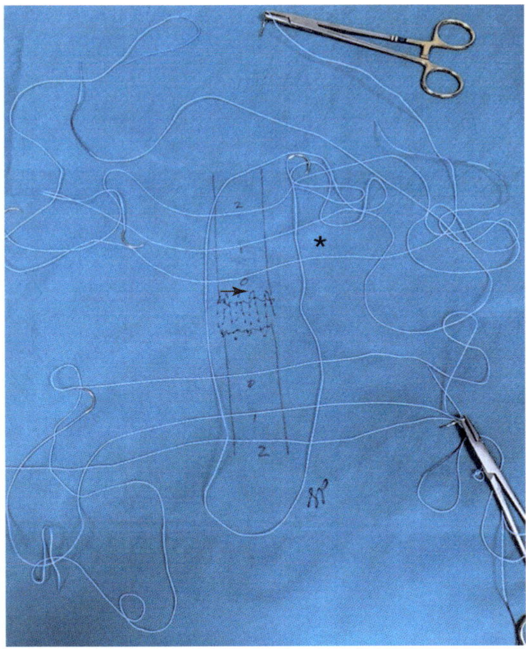

Fig. 10.1 The two ends of the Achilles tendon rupture are drawn. Three (No. 2 Orthocord) sutures are passed on each side of the tendon in the same order (0, 1, 2). Once these are tied down, a box (No. 2 Orthocord) suture (*) is passed from the proximal to distal and tied proximally, then a 0 Vicryl (←) is used to approximate the tendon edges

are passed transversely through the tendon from proximal to distal. Then the ankle is plantarflexed and three No. 2 Orthocord are passed similarly in the distal stump (Fig. 10.4a, b). The stumps are retracted, and the deep fascial compartment is opened (Fig. 10.5). Then the ankle is maintained in plantarflexion, and the sutures are tied from the farthest from the tear to the nearest (Fig. 10.6). Then a No. 2 Orthocord is used as a running box suture, starting on the medial side from proximal to distal then from distal to proximal on the lateral side then back to proximal medial, where it is tied (Fig. 10.7). Then a running 0 Vicryl suture is used to approximate the proximal and distal edges of the tear (Fig. 10.8). The wound is thoroughly irrigated, then the paratenon is closed using 2-0 Vicryl sutures, followed by staples for the skin (Fig. 10.9). A sterile dressing is applied, followed by a bulky Jones splint in a neutral foot position and slight ankle plantarflexion.

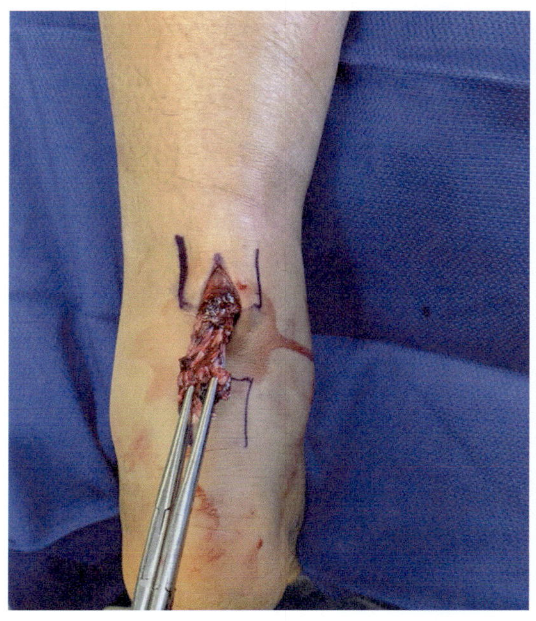

Fig. 10.3 The proximal stump of the Achilles tendon is identified, freed, and grasped with Alice clamps (Akoh CC, Fletcher A, Sharma A, Parekh SG. Clinical Outcomes and Complications Following Limited Open Achilles Repair Without an Instrumented Guide. Foot & Ankle International)

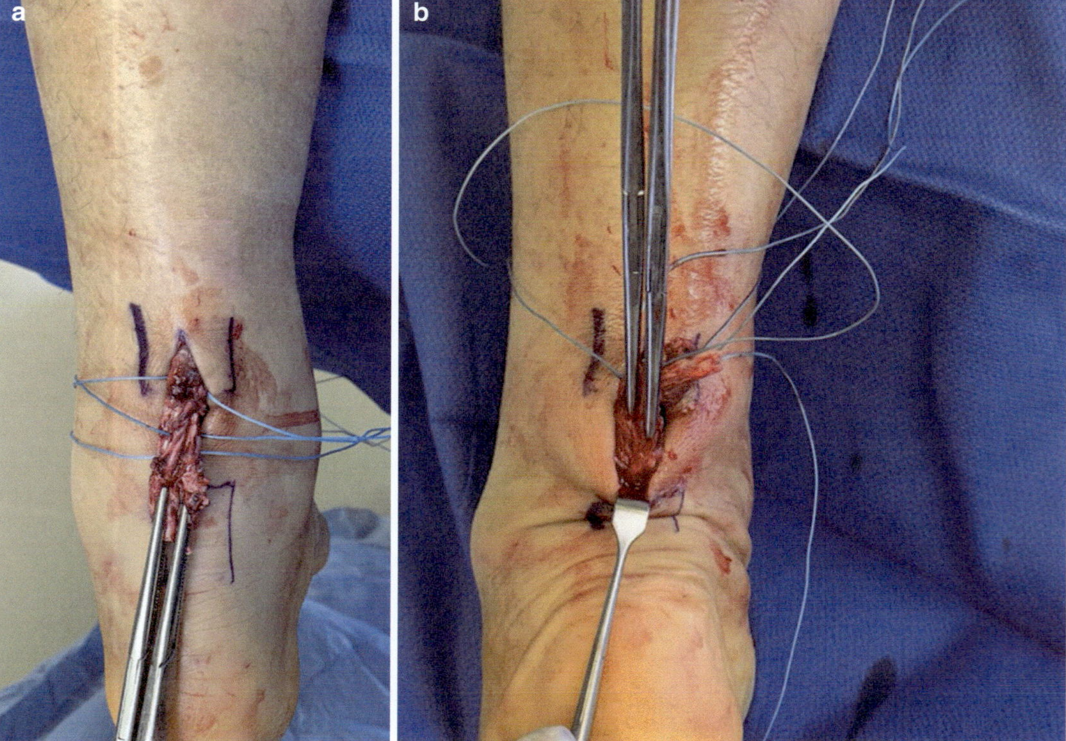

Fig. 10.4 (**a**) Three No. 2 Orthocord sutures were passed in the proximal stump. (**b**) The ankle is plantarflexed, and the distal stump is grasped with Alice clamps, then three No. 2 Orthocord sutures are passed through the distal stump (Akoh CC, Fletcher A, Sharma A, Parekh SG. Clinical Outcomes and Complications Following Limited Open Achilles Repair Without an Instrumented Guide. Foot & Ankle International)

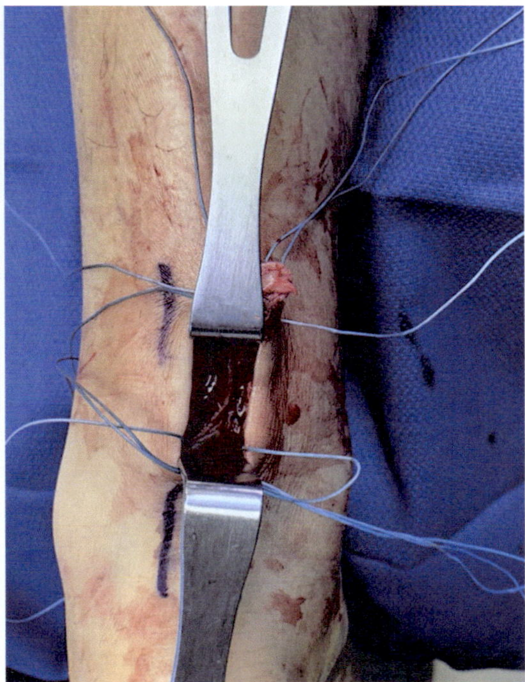

Fig. 10.5 The two ends of the Achilles tendon are retracted, and the deep fascial compartment is opened centrally (Akoh CC, Fletcher A, Sharma A, Parekh SG. Clinical Outcomes and Complications Following Limited Open Achilles Repair Without an Instrumented Guide. Foot & Ankle International)

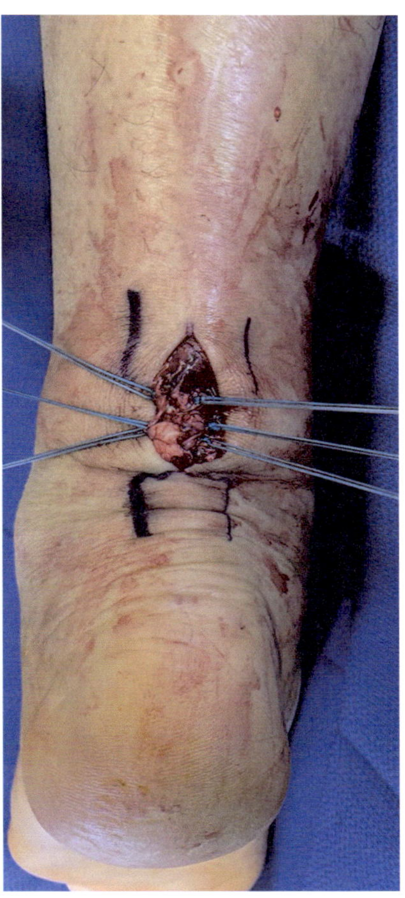

Fig. 10.6 The sutures were tied on the medial and lateral sides simultaneously with the ankle in plantarflexion (Akoh CC, Fletcher A, Sharma A, Parekh SG. Clinical Outcomes and Complications Following Limited Open Achilles Repair Without an Instrumented Guide. Foot & Ankle International)

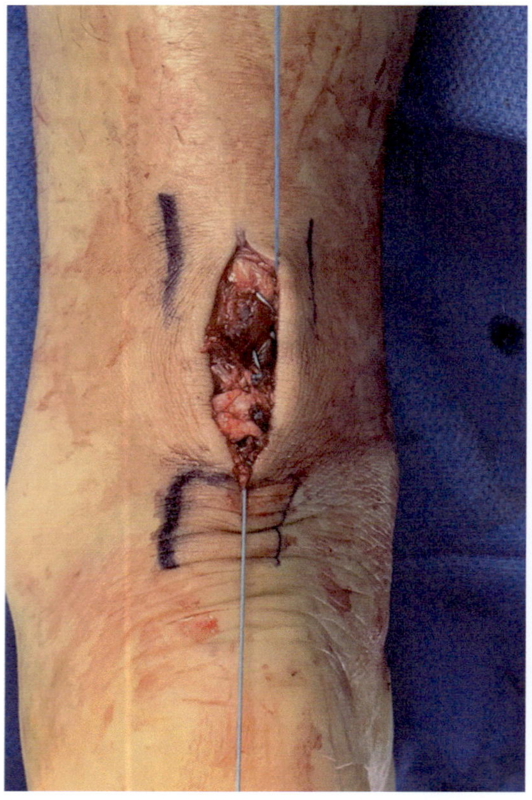

Fig. 10.7 A running box suture is passed across the tendon rupture from proximal to distal, then tied down proximally

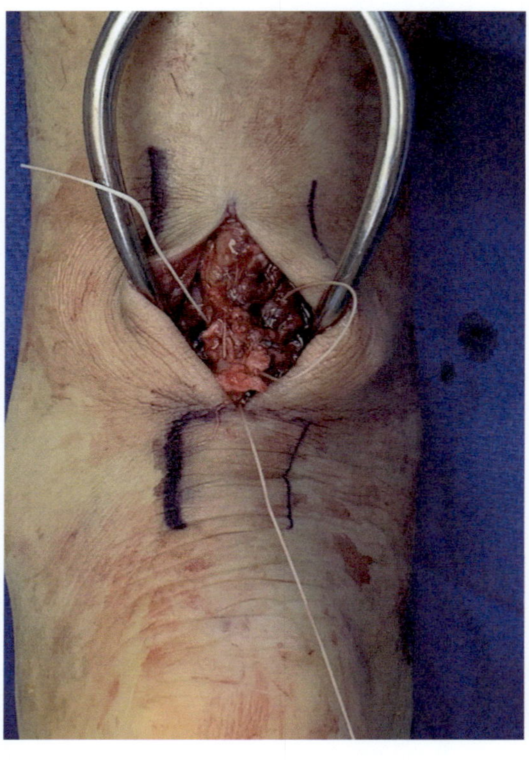

Fig. 10.8 A running 0 Vicryl suture is used to approximate the proximal and distal edges of the tear (Akoh CC, Fletcher A, Sharma A, Parekh SG. Clinical Outcomes and Complications Following Limited Open Achilles Repair Without an Instrumented Guide. Foot & Ankle International)

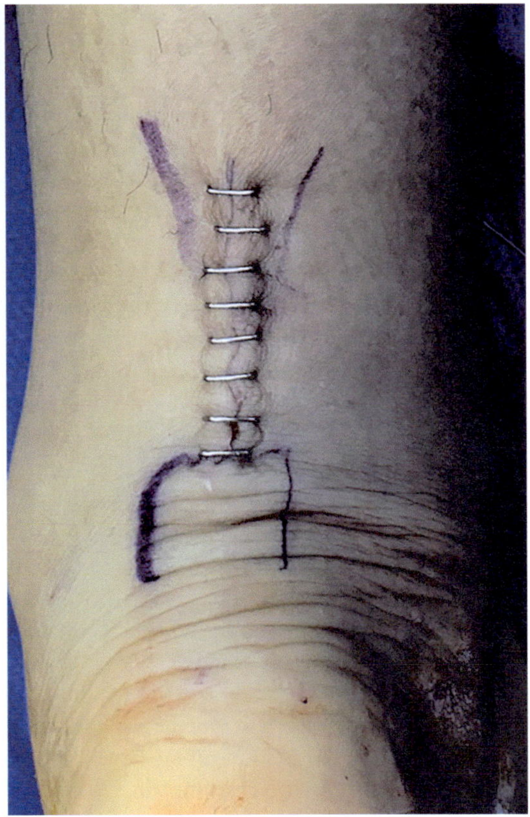

Fig. 10.9 Final closure of the wound

Rehabilitation

The patient is kept in the postoperative splint for 2 weeks. All patients are given aspirin 325 mg twice daily for a month as thromboprophylaxis. Skin staples are removed in the clinic, and the patient is transitioned to a pneumatic walking boot with 5/16-inch heel lifts. Weight-bearing as tolerated is allowed. Each heel lift is removed on a weekly basis up to week 6, then the patient is weaned from their boot to regular shoe by week 8. The rehabilitation protocol is divided into three phases. Phase 1, from 2 to 6 weeks, includes active ankle range of motion with dorsiflexion limited to neutral, closed-chain strengthening exercises, and gait training. Phase 2, from 6 to 10 weeks, includes proprioceptive exercises, open chain exercises, and progression to standing bilateral heel raises. Phase 3, after 12 weeks, includes oriented sports-specific and polymetric training. The decision to discharge patients from therapy depends on their ability to perform sports-specific activities (repetitive single-leg hops, normal toe-off phase during sprinting, adequate proprioception, etc.).

Outcomes

Recovery and Return to Play

Research studies analyzing athletes in the NFL, NBA, MLB, and professional soccer leagues who suffer an Achilles tendon rupture provide valuable data on the rate of returning to sport and recovery timeline after this debilitating injury. In the NFL, acute Achilles tendon tear is an uncommon but potentially devastating pathology since 36% of players who sustain this injury never return to play [4]. The recovery time for NFL athletes was between 11 and 12 months on average [4, 22]. Specifically, the running back position had the longest duration for recovery at an average of 11.9 months [4, 21]. When compared to orther orthopaedic procedures, the achilles tendon repair had the second lowest return to play rate following knee surgeries (patellar tendon repair and ACL reconstruction) [23].

In the NBA, the average time for recovery after surgery for Achilles tendon ruptures was 10.5 months (range: 5 months to 16 months) [22]. NBA players in general have the lowest return-to-play rates following repair for Achilles tendon ruptures (range: 61.0–79.5%) when compared to return-to-play rates after other orthopedic procedures [24]. NBA athletes with a mean age $\geq$ 30 years and a BMI $\geq$27 kg/m^2 were less likely to return to play [25].

In the MLB, players demonstrated a 61.9% return-to-play rate [14]. Among the world's best soccer leagues, the average return-to-play rate was near 95%, and the average duration of recovery was 9 months for professional soccer players [26]. Among Major League Soccer players, the average return-to-play rate was near 77% [27].

Athletic Performance

Athletes in the NFL, NBA, MLB, and professional soccer leagues who suffer an Achilles tendon rupture often experience a decrease in athletic performance. Returning NFL athletes demonstrated more than a 50% decrease in their performance based on their power ratings as compared to preinjury seasons [4, 22]. Athletes at the linebacker position had the greatest rate of performance reduction, with a 95% decline [4, 21]. There was a significant decrease in the number of games played by NFL athletes who sustained this injury when comparing three seasons before and after the recovery period (11.7 games vs. 6.2 games) [4].

In the NBA, athletes who sustained Achilles tendon pathology have decreased their player efficiency ratings (range: 2.9–4.4), number of games played (range: 23.2–28.6), and number of minutes played per game (range:4.4–6.5) [23].

In the MLB, players demonstrated no significant differences in batting average, stolen bases, on-base percentage, home runs, most valuable player awards, and all-star game appearances after injury overall. Upon subgroup analysis, it was found that Achilles injuries to the power-generating leg were associated with decreased plate appearances, triples, and speed score, with a greater percentage of at-bats with strikeouts [14]. No significant differences were found for MLB player performance, number of games played, and number of minutes played per game between preinjury and postinjury time periods [28].

Among the world's best soccer leagues, 18% of players who suffered an Achilles injury performed worse in their first two seasons following their return to sport than in their preinjury level [26]. In the MLS, players completed fewer seasons (2.5 seasons vs 4.5 seasons) and fewer games per season (13.4 games vs. 23.2 games) after recovery when compared with players who did not suffer an Achilles rupture [27].

Achilles Rerupture and Surgical Complications

Approximately 15% of NFL players who recovered from an Achilles rupture experienced a subsequent rerupture of the ipsilateral Achilles tendon within 2 years of their surgery [2]. Among the world's best soccer leagues, 6% of players sustained a rerupture of the ipsilateral Achilles tendon [26].

In addition to Achilles tendon rerupture, sural nerve hypoesthesia, and infection, professional athletes who undergo Achilles tendon repair are susceptible to surgical complications. With an incidence of 24%, venous thromboembolism is a common complication that arises from the operative management of Achilles tendon rupture [29]. The current literature reports controversial data regarding the overall incidence of symptomatic venous thromboembolic events after an Achilles tendon injury, and there is no consensus on whether prophylaxis is warranted [30, 31]. Also, it is still debatable whether an antiplatelet or anti-coagulant agent is the ideal choice to decrease this risk [32]. Wound-healing complications are also important risks associated with surgical repair that should be taken into consideration. When compared with the percutaneous approach, open procedures for tendon repair have demonstrated delayed wound healing in 28.6% of patients [33].

References

1. Malvankar S, Khan WS. Evolution of the Achilles tendon: the athlete's Achilles heel? Foot (Edinb). 2011;21(4):193–7. https://doi.org/10.1016/j.foot.2011.08.004. Epub 2011 Sep 6
2. Yang J, Hodax JD, Machan JT, Krill MK, Lemme NJ, Durand WM, Hoffman JT, Hewett TE, Owens BD. Factors affecting return to play after primary Achilles tendon tear: a cohort of NFL players. Orthop J Sports Med. 2019;7(3):2325967119830139. https://doi.org/10.1177/2325967119830139. PMID: 30886876; PMCID: PMC6415485
3. Kannus P, Jozsa L. Histopathological changes preceding spontaneous rupture of a tendon: a controlled study of 891 patients. J Bone Joint Surg Am. 1991;73:1507–25.
4. Parekh SG, Wray WH, Brimmo O, Sennett BJ, Wapner KL. Epidemiology and outcomes of Achilles tendon ruptures in the National Football League. Foot Ankle Spec. 2009;2(6):283–6. https://doi.org/10.1177/1938640009351138.
5. Del Buono A, Chan O, Maffulli N. Achilles tendon: functional anatomy and novel emerging models of imaging classification. Int Orthop. 2013;37(4):715–21. https://doi.org/10.1007/s00264-012-1743-y.

6. Raikin SM, Garras DN, Krapchev PV. Achilles tendon injuries in a United States population. Foot Ankle Int. 2013;34(4):475–80. https://doi.org/10.1177/1071100713477621.

7. Leppilahti J, Puranen J, Orava S. Incidence of Achilles tendon rupture. Acta Orthop Scand. 1996;67(3):277–9.

8. Van der Linden PD, Sturkenboom MC, Herings RM. Increased risk of Achilles tendon rupture with quinolone antibacterial use, especially in elderly patients taking oral corticosteroids. Arch Intern Med. 2003;163(15):1801–7.

9. Mahler F, Fritschy D. Partial and complete ruptures of the Achilles tendon and local corticosteroid injections. Br J Sports Med. 1992;26(1):7–14.

10. Jozsa L, Balint JB, Kannus P, Reffy A, Barzo M. Distribution of blood groups in patients with tendon rupture: an analysis of 832 cases. J Bone Joint Surg Br. 1989;71(2):272–4.

11. White DW, Wenke JC, Mosely DS, Mountcastle SB, Basamania CJ. Incidence of major tendon ruptures and anterior cruciate ligament tears in US Army soldiers. Am J Sports Med. 2007;35(8):1308–14.

12. Krill MK, Borchers JR, Hoffman JT, Krill ML, Hewett TE. Effect of position, time in the season, and playing surface on Achilles tendon ruptures in NFL games: a 2009-10 to 2016-17 review. Phys Sportsmed. 2017;45(3):259–64. https://doi.org/10.1080/00913847.2017.1343652. Epub 2017 Jun 22

13. Lemme NJ, Li NY, Kleiner JE, Tan S, DeFroda SF, Owens BD. Epidemiology and video analysis of Achilles tendon ruptures in the National Basketball Association. Am J Sports Med. 2019;47(10):2360–6. https://doi.org/10.1177/0363546519858609.

14. Saltzman BM, Tetreault MW, Bohl DD, Tetreault D, Lee S, Bach BR Jr. Analysis of player statistics in Major League Baseball players before and after Achilles tendon repair. HSS J. 2017;13(2):108–18. https://doi.org/10.1007/s11420-016-9540-6.

15. Chiodo CP, Glazebrook M, Bluman EM, Cohen BE, Femino JE, Giza E, Watters WC 3rd, Goldberg MJ, Keith M, Haralson RH 3rd, Turkelson CM, Wies JL, Raymond L, Anderson S, Boyer K, Sluka P, American Academy of Orthopaedic Surgeons. Diagnosis and treatment of acute Achilles tendon rupture. J Am Acad Orthop Surg. 2010;18(8):503–10.

16. Park SH, Lee HS, Young KW, Seo SG. Treatment of acute Achilles tendon rupture. Clin Orthop Surg. 2020;12(1):1–8. https://doi.org/10.4055/cios.2020.12.1.1.

17. Schepsis AA, Jones H, Haas AL. Achilles tendon disorders in athletes. Am J Sports Med. 2002;30(2):287–305.

18. Rettig AC, Liotta FJ, Klootwyk TE, Porter DA, Mieling P. Potential risk of rerupture in primary Achilles tendon repair in athletes younger than 30 years of age. Am J Sports Med. 2005;33(1):119–23. https://doi.org/10.1177/0363546504268720.

19. Bhandari M, Guyatt GH, Siddiqui F. Treatment of acute Achilles tendon ruptures: a systematic overview and metaanalysis. Clin Orthop Relat Res. 2002;400:190–200.

20. Heckman DS, Gluck GS, Parekh SG. Tendon disorders of the foot and ankle, part 2: Achilles tendon disorders. Am J Sports Med. 2009;37(6):1223–34. https://doi.org/10.1177/0363546509335947.

21. Akoh CC, Fletcher A, Sharma A, Parekh SG. Clinical outcomes and complications following limited open Achilles repair without an instrumented guide. Foot Ankle Int. 2021;42(3):294–304. https://doi.org/10.1177/1071100720962493.

22. Johns W, Walley KC, Seedat R, Thordarson DB, Jackson B, Gonzalez T. Career outlook and performance of professional athletes after Achilles tendon rupture: a systematic review. Foot Ankle Int. 2021;42(4):495–509. https://doi.org/10.1177/1071100720969633.

23. Mai HT, Alvarez AP, Freshman RD, et al. The NFL orthopaedic surgery outcomes database (NO-SOD): the effect of common orthopaedic procedures on football careers. Am J Sports Med. 2016;44(9):2255–62.

24. Allahabadi S, Su F, Lansdown DA. Systematic review of orthopaedic and sports medicine injuries and treatment outcomes in Women's National Basketball Association and National Basketball Association Players. Orthop J Sports Med. 2021;9(2):2325967120982076. https://doi.org/10.1177/2325967120982076.

25. Minhas SV, Kester BS, Larkin KE, Hsu WK. The effect of an orthopaedic surgical procedure in the National Basketball Association. Am J Sports Med. 2016;44(4):1056–61. https://doi.org/10.1177/0363546515623028.

26. Grassi A, Rossi G, D'Hooghe P, et al. Eighty-two per cent of male professional football (soccer) players return to play at the previous level two seasons after Achilles tendon rupture treated with surgical repair. Br J Sports Med. 2020;54:480–6.

27. Sochacki KR, Jack RA II, Hirase T, et al. There is a high return to sport rate but with reduced career lengths after Achilles tendon repair in Major League Soccer players. J ISAKOS: Joint Disorders & Orthopaedic Sports Medicine. 2019;4:15–20.

28. Trofa DP, Miller JC, Jang ES, Woode DR, Greisberg JK, Vosseller JT. Professional athletes' return to play and performance after operative repair of an Achilles tendon rupture. Am J Sports Med. 2017;45(12):2864–71. https://doi.org/10.1177/0363546517713001.

29. Makhdom AM, Cota A, Saran N, et. al. Incidence of symptomatic deep venous thrombosis after Achilles tendon rupture. J Foot Ankle Surg. 2013;52:584–7.

30. Patel A, Ogawa B, Charlton T, Thordarson D. Incidence of deep vein thrombosis and pulmonary embolism after Achilles tendon rupture. Clin Orthop Relat Res. 2012;470(1):270–4. https://doi.org/10.1007/s11999-011-2166-6. Epub 2011 Nov 2. PMID: 22045072; PMCID: PMC3237970

31. Pedersen MH, Wahlsten LR, Grønborg H, Gislason GH, Petersen MM, Bonde AN. Symptomatic venous thromboembolism after Achilles tendon

rupture: a Nationwide Danish Cohort Study of 28,546 patients with Achilles tendon rupture. Am J Sports Med. 2019;47(13):3229–37. https://doi.org/10.1177/0363546519876054. Epub 2019 Oct 1

32. Braithwaite I, Dunbar L, Eathorne A, Weatherall M, Beasley R. Venous thromboembolism rates in patients with lower limb immobilization after Achilles tendon injury are unchanged after the introduction of prophylactic aspirin: audit. J Thromb Haemost. 2016;14(2):331–5. https://doi.org/10.1111/jth.13224. Epub 2016 Jan 26

33. Van Maele M, Misselyn D, Metsemakers WJ, et al. Is open acute Achilles tendon rupture repair still justified? A single center experience and critical appraisal of the literature. Injury. 2018;49:1947–52.

Achilles Tendon Sleeve Avulsion Injuries: Diagnosis and Management

Eric Z. Lukosius and Karl M. Schweitzer Jr.

Background

The classic Achilles tendon rupture occurs in a watershed area about 2–6 cm proximal to the Achilles calcaneal insertion, leaving reasonably sized proximal and distal tendon stumps for end-to-end repair [1]. An Achilles sleeve avulsion rupture is a rare variant, thought to be less than 10% of all operative Achilles tendon ruptures, that occurs at the level of the Achilles tendon calcaneal insertion [2–4].

Bibbo et al. [5] were the first to formally describe this specific "sleeve avulsion" injury in a case series of six patients, with the majority of patients describing prodromal symptoms at the posterior heel and exhibiting insertional Achilles tendinopathic changes at the time of surgery, including a calcaneal enthesophyte, Achilles tendinosis and calcifications, and a Haglund's prominence. A small osseous fragment usually avulses with the central slip of the Achilles tendon insertion, which is part of the baseline insertional tendinopathy that is present in most of these patients. In terms of the rupture pattern, this can be equated to sleeve avulsion fractures at the inferior patellar pole at the knee in skeletally immature patients.

As mentioned above, patients presenting with this injury pattern commonly have a history of insertional Achilles tendinopathy. The retrocalcaneal bursitis, insertional tendinosis, and enthesopathy associated with this process can weaken the central Achilles tendon insertion, which is commonly the component that avulses in this pattern, leaving intact medial and lateral Achilles fibers at the posterior calcaneus. Other variants on this injury spectrum include (1) a large posterior calcaneal avulsion fracture, which can be repaired indirectly via open reduction and internal fixation of the large osseous fragment back to the native calcaneus and (2) a complete, Achilles insertional rupture, where the entire Achilles tendon ruptures off the posterior calcaneus, for which the tendon can be repaired back to bone. Various classification systems for avulsion fractures of the calcaneal tuberosity have been proposed, with varying patterns based on bone quality/density, mechanism of injury, and the manner in which the Achilles tendon fibers transmit force to the calcaneal insertion [6, 7].

In the case of an Achilles tendon sleeve avulsion injury, there is not an adequate distal tendon stump to primarily repair to the proximal stump, in end-to-end fashion. Often, the avulsed osseous fragment is too small to repair back to the native bone. Nonetheless, this specific injury pattern must be recognized and repaired for the most

E. Z. Lukosius (✉)
Department of Orthopaedic Surgery, Duke University Medical Center, Durham, NC, USA
e-mail: eric.lukosius@duke.edu

K. M. Schweitzer Jr.
Department of Orthopaedic Surgery, Duke University Medical Center, Durham, NC, USA

Duke Orthopaedics of Raleigh, Raleigh, NC, USA
e-mail: karl.schweitzer@duke.edu

optimal return to function and outcome [3, 4] and also to help counsel patients on injury specifics, anticipated healing times, and prognosis.

Anatomy and Biomechanics

The Achilles tendon is the largest and strongest tendon in the human body, which is formed by the confluence of the soleus muscle and the medial and lateral heads of the gastrocnemius muscle. The soleus tendon contributes the greatest amount of fibers to the Achilles tendon. As the Achilles courses distally toward the calcaneus, its fibers rotate internally, such that the medial fibers (i.e., medial gastrocnemius head) rotate to a more superficial or posterior position and the lateral fibers (i.e., lateral gastrocnemius head and soleus) end up deeper or more anterior [8, 9]. Lohrer et al. [10], in an anatomic, cadaveric study, demonstrated a consistently broad insertion of the Achilles tendon that resembles a crescent shape, extending around the posterior calcaneus both medially and laterally.

Although slight variations have been described in prior cadaveric work, Ballal et al. [8], in a more recent cadaveric, dissection study, demonstrated the various fascicle contributions to the Achilles tendon and the respective insertional footprint on the posterior calcaneus (Fig. 11.1). In all 12 fresh-frozen specimens, the medial head of the gastrocnemius tendon fascicles inserted across the entire width of the inferior facet, making up the superficial tendon insertion, with a mean footprint width of 28.3 mm (range, 24–34 mm) and mean height of 7.8 mm (range, 6–10 mm). The deep tendon insertion is formed from contributions from the lateral head of the gastrocnemius and soleus tendon fascicles. The lateral head of the gastrocnemius tendon fascicles insert at the lateral part of the middle facet with a mean width of 14.4 mm (range, 12–19 mm) and a mean height of 10 mm (range, 7–12 mm). Finally, the soleus tendon fascicles insert at the medial aspect of the middle facet, with an insertional footprint of a mean width of 18.2 mm (range, 15–28 mm) and a mean height of 15 mm (range, 13–17 mm).

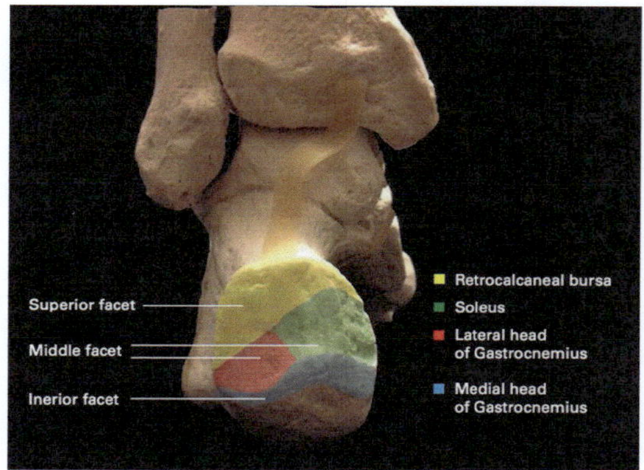

Fig. 11.1 Achilles tendon insertional footprint of its various fascicles at the posterior calcaneus facets (from Fig. 6 in Ballal MS, Walker CR, Molloy AP. The anatomical footprint of the Achilles tendon: a cadaveric study. *Bone Joint J* 2014;96:1346)

Huh et al. [3] reported that all patients in their study, at the time of surgery, were found to have a central Achilles tendon avulsion, with intact medial and lateral fascicle bands. In the majority of cases, a single osseous fragment, or a small group of them, was found attached to this central tendon avulsion, the donor site for which was the central portion of the calcaneal insertion footprint (i.e., central portions of the middle and inferior calcaneal facets), not the posterior tuberosity, as would occur with a posterior tuberosity (extra-articular) or tongue-type (intra-articular) calcaneal fracture. In two cases, Huh et al. [3] noted a coronal sheer, an avulsion pattern that involved an avulsion of, primarily, the posterocentral Achilles fascicles, which would essentially represent tendon fibers from the medial gastrocnemius head.

As previously mentioned, the nature of an Achilles sleeve avulsion rupture can be a challenge to repair—there is inadequate tendon present distally for a tendon-to-tendon repair and insufficient, avulsed calcaneal bone present to allow for open reduction and internal fixation back to the posterior tuberosity. Furthermore, the majority of these patients present with prodromal symptoms and clinical and radiographic findings consistent with baseline insertional Achilles tendinopathy, such as retrocalcaneal bursitis, Achilles tendinosis, enthesopathy, and an impinging Haglund's prominence, which should be addressed concomitantly to sleeve avulsion repair, including debridement, decompression, and incorporation into the overall reconstruction, to best address all the relevant and symptomatic features of this process for the patient.

The Achilles tendon-calcaneal bone insertion site, like other tendon-bone attachments in the human body, such as the rotator cuff tendon complex-proximal humerus in the shoulder, has a complex anatomy and structure, grossly and histologically [9, 11]. This attachment site consists of bone, fibrocartilage (both mineralized and nonmineralized), and tendon. This area allows for force transmission between tendon and bone, but also a stress absorber during mechanical loading [9, 11]. Leung et al. [12], in an Achilles tendon-calcaneal bone model and a comparative study of 47 adolescent Chinese goats, found that superior histological healing and biomechanical properties (i.e., loading, strength) were demonstrated with homogenous tissue repair types, such as bone-to-bone and tendon-to-tendon, compared to tendon-to-bone interface. Morphologically, the latter, heterogenous repair, showed slower tissue remodeling, inadequate regeneration within the fibrocartilaginous region, and excessive fibrous or scar tissue formation at the actual healing site at the bone-tendon interface [11].

Presentation and Diagnosis

With only a few subtle differences, a patient with an acute Achilles sleeve avulsion rupture presents much like a patient with a standard, midsubstance Achilles tear. The report of "feeling a pop" or the sensation of "being kicked in the back of the ankle" is common during the acute event, with subsequent bruising, pain, weakness, and gait dysfunction, which should prompt presentation to an appropriate medical provider. Unique to this injury, the patient will typically report a history of insertional Achilles tendon discomfort and prodromal symptoms. Huh et al. [3] reported that 73% of patients had prodromal insertional Achilles symptoms, and Schipper et al. [4] reported prodromal symptoms in 44% and 92%

of their general population and professional athlete cohorts, respectively. In both studies, this specific injury was highly male predominant [3, 4]. In addition, Huh et al. [3] reported in their case series that 91% of patients who had repair of this injury were either overweight or obese. Interestingly, obesity was previously shown to be an independent risk factor for Achilles tendinopathy [11].

On examination, there can be localized tenderness about the posterior heel and distal Achilles. A central palpable gap, weak ankle plantarflexion, and positive Thompson test may still be present despite this typically being a "partial" injury at the insertional region. In short, the examination alone of a patient with an acute Achilles sleeve avulsion injury does not always allow the evaluating medical provider to discern it from the more common, midsubstance rupture. However, given the patient's reported history, in conjunction with examination and relevant imaging, the specific diagnosis becomes quite clear.

As such, standard ankle radiographs, in particular the lateral view, are critical to obtain in any patient with a concern for an Achilles rupture, no matter what the subtype is. There is commonly a loss of the normal posterior ankle soft tissue contours and shadowing, also known as an obliteration of the Kager triangle, with most any Achilles tendon rupture, including a sleeve-avulsion variant. More important to recognize here are baseline enthesopathic changes at the posterior calcaneus. These can include a posterior enthesophyte with associated calcifications, commonly seen with insertional Achilles tendinopathy, and a more proximally located osseous, avulsion fragment or "fleck sign," representative of the sleeve avulsion or partial, insertional avulsion injury (Fig. 11.2).

To reemphasize, obtaining a lateral ankle radiograph is critical as 36% (4/11) of cases reported by Huh et al. [3] were first identified at the time of surgery and required an intraoperative adjustment in the repair plan. These misses were due to inadequate preoperative imaging in three cases, and in one case, the avulsion fleck on the lateral ankle radiograph was not recognized by the treating surgeon and only later appreciated

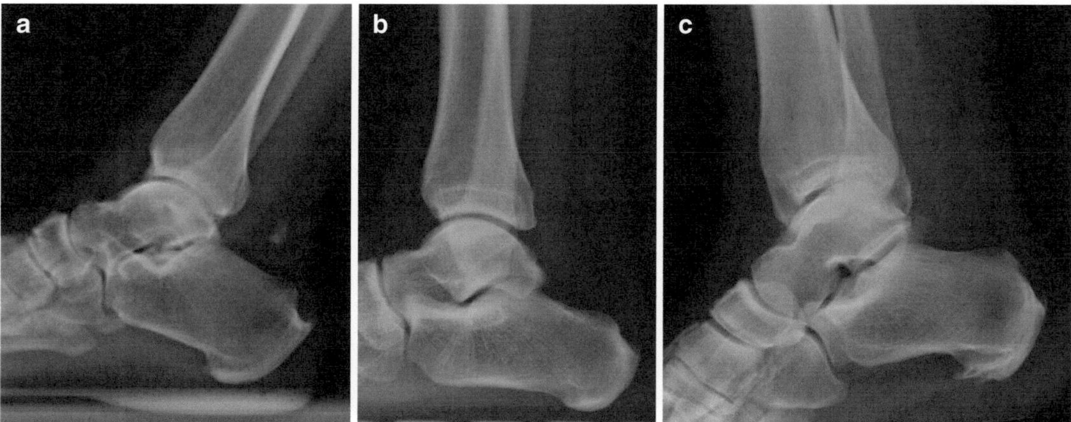

Fig. 11.2 Lateral ankle radiographs demonstrating various appearances of an Achilles sleeve avulsion injury, from a single osseous fragment (**a**) to multiple bony pieces (**b**), and more subtle avulsion "flecks" (**c**) seen retracted within the posterior ankle soft tissues, along with corresponding insertional/enthesopathic changes seen at the posterior calcaneus and Haglund's deformity

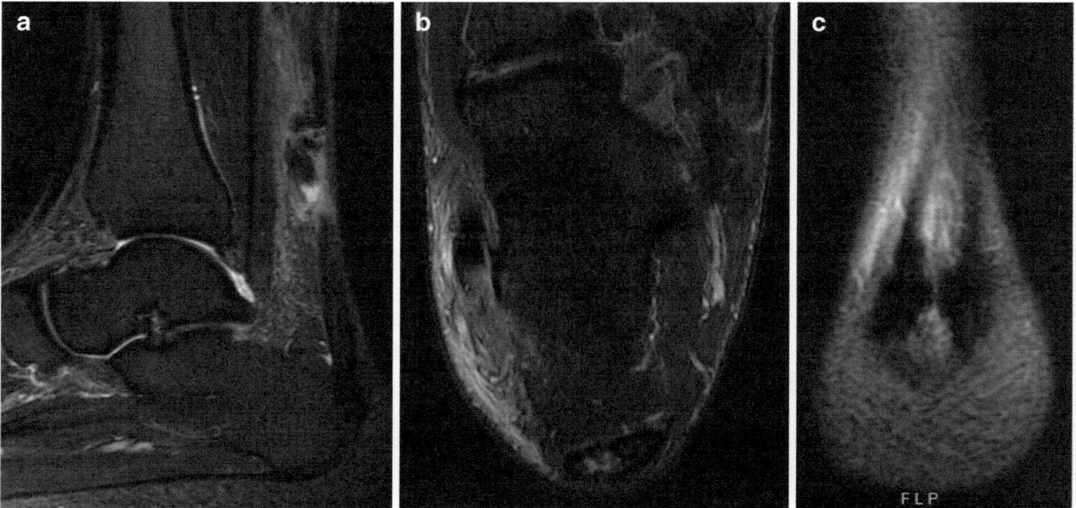

Fig. 11.3 MRI ankle T2 FS sagittal (**a**), axial (**b**), and coronal (**c**) sequences shown in a patient with an acute Achilles tendon sleeve avulsion. The sagittal view demonstrates the retracted central Achilles tendon slip, and the axial and coronal views show the same, with the central tendon void surrounded by intact medial and lateral Achilles tendon fascicles

following the case [3]. When the above clinical history, examination, and radiographic findings are identified, obtaining an ankle MRI to further diagnose and characterize this injury pattern is quite useful for the treating surgeon for preoperative planning purposes (Fig. 11.3).

Nonoperative Management

Unlike midsubstance Achilles ruptures, there is no substantial evidence supporting the nonsurgical management of patients with Achilles sleeve avulsion injuries. Thus, unless the patient is medically inappropriate for surgery, of low functional demand, or otherwise contraindicated for surgery, an Achilles sleeve avulsion injury is best managed surgically in order to optimize the healing potential and to restore the tension in the gastrosoleus-Achilles complex via a tendon-to-bone repair. If nonoperative care is selected, then functional bracing in an ankle foot orthosis (AFO) with an appropriate rehabilitation program can help patients make progress on muscle strengthening, function, and gait.

Surgical Management and Outcomes

Patients with Achilles tendon sleeve avulsion injuries are generally managed surgically in order to achieve the most optimal and defined outcome. Given the relative rarity of this specific injury, there is a paucity of evidence-based literature to support one technique over another. A repair of this specific injury pattern has been accomplished via transcalcaneal drill tunnels, suture anchors, or a combination thereof [3–5, 13–17]. Both open and less-invasive approaches have been described. The theoretic advantages and disadvantages of a transosseous drill tunnel include low cost and reduced infection risk, given there are no implants or anchors used, in exchange for being a more technically demanding procedure, with potential iatrogenic pain experienced due to exposure over the plantar fascial origin or plantar nerve injury. On the other hand, suture anchor repairs are thought to be stronger, perhaps allowing for earlier rehabilitation, and are less technically demanding procedures, albeit with associated implant costs.

Bibbo et al. [5] reported on their results in treating a series of patients with Achilles tendon sleeve avulsion injuries using a transcalcaneal suture repair technique via a longitudinal posterior incision. Results were favorable with patients, ranging from lower-demand to recreational and professional athletes, being able to return to full activity and sport. No significant difference was found in peak plantarflexion strength and AOFAS ankle/hindfoot scores between the operative and nonoperative legs.

Bibbo [14] later reported on a modified, less-invasive technique, utilizing two smaller incisions, mostly intended for patients with soft tissue limitations and/or medical comorbidities that limit wound healing. In this dual-incision approach, a 3–4 cm incision is made over the posteromedial calcaneus in order to mobilize the free avulsed tendon stump and also to resect the Haglund's prominence and prepare the bone for tendon reattachment. The Achilles tendon stump is bluntly mobilized, keeping the paratenon intact. In order to achieve more tendon length, a second incision of similar length is made midline over the gastrocnemius aponeurosis, where a V-Y fascial advancement is performed. Distal traction is maintained on the Achilles stump, while the length achieved from the proximal advancement is set, followed by the placement of nonabsorbable suture in a modified Bunnell fashion through the ruptured Achilles stump. These sutures are then passed through calcaneal drill tunnels and tied over the plantar fascia distally through a small incision at an appropriate tension.

Pavlou et al. [13] also reported on their technique for Achilles sleeve avulsion repair using a transcalcaneal approach for fixation. Their modification was to use an ACL passing pin to aid in the passage of the sutures sewn through the ruptured Achilles tendon stump. They further augmented this repair using suture anchors placed in the posterior calcaneus.

Huh et al. [3], in a level IV retrospective case series, reported their findings and outcomes on 11 consecutive patients (10 males and 1 female), mean age of 44 years, with Achilles tendon sleeve avulsion injuries treated using a suture anchor repair at a mean follow-up of 38.4 months. They found that these injuries occurred primarily in patients with the above listed demographics, with preexisting insertional Achilles tendinopathy during athletics. The surgical technique utilized

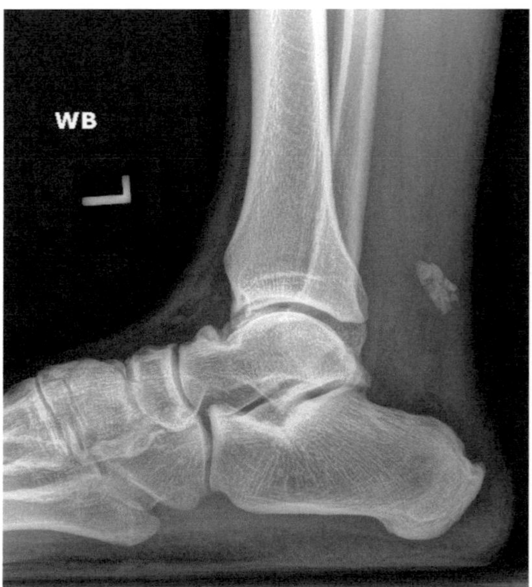

Fig. 11.4 Lateral ankle radiograph demonstrating the retracted, large avulsed bony fragment from the posterior calcaneus and baseline insertional Achilles tendinopathic changes

included a posterior longitudinal incision over the Achilles tendon, centered over the palpable tendon defect, with distal exposure of the posterior calcaneus to access the insertional tendinopathy component. The paratenon was incised longitudinally and the Achilles sleeve avulsion rupture exposed. The ruptured tendon component was bluntly mobilized proximally and traction held on the tendon stump with an Allis clamp. The avulsed osseous fragments were excised from the ruptured central tendon stump. Distally, the insertional Achilles pathology was debrided with rongeur and Haglund's deformity resected with a microsagittal saw or osteotome. Two, double-loaded suture anchors (3.5 mm or 5.5 mm) were placed in the posterior calcaneus at a level 1 cm proximal to the distal Achilles tendon insertion. A pair of nonabsorbable sutures from each anchor was each passed through the ruptured central Achilles tendon stump, and the other two pairs of sutures were passed through the intact medial and lateral Achilles tendon slips. These sutures were tied with the ankle in maximal plantarflexion, and then the repaired central tendon slip was sewn in a side-to-side fashion to the medial and lateral Achilles bands.

Huh et al. [3] reported that 10 out of 11 patients were completely satisfied with their surgical outcome, and only one reported complication, which was delayed wound healing treated with local wound care. Ten patients returned to their full preoperative work and recreational/sporting activity levels. One patient was unable to perform a sustained single-limb heel rise on the operative extremity.

In a larger, retrospective case series, Schipper et al. [4] reported on their surgical outcomes on 16 general population patients and 12 professional athletes with Achilles sleeve avulsion injuries, at a mean follow-up of 8.1 years for the former group. A 4–5 cm incision was utilized over the posteromedial Achilles/heel and the ruptured Achilles tendon portion mobilized bluntly. The Haglund's prominence was resected and the tendon end debrided, along with the removal of any small, avulsed bony fragments. The Achilles sleeve avulsion was repaired using either transosseous bone tunnels or two suture anchors based on surgeon preference. A gastrocnemius recession was used only if the tendon end was not reducible to the posterior calcaneus, and a flexor hallucis longus (FHL) tendon transfer was used if greater than 50% of the Achilles tendon width was debrided.

In the general population group, the median patient age was 47.5 years and the majority ($n = 12$, 75%) were male [4]. A prior history of Achilles pain was reported in 43.8% of patients, but 75% of patients had radiographic changes consistent with insertional Achilles tendinopathy. The majority of patients (81.3%) had a Haglund's excision. Seven out of 16 (43.8%) general population patients had an FHL tendon transfer, and three out of 16 (18.8%) had a gastrocnemius recession. A transosseous tunnel suture repair was performed in 13 out of 16 patients, while the other three patients had suture anchor repair. There were no reruptures, and two patients had postoperative infections requiring surgical debridement.

The professional athlete cohort had a median age of 27.9 years, with all patients reporting at least a 5-month history of preceding insertional Achilles tendon symptoms and 91.7% of patients with at least 9 months of prodromal Achilles pain

[4]. All professional athletes had a Haglund's excision, while one underwent an FHL tendon transfer. Six athletes (50%) had suture anchor repair, and the other half had transosseous suture repair. There were no reruptures, and one patient had a wound dehiscence requiring a skin graft to heal. All athletes returned to play at a mean of 13.4 months.

Yang et al. [15] reported on a modified transosseous suture repair technique on 11 patients with Achilles tendon sleeve avulsions. In this technique, following a debridement of the ruptured Achilles tendon end, two whip stitches using heavy nonabsorbable sutures were passed through the medial and lateral sides of the tendon. The Haglund's deformity was removed, along with the removal of the main portion of insertional bone spurs, maintaining a 5 mm portion of the bone spur. Three bone tunnels were placed through this bone spur base, and after further preparation, the sutures were passed through these tunnels and tied, allowing a reduction of the Achilles tendon stump back to its native insertion. There were no reruptures or infections. All patients had their preinjury insertional Achilles tendinopathy symptoms relieved. Patients returned to work and sport at 2.8 and 12.3 months postoperatively, respectively.

In order to minimize wound and infectious complications, less-invasive techniques have been developed and utilized for the repair of these insertional Achilles injuries. Case series on these techniques utilize smaller incisions, percutaneous passage of sutures through the Achilles stump, and suture anchor fixation with good results and minimal complications [16, 17].

Surgeon Preferred Surgical Technique—Case Example

The patient is a 39-year-old personal trainer who reports feeling a "pop" while changing from running backward to forward during a pickup basketball game, with immediate posterior heel and Achilles pain in the left ankle. He reports some prodromal pain in this area of the preceding 4–6 months and has a prior history of a right Achilles sleeve avulsion repair performed by my partner 5 years prior to this injury. His examination is consistent with an Achilles tendon rupture, with a negative Thompson test and a loss of normal resting plantarflexion tone to the ankle. A lateral radiograph shows a moderately sized avulsion fracture fragment retracted proximally in the posterior ankle soft tissues (Fig. 11.4). Given his prior history of this exact injury on the contralateral side, along with the diagnostic radiographic features, we did not feel the need to obtain an MRI. The patient, having done well on the right side, elected to proceed with surgical repair in a similar fashion on the left Achilles tendon.

In the prone position, under monitored anesthesia care and regional block, after the inflation of a well-padded thigh tourniquet and the administration of intravenous (IV) antibiotics, we perform a longitudinal incision over the posterior Achilles/heel. The paratenon is incised longitudinally and careful medial and lateral flaps raised. The central Achilles tendon rupture with associated avulsed osseous fragment are identified with the donor site located at the posterior calcaneus, along with intact bordering Achilles tendon slips on either side, confirming the diagnosis of an Achilles sleeve avulsion injury (Fig. 11.5). The central tendon slip is mobilized, and the attached bony fragment is carefully excised from the central tendon slip, followed by placement of a flat, braided suture (SutureTape, Arthrex, Inc.; Naples, FL) on either side of the tendon in a running Krackow fashion. Depending on the size of the central tendon slip, there are two to four SutureTape limbs exiting out of the central tendon slip (Fig. 11.6a).

Attention is turned distally at the posterior calcaneus, and the Achilles is gently debrided of any degenerative tissue and split into medial and lateral flaps, overall leaving these slips intact but allowing for the exposure of the Haglund's prominence and enthesopathic changes. A retrocalcaneal bursectomy is performed, followed by a careful resection of the Haglund's deformity and enthesophytes using a microsagittal saw (Fig. 11.6b). The resection is confirmed to be appropriate under lateral fluoroscopy, and the edges are smoothed with a rasp and saw blade to contour smoothly.

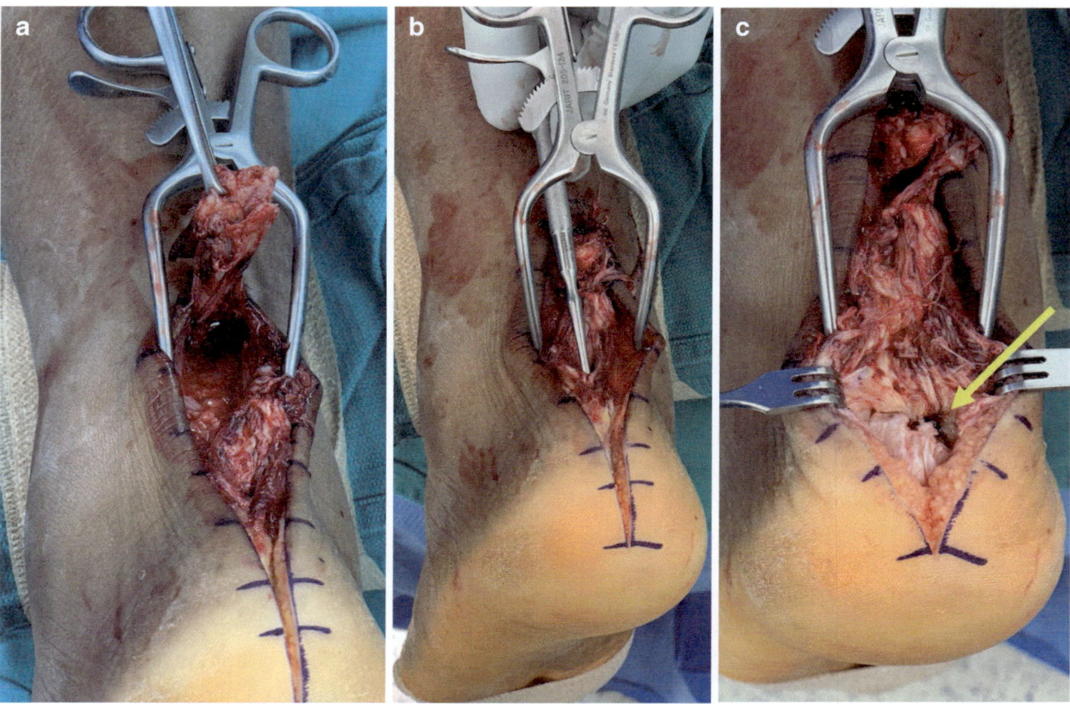

Fig. 11.5 Intraoperative photographs demonstrating the appearance of a typical, acute Achilles sleeve avulsion injury. The Allis clamp is holding the avulsed bony fragment and associated central Achilles rupture (**a**). The Freer elevator is placed into the void where the central Achilles avulsion injury occurred (**b**). More distal exposure on the calcaneus demonstrates the Achilles sleeve avulsion donor site (arrow) at the posterolateral calcaneus (**c**)

We feel that this insertional Achilles work is critical for several reasons. From a pain and function standpoint, it allows for a more comprehensive approach to relieve the posterior heel pain in excising inflamed retrocalcaneal bursa, along with resecting the symptomatic Haglund's prominence and posterior calcaneal enthesophytes. The remaining posterior calcaneal bone surface after resection provides a large flat area for suture anchor reconstruction, along with a bleeding bone surface for the debrided Achilles tendon to heal back to, which is critical given the insertional pattern of this injury. Furthermore, this resection decompresses the posterior heel, which reduces tissue bulk and allows for a tension-free soft tissue closure.

A commercially available knotless suture anchor system is utilized (SpeedBridge™, Arthrex, Inc.; Naples, FL), and four drill holes in the shape of a square or rectangle are carefully positioned and placed on the resected flat posterior calcaneal surface. Two SwiveLock® 4.75 mm anchors loaded with FiberTape® and #2 FiberWire® are placed in the proximal row (Fig. 11.6c). In order to separately reduce and fixate the avulsed central Achilles slip, a fifth, more central drill hole is made in the middle of the prior drill hole pattern. The SutureTape limbs from the central Achilles tendon are passed through an additional 4.75 mm SwiveLock® anchor and the appropriate tension set with the ankle held in plantarflexion and fixated into the calcaneus. An alternative reconstruction option that we have utilized is to pass the SutureTapes through the Swivelock® anchors of the distal row of the reconstruction, along with the FiberTape®

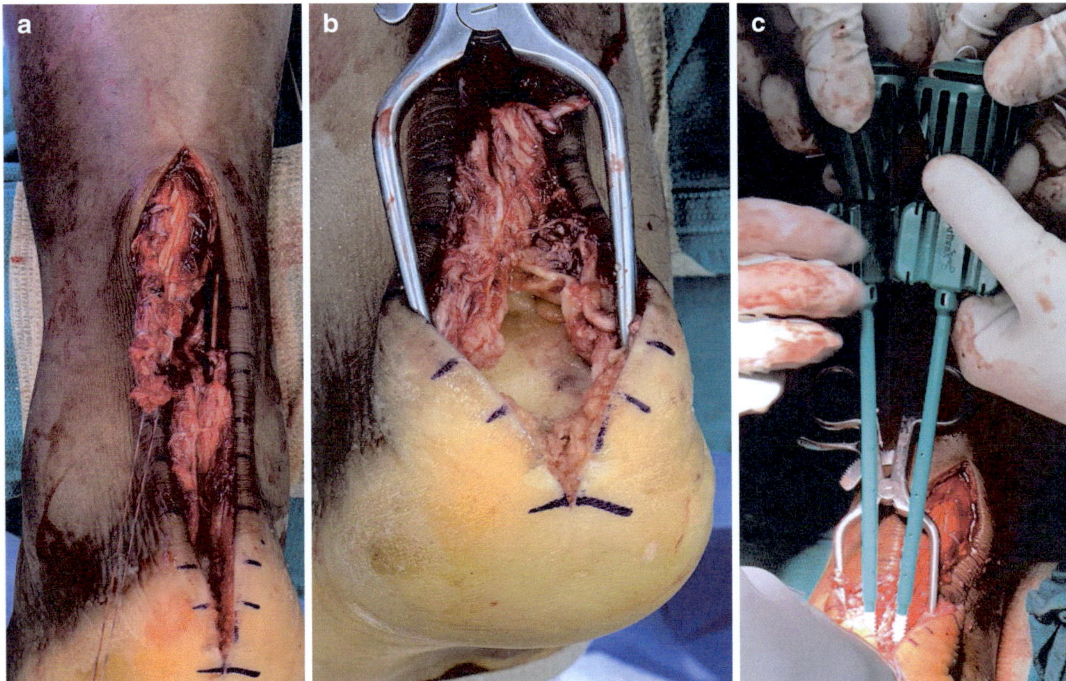

Fig. 11.6 The ruptured Achilles slip is sewn in a running Krackow fashion using SutureTape (**a**). The posterior calcaneus with Haglund's deformity and enthesophytes are decompressed in an oblique fashion using a microsagittal saw (**b**) to create a flat bleeding surface for tendon-to-bone reconstruction. The proximal row of anchors are placed after drilling and tapping (**c**)

sutures, avoiding a fifth drill hole if the resected osseous surface area is limited.

With the correct tension set, the central Achilles tendon is sewn side to side to the intact medial and lateral bands, and then the SpeedBridge™ construct is finalized by passing the FiberTape® suture through each side of the Achilles tendon, crossed and secured distally in a knotless fashion through the distal row of the SwiveLock® anchors. The tourniquet is released and hemostasis achieved, and after a thorough irrigation, the paratenon is reapproximated and closed over the reconstruction (Fig. 11.7). A standard closure is performed, followed by the placement of a well-padded short leg splint with the ankle in resting plantarflexion.

The patient is maintained non-weight-bearing in this splint for 2 weeks, followed by suture removal and placement in a short leg cast for an additional week to ensure complete wound healing. At 3 weeks postoperatively, the patient is allowed weight-bearing to tolerance in a cam boot with a series of heel lifts, which are gradually removed, with the goal of having the patient plantigrade in the boot by 6 weeks postoperatively. Physical therapy is initiated around 3–4 weeks postoperatively and range of motion and progressive strengthening exercises performed with the goal of weaning to a sneaker by 8–10 weeks from the time of surgery. Running, jumping, and other higher impact-activities are initiated at 3–4 months.

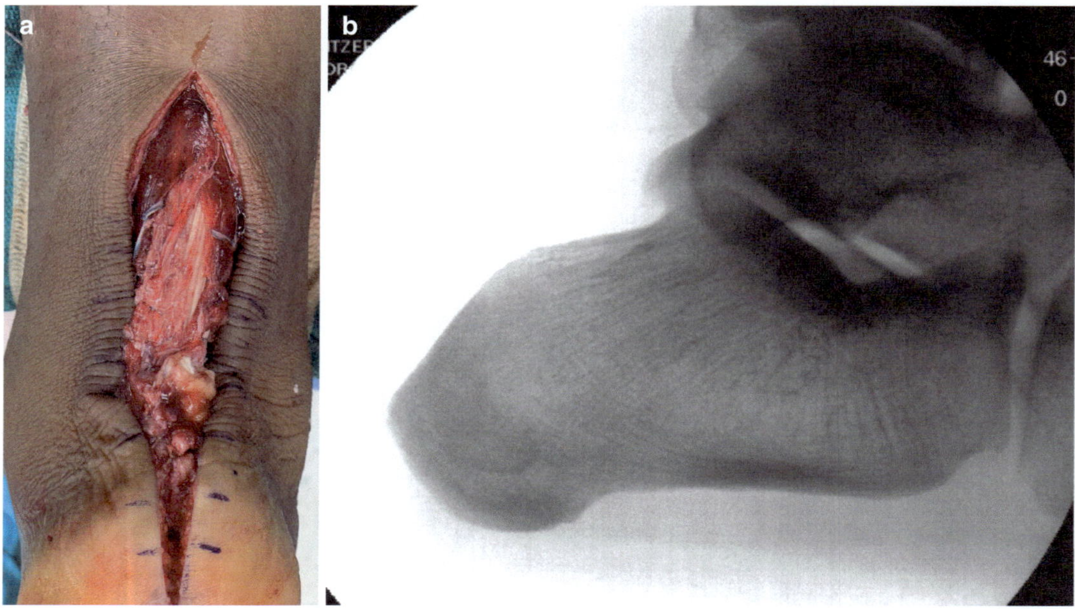

Fig. 11.7 Intraoperative photograph showing the final reconstruction as the paratenon is closed from proximal to distal (**a**). Final lateral ankle fluoroscopic view showing adequate decompression of the posterior calcaneus (**b**)

References

1. Chen TM, Rozen WM, Pan W, Ashton MW, Richardson MD, Taylor GI. The arterial anatomy of the Achilles tendon: anatomical study and clinical implications. Clin Anat. 2009;22:377–85.
2. Weinfeld SB. Achilles tendon disorders. Med Clin North Am. 2014;98:331–8.
3. Huh J, Easley ME, Nunley JA II. Characterization and surgical management of Achilles tendon sleeve avulsions. Foot Ankle Int. 2016;37:596–604.
4. Schipper ON, Anderson RB, Cohen BE. Outcomes after primary repair of insertional ruptures of the Achilles tendon. Foot Ankle Int. 2018;39:664–8.
5. Bibbo C, Anderson RB, Davis WH, Agnone M. Repair of the Achilles tendon sleeve avulsion: quantitative and functional evaluation of a transcalcaneal suture technique. Foot Ankle Int. 2003;24:539–44.
6. Beavis RC, Rourke K, Court-Brown C. Avulsion fracture of the calcaneal tuberosity: a case report and literature review. Foot Ankle Int. 2008;29:863–6.
7. Lee SM, Huh SW, Chung JW, Kim DW, Kim YJ, Rhee SK. Avulsion fracture of the calcaneal tuberosity: classification and its characteristics. Clin Orthop Surg. 2012;4:134–8.
8. Ballal MS, Walker CR, Molloy AP. The anatomical footprint of the Achilles tendon: a cadaveric study. Bone Joint J. 2014;96:1344–8.
9. Benjamin M, Toumi H, Ralphs JR, Bydder G, Best TM, Milz S. Where tendons and ligaments meet bone: attachment sites ('entheses') in relation to exercise and/or mechanical load. J Anat. 2006;208:471–90.
10. Lohrer H, Arentz S, Nauck T, Dorn-Lange NV, Konerding MA. The Achilles tendon insertion is crescent-shaped: an in vitro anatomic investigation. Clin Orthop Relat Res. 2008;466:2230–7.
11. Holmes GB, Lin J. Etiologic factors associated with symptomatic Achilles tendinopathy. Foot Ankle Int. 2006;27:952–9.
12. Leung KS, Chong WS, Chow DHK, Zhang P, Cheung WH, Wong MWN, Qin L. A comparative study on the biomechanical and histological properties of bone-to-bone, bone-to-tendon, and tendon-to-tendon healing: an Achilles tendon-calcaneus model in goats. Am J Sports Med. 2015;43:1413–21.
13. Pavlou G, Roach R, Salehi-Bird S. Repair of the Achilles tendon sleeve avulsion: a transcalcaneal suture technique. Foot Ankle Int. 2009;30:65–7.
14. Bibbo C. Technique tip: limited dual incision technique for repair of Achilles sleeve avulsions. Foot Ankle Int. 2004;25:513–5.
15. Yang YP, Wang DY, Wei LW, An N, Tao LY, Jiao C, Guo QW, Hu YL. Repair of Achilles sleeve avulsion: a new transosseous suture technique. J Orthop Surg Res. 2020;15:224–30.
16. Longo UG, Candela V, Berton A, Di Naro C, Stelitano G, Maffulli N, Denaro V. Less invasive fixation of acute avulsions of the Achilles tendon: a technical note. Medicina. 2020;56:715–22.
17. Liu CY, Wu TC, Yang KC, Li YC, Wang CC. Ultrasonography-guided minimally invasive surgery for Achilles sleeve avulsions. Foot Ankle Int. 2021;42:544–53.

Rehabilitation of Achilles Tendon Tears (Operative and Nonoperative)

12

Sachin Allahabadi, Christopher Antonelli, Sarah Lander, and Brian C. Lau

Introduction

Acute Achilles tendon ruptures treated with operative or nonoperative management require an appreciation and close adherence to the rehabilitation process, which is a critical component of recovery and an ultimate return to function for the patient. The goals of rehabilitation include protecting the tendon and/or repair while also recovering the range of motion (ROM) and enhancing strength. Compliance with empirical rehabilitation protocols is crucial to provide optimal conditions for tendon healing and regeneration while maximizing the ability to return to activities.

Traditional rehabilitation programs were designed with an aim to minimize complications after Achilles rupture and repair. For example, therapy protocols sought to minimize rerupture, repair or rupture site gapping, and wound break-

down. Until the late 1980s, the majority of Achilles injuries were therefore managed with prolonged immobilization up to 12 weeks, with hopes of allowing for tendon healing and recovery [1, 2]. However, prolonged immobilization has been associated with a multitude of complications, including muscle atrophy, arthrofibrosis, adhesions, articular cartilage degeneration, as well as deep vein thrombosis [3–7]. Prolonged immobilization with the rationale of protecting the tendon has been proven to be counterproductive. Immobilization negatively impacts the tendon, resulting in lower strain to failure and lower tensile strength with altered physiologic characteristics [8, 9]. The literature has also revealed that prolonged immobilization is associated with a lower force-generating capacity per unit area, interstitial fibrosis, as well as a decrease in muscle size [10–12]. On a basic science level, Bring et al., in a rat model, demonstrated that prolonged immobilization compromised the upregulation of repair gene expression, thus halting the healing process [13]. Therefore, prolonged immobilization, even with more recent protocols of 6 weeks, is not ideal for successful rehabilitation and function.

To counter the shortcomings of prolonged immobilization, early functional rehabilitation protocols have been evaluated. A landmark study published in the *Journal of Bone & Joint Surgery* in 2010 by Willits et al. demonstrated similar outcomes in strength, range of motion, and calf circumference between operatively and

S. Allahabadi
Department of Orthopaedics, University of California San Francisco Medical Center,
San Francisco, CA, USA
e-mail: sachin.allahabadi@ucsf.edu

C. Antonelli
Physical Therapy, Duke Sport Science Institute, Duke University, Durham, NC, USA
e-mail: Christopher.antonelli@duke.edu

S. Lander · B. C. Lau (✉)
Division of Sports Medicine, Department of Orthopaedics, Duke Sport Science Institute, Duke University, Durham, NC, USA
e-mail: Sarah.lander@duke.edu; Brian.lau@duke.edu

© The Author(s), under exclusive license to Springer Nature Switzerland AG 2023
S. B. Adams (ed.), *The Achilles Tendon*, https://doi.org/10.1007/978-3-031-45594-0_12

nonoperatively managed Achilles ruptures using an accelerated functional rehabilitation protocol [14]. The authors' protocol permitted weight-bearing and active motion at 2 weeks with progression to weight-bearing as tolerated by 4 weeks and no heel lifts at 6 weeks [14]. More recently, early functional rehabilitation has been defined by the inclusion of weight-bearing and specific motion exercises within the first 2 weeks after an acute Achilles tendon repair or rupture [15, 16]. Early mobilization has been well documented to be a key aspect of rehabilitation [14, 17, 18]. A few concerns of early mobilization are gap formation at the repair site and the lengthening of the tendon, which can cause functional weakness due to an increased excursion of the tendon in order to provide the appropriate tension [19]. However, a meta-analysis of randomized controlled trials comparing early functional rehabilitation to delayed regimens determined early functional rehabilitation as a safe and effective postoperative management option, including superior patient-reported outcomes [20]. Recent data and protocols have targeted early functional rehabilitation.

Rehabilitation Protocols

The conservative treatment of acute Achilles injuries has gained support due to the implementation of functional rehabilitation. While previous evidence suggested that surgery resulted in lower rerupture rates than conservative treatment, more recent studies have shown that functional rehabilitation provides similar rerupture rates and functional outcomes while minimizing general complications of surgery [21].

The goal of functional rehabilitation is to restore the range of motion, optimize strength and balance, normalize gait mechanics, and maximize function to allow for a return to the prior level of activity. A 2012 meta-analysis by Soroceanu et al. found that functional rehabilitation with an early range of motion led to equal rerupture rates for surgical and nonsurgical patients [21, 22]. Furthermore, there were no dif-

ferences in calf circumference, strength, or functional outcomes when a functional rehabilitation protocol was used without surgery. Typically, reported functional rehabilitation protocols include early weight-bearing and mobilization with favorable outcomes [21–23]. Early weight-bearing is widely accepted in functional rehabilitation and does not appear to increase the risk for rerupture [22, 23]. Willits et al. demonstrated that at 1 and 2 years postinjury, the affected limb in both operative and nonoperative treatment that received functional rehabilitation was able to achieve at least 80% of the plantarflexion strength compared to the nonaffected limb in isokinetic testing [14, 24].

Currently, the optimal rehabilitation protocol remains unclear. Various studies that investigate on functional rehabilitation report varying lengths of immobilization time, different times to begin weight-bearing, and different orthoses. A 2015 study by Hutchison and colleagues reported on 273 acute Achilles tendon rupture cases, 211 of which were treated conservatively and 62 operatively with identical rehabilitation protocols [25]. Both groups underwent immediate weight-bearing in a fixed equinus position with immobilization until week 10 of the protocol [25]. The rerupture rate was only 1.1% (3 patients) for all cases with this protocol, with no differences between operative and nonoperative groups [25]. In 2014, Barfod and colleagues found that immediate weight-bearing and controlled early mobilization led to higher quality of life and good functional outcomes when compared to non-weight-bearing [26]. Based on the results of this study, a combination of both early weight-bearing and controlled early mobilization may lead to the best outcomes with functional rehabilitation [26]. The focus of the rehabilitation following an acute Achilles tendon rupture will be to restore the range of motion, maximize strength and power, normalize gait mechanics, and return the patient to their prior level of function. An understanding of peak stress, force, and strain on the Achilles tendon is essential to the rehabilitation specialist to ensure a safe and compliant rehabilitative process.

Nonoperative Functional Rehabilitation

The nonoperative management of Achilles ruptures has led to favorable outcomes and comes with the benefit of avoiding the complications of surgery. Compliance with and adherence to the functional rehabilitation protocol are paramount to minimize the risks of tendon elongation and residual calf weakness. Currently available evidence has shown that when the protocol is adhered to, there is not a significant clinical difference in outcomes between operative and nonoperative treatment.

Similar to the operative rehabilitation protocol, nonoperative functional rehabilitation includes early weight-bearing and early range of motion. A highly studied nonoperative functional rehabilitation protocol was described by Willits and colleagues [14]. The Glazebrook/Rubinger Achilles (GAPNOT) protocol for nonoperative treatment is a standardized and accelerated protocol modified from the Willits study [14, 24]. Patients with an acute Achilles tendon rupture are ideal for nonoperative management if there is a confirmed diagnosis of the injury within 2 days of injury and if the patient had minimal weight-bearing activities within that period. Patients are initially immobilized in maximum plantarflexion for 2 weeks while remaining non-weight-bearing. Following the period of immobilization, patients are then placed in a boot with heel lifts to remain in a plantarflexion position. The initiation of ROM begins, and modalities for pain, swelling, and neuromuscular reeducation are utilized. Light strengthening exercises begin at 4 weeks postinjury and progressively continue until 100% strength is regained. Weight-bearing is progressed 25% each week from weeks 2–6, with full weight-bearing being achieved at the 6-week mark. ROM beyond neutral dorsiflexion is avoided from weeks 2 to 8 to reduce the risk of tendon elongation. Weaning from the boot begins at week 8, with gait training being initiated with the full weight-bearing status. Tendon elongation is most likely to occur during the 10-week to 16-week mark as patients begin walking more and gaining more confidence with daily activities. Care is to be made with closed kinetic chain strengthening, stair navigation, and ambulation to protect against tendon elongation. Light jogging and skipping activities can begin at 16 weeks postinjury if the patient can perform 25 consecutive single-leg heel raises. Return-to-sport activities begin at the 6-month mark while minimizing jumping, cutting, and sprinting. A return to running and jumping sports begins at the 9-month mark if the patient has regained 100% strength.

Weeks 0–2
Immobilization in maximum plantarflexion and non-weight-bearing.

Weeks 2–4
Physical therapy typically begins. At the 2-week mark, the patient is placed in an Achilles-specific boot with a 40° heel lift. Protected weight-bearing begins at weeks 2–3, beginning with 25% weight-bearing. Weight-bearing status is increased by 25% each week until week 6, when the patient will become 100% weight-bearing. Active ankle ROM begins in all planes, with dorsiflexion being limited to neutral. At 3 weeks, seated heel raises can begin ensuring that the ankle does not go beyond neutral. Hip and knee strengthening can be performed with no ankle involvement. The use of modalities can be used for pain, swelling, and muscle reeducation (cryotherapy, compression, electrical muscle stimulation, blood flow restriction training). Non-weight-bearing cardiovascular activities and aquatic therapy can be performed if patients adhere to weight-bearing precautions.

Weeks 4–6
At 4 weeks, the weight-bearing progression continues to 75% weight-bearing. An ankle range of motion in all planes and joint mobilizations, ensuring the ankle does not go beyond neutral, can be performed. Light plantarflexion strengthening exercises can be performed ensuring the ankle does not go beyond neutral. Non-weight-bearing cardiovascular activities can be performed. Continued focus on swelling and pain management. Appropriate hip and knee strengthening can be performed.

Weeks 6–8

The weight-bearing progression achieves full weight-bearing status in the boot at 6 weeks. Weaning from the boot typically begins at the 8-week mark. The patient can gradually begin removing heel lifts from the boot between weeks 6 and 8. Resisted plantarflexion, including standing bilateral heel raises (Fig. 12.1), can begin during this stage of recovery, as well as weighted-resisted exercises, as long as the ankle does not go beyond neutral. Gait training is initiated due to full weight-bearing status.

Weeks 8–12

This is a very vulnerable phase for the tendon. Weaning from the boot can begin at week 8 typically over a 2–5-day process—though this is very patient dependent. Sudden or increased loading of the tendon with activities of daily living and exercise could result in a rerupture. Avoid stretching the Achilles tendon beyond neutral as normal daily activities will lengthen the tendon. There is continued focus on plantarflexion strengthening while minimizing dorsiflexion beyond neutral.

Standing heel raise progressions can be implemented, starting with bilateral heel raises and progressing toward unilateral heel raises (Fig. 12.2) as able. Closed kinetic chain calf strengthening exercises can begin with care placed to not dorsiflex beyond neutral (Fig. 12.3). Balance and proprioception therapeutic exercises are to be performed. General lower extremity strength training continues to be emphasized.

Weeks 12–16

Often, patients are unable to perform a single-leg heel raise until 4 months postinjury. Rehabilitation continues to focus on plantarflexion strengthening, with double-leg heel raises progressing to single-leg heel raises. Progressive gastrocnemius-soleus loading is performed to improve strength and enhance the mechanical and structural properties of the Achilles tendon. Gait training is performed to normalize gait mechanics. General lower extremity strengthening, endurance, and stability are performed to prepare the patient for a return to higher-level activities when able (Figs. 12.4, 12.5, and 12.6).

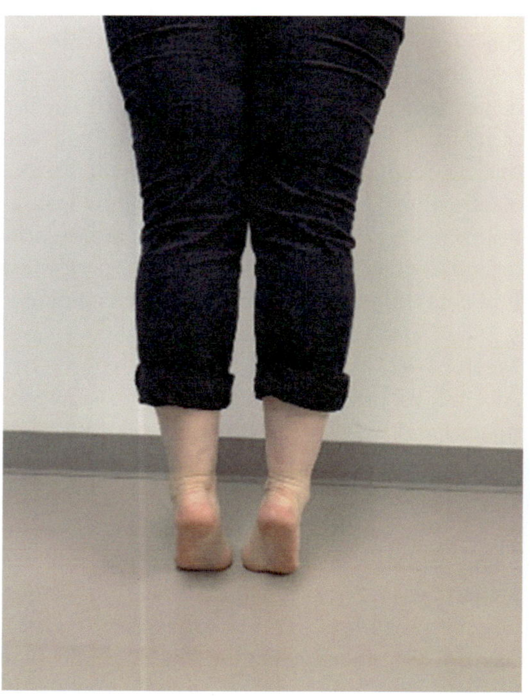

Fig. 12.1 Standing bilateral lower extremity heel raise

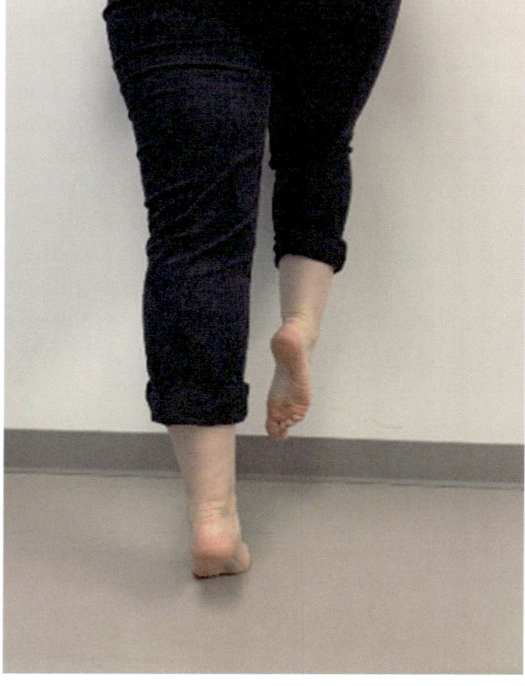

Fig. 12.2 Standing single lower extremity heel raise

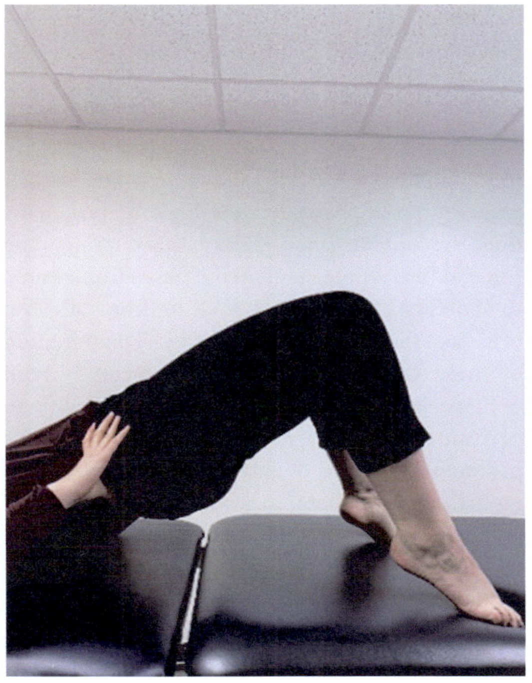

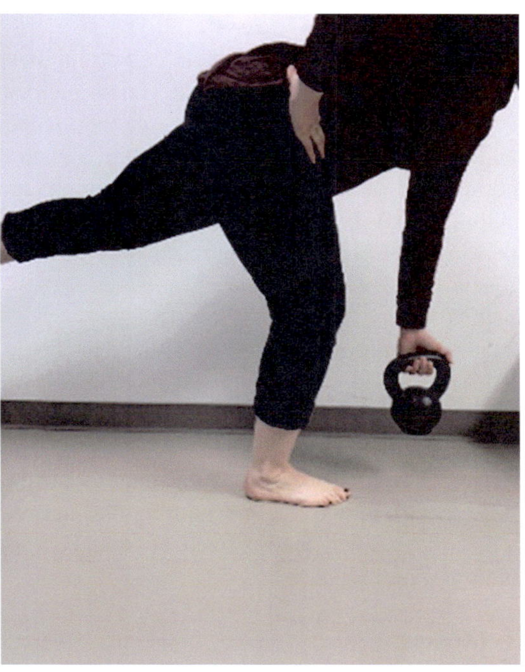

Fig. 12.3 Hook-lying bridge with heel raise to improve plantarflexion strength

Fig. 12.5 Single-leg deadlift to improve lower extremity stability and posterior chain strength

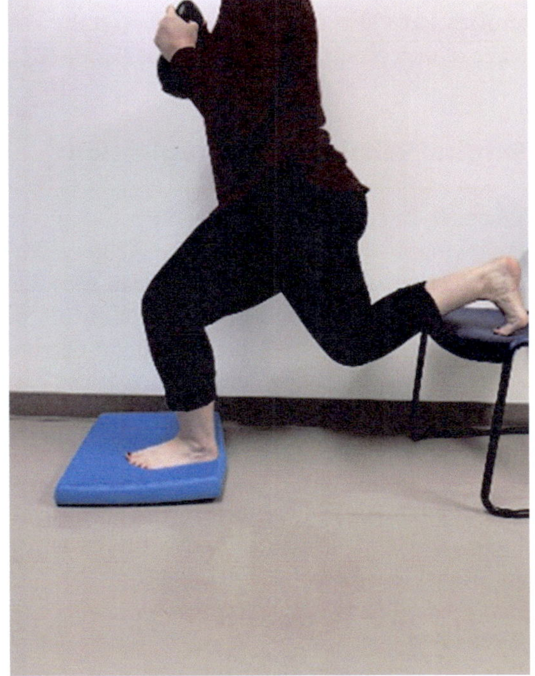

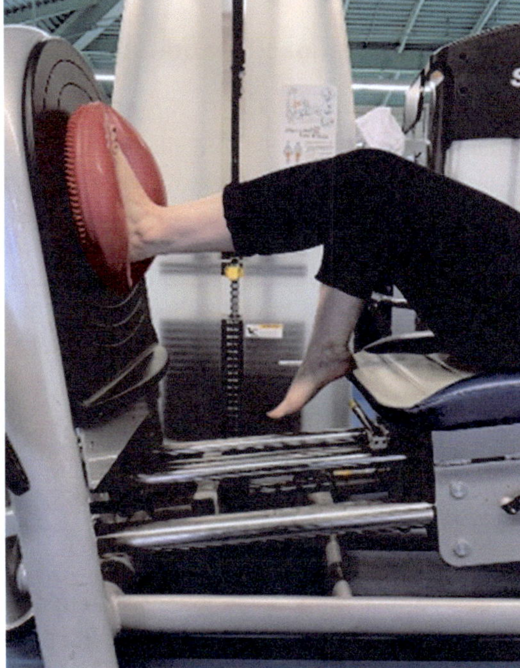

Fig. 12.4 Functional lower extremity exercise on a foam pad to improve dynamic stability and single-leg strength

Fig. 12.6 Unilateral leg press on uneven surface to improve dynamic stability and lower extremity strength

Weeks 16–24

There is continued emphasis on calf strengthening with various heel-raise combinations. Furthermore, lower extremity strengthening, endurance, and stability should remain a central component of the program. Light jogging and skipping may be initiated if patients are able to perform 25 consecutive heel raises.

6–9 Months

A gradual return to sports activities can begin, but it is advised to avoid contact sports and high-intensity activities such as sprinting, cutting, and jumping. There is continued emphasis on calf strengthening and balance. At 9 months postinjury, sprinting, cutting, and jumping are permitted if the patient has regained at least 80% of their noninjured leg.

9–12 Months

Return to sports that involve running and jumping if the patient has regained 100% strength.

The authors' suggested nonoperative rehabilitation protocol is summarized in Table 12.1.

Surgical Functional Rehabilitation

Immediate full weight-bearing leads to higher patient satisfaction, earlier ambulation, and earlier return to preinjury activity. There is also increased calf muscle strength, reduced calf muscle atrophy and tendon elongation, less severe adhesions, and less use of resources, including outpatient visits and physical therapy [23]. The recommended postsurgical rehabilitation is immediate full weight-bearing with the ankle fixed at 30° of plantarflexion with an orthosis. The range of motion begins at 3 weeks postsurgery with dorsiflexion to 0° and full plantarflexion. Plantarflexion is reduced by 10° each week from weeks 3 to 6 until a neutral position is achieved. At 7 weeks postsurgery, there is full weight-bearing without an orthosis, full free range of motion, and progressive strengthening [21, 23]. Heel-raising and heel-lowering strengthening exercises can improve the mechanical and structural properties of the tendon. Improving calf strength is imperative for positive functional outcomes and full return to preinjury activities. Progressive load to the Achilles tendon needs to be applied to improve tendon health. Heel raise and lowering progressions are basic staples in functional rehabilitation, and appropriate knowledge of progressive tendon loading principles must be implemented. Peak stress, strain, and force to the Achilles tendon increases from seated to standing heel raises as well as from bilateral heel raises to unilateral heel raises. The initiation of these exercises is often implemented about 6–8 weeks postoperatively [27]. The ability to perform a single-legged heel raise at 12 weeks postoperatively has demonstrated improved self-reported patient outcomes and physical activity levels [27]. Calf circumference that is equal to or less than 5 mm in the operative leg compared to the nonoperative leg, when measured 10 cm distal to the tibial tuberosity, can also be used as a metric for return to activity [28]. Peak Achilles tendon stresses have been observed in the early concentric phase of a heel raise as the gastrocnemius-soleus complex accelerates the body upward. Similar peak Achilles tendon stresses have also been observed during the late stage of the eccentric phase of heel lowering [27].

Surgical Rehabilitation Progression

Weeks 0–2

Following a surgical repair of the Achilles tendon, the best available evidence recommends that the patient be immobilized in a boot at 30° of plantarflexion. They will be full weight-bearing as this leads to higher patient satisfaction and earlier return to preinjury level [21, 23, 25, 26]. Rehabilitation can begin to focus on pain and swelling management. Rehabilitation can also begin with hip, quadriceps, and hamstring strengthening if tolerable. Active toe curls are performed to encourage circulation.

Weeks 3–6

The patient remains full weight-bearing within the boot. Continued focus on pain and swelling management is important during this phase.

Table 12.1 Functional rehabilitation protocol for Achille tendon ruptures managed nonoperatively

Time from surgery (week)	Weight-bearing	Immobilization	ROM	Strengthening/activity	Rehabilitation adjuncts
0–2	Non-weight-bearing	Immobilized in cast in maximal plantarflexion.	None	None at ankle; hip/knee exercises.	None.
2–4	Weeks 2–3: 25% WB Weeks 3–4: 50% WB	Achilles-specific walking boot with maximum plantarflexion heel lifts.	AROM/PROM PF and DF to neutral; inversion/eversion below neutral	Submaximal isometrics, excluding DF; seated heel raises.	Cryotherapy; electrical stimulation; blood flow restriction training; soft tissue massage; aquatic exercises; non-weight-bearing cardiovascular exercises.
4–6	Weeks 4–5: 75% WB Weeks 5–6: 100% WB	Achilles-specific walking boot with maximum plantarflexion heel lifts.	AROM/PROM PF and DF to neutral; inversion/eversion below neutral	Submaximal isometrics, excluding DF; seated heel raises; light resistance tubing for PF, inversion, and eversion.	Cryotherapy; electrical stimulation; blood flow restriction training; soft tissue massage; aquatic exercises; light weight-bearing cardiovascular exercises without extending the ankle beyond neutral.
6–8	WBAT	Begin removing heel lifts from boot—remove one lift daily as tolerated. Wean from boot at 8 weeks. Leave one to two lifts in regular shoe as needed.	AROM/PROM PF and DF to neutral; inversion/eversion below neutral	Gait training; graduated resistance exercises; progressive resistive tubing as tolerated; weight-resisted exercises: do not go past neutral; balance/proprioception.	Cryotherapy; electrical stimulation; blood flow restriction training; soft tissue massage; aquatic exercises; WBAT cardiovascular exercises without extending the ankle beyond neutral.
8–12	WBAT	Always wear shoes; minimize being barefoot/in socks.	AROM/PROM PF and DF to neutral; inversion/eversion below neutral	Continue to progress in strength, balance, and proprioception. Add standing double-heel raises and progress to single-heel raises when tolerated.	Cryotherapy; electrical stimulation; blood flow restriction training; soft tissue massage; aquatic exercises; add stationary bike, elliptical, and treadmill walking as tolerated.
12–16	WBAT	Normal shoe wear.	Full	Continue to progress in strength, balance, and proprioception. Avoid squats, lunges, etc. due to excessive stretch on the tendon.	Modalities, manual therapy as needed.
16–24	WBAT	Normal shoe wear.	Full	Increase dynamic weight-bearing exercises as tolerated. Initiate skipping and jogging if appropriate.	Modalities, manual therapy as needed.

(continued)

Table 12.1 (continued)

Time from surgery (week)	Weight-bearing	Immobilization	ROM	Strengthening/activity	Rehabilitation adjuncts
24–36	WBAT	Normal shoe wear.	Full	Return to normal sporting activities that do not involve cutting, sprinting, or jumping if the patient has regained 80% strength.	Modalities, manual therapy as needed.
36–52	WBAT	Normal shoe wear.	Full	Return to sports that involve running/jumping if the patient has regained 100% strength.	Modalities, manual therapy as needed.

WB weight-bearing, *WBAT* weight-bearing as tolerated, *ROM* range of motion, *AROM* active range of motion, *PROM* passive range of motion, *PF* plantarflexion, *DF* dorsiflexion

During this postoperative phase, the patient will reduce the plantarflexion angle by 10° each week until they achieve 0° of dorsiflexion. Active plantarflexion is initiated during this phase of rehabilitation. Passive dorsiflexion to 0° is also performed. Low-grade talocrural and calcaneal mobilizations can be performed to minimize stiffness secondary to the boot. Submaximal isometrics can be initiated in plantarflexion, dorsiflexion, inversion, and eversion and can then be progressed to seated heel raises and resistive tubing as tolerated (Fig. 12.7). Patients generally begin with three sets of ten repetitions, and the exercise volume is increased based on patient tolerance [28]. Towel scrunches for foot intrinsic musculature can also be performed (Fig. 12.8). Weight shifts and single-leg balance can be performed when they achieve 0° of dorsiflexion. When wounds are healed, aquatic therapy can be initiated as appropriate to continue to progress in rehabilitation. The stationary bike can be utilized in the boot with light resistance. Modalities for pain/swelling, soft tissue mobilization, and scar mobilization continue as needed.

Weeks 7–12

Weaning from the boot is initiated at the 7-week mark. Manual therapy for ankle mobilizations and full progressive ROM in all planes continue to be performed with the goal of full dorsiflexion ROM by 12 weeks postoperatively. Gait training can be performed on land with the use of supple-

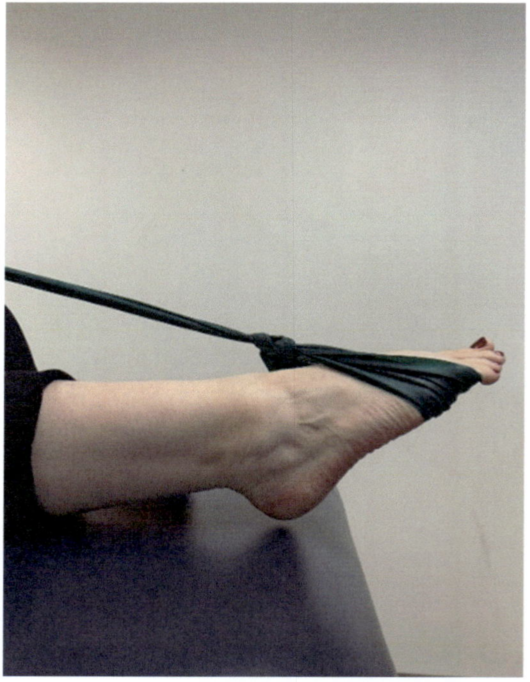

Fig. 12.7 Plantarflexion with resistance tubing

mental gait training equipment such as aquatic therapy and an antigravity treadmill such as the Alter-G® (AlterG, Inc., Fremont, CA, USA) to improve mechanics as needed. Progressive single-leg balance and proprioceptive therapeutic exercises are continued (Fig. 12.9). Continued focus on progressive calf and ankle strengthening with the goal of working toward standing bilat-

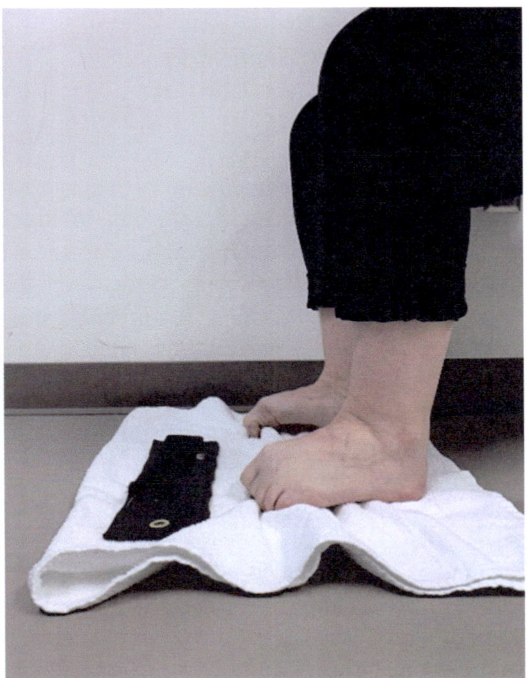

Fig. 12.8 Towel scrunches

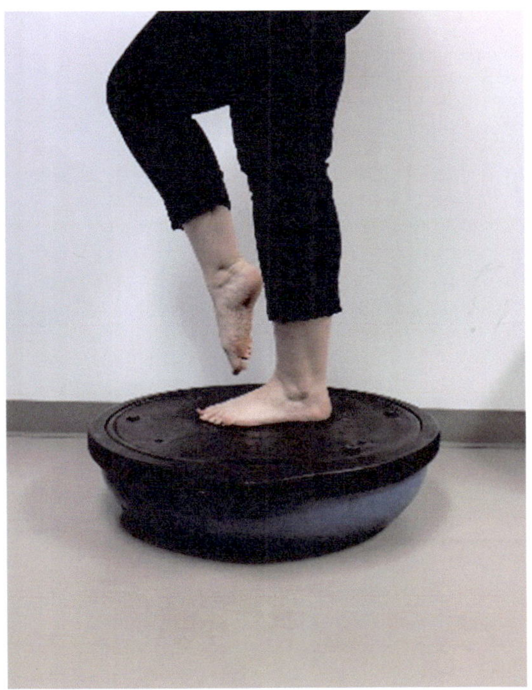

Fig. 12.9 Use of a balance tool to improve single-leg balance, stability, strength, and proprioception

eral heel raises and progressing toward single-leg calf raises as tolerated (Figs. 12.1 and 12.2). Patients generally begin with three sets of ten repetitions, and the exercise volume is increased based on patient tolerance. Volume can be progressed until multiple sets of 25 repetitions [28]. General lower extremity open kinetic chain and closed kinetic chain strengthening exercises are to be continued, with care being taken to not work beyond 0° of dorsiflexion to protect against early tendon elongation. Stationary bikes can be used with increased resistance. Aquatic therapy can continue as a supplemental rehabilitation tool for gait training, balance, strengthening, cardiovascular endurance, etc. Modalities for pain/swelling, soft tissue mobilization, and scar mobilization continue as needed.

Weeks 12–24

The patient should have full ROM in all planes. Manual therapy techniques can be continued to improve joint mobility and ROM as needed. Continued focus on single-leg calf strength emphasizing eccentric calf strength occurs in this phase. Further dynamic balance and stability are introduced (Fig. 12.10). General lower extremity strengthening is continued during this phase to prepare for a return to higher-level activities. A return-to-run program can be initiated at a minimum of 12 weeks postoperatively if the patient can perform 25 single-leg heel raises [24, 28]. Power, agility, and plyometric drills can be performed as needed. Sports-specific drills can begin during this phase, depending on sports demands.

Weeks 24+

The patient can return to sport during this phase of their rehabilitation. There is continued emphasis on single-leg calf strength and power production, as well as global lower extremity strength. Progressive agility, power, and plyometric drills continue to be performed. Further sports-specific exercises are performed. Return-to-sports testing can be performed if appropriate.

The authors' suggested rehabilitation protocol after surgical repair is summarized in Table 12.2.

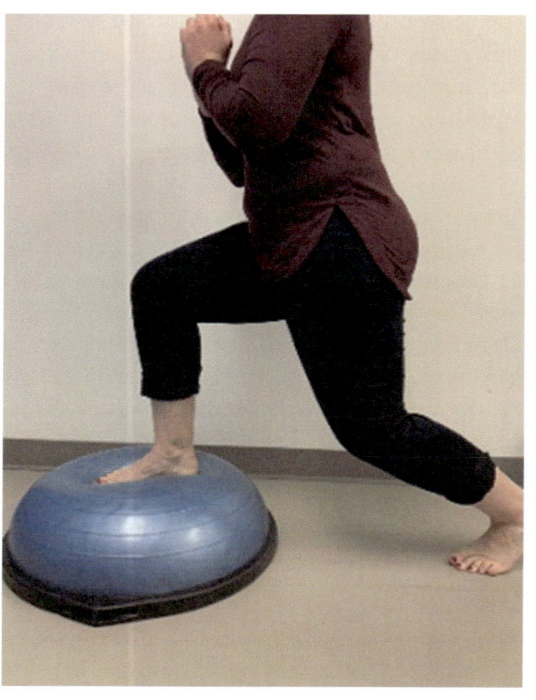

Fig. 12.10 Lunge onto an uneven surface, focusing on single-leg strength and stability

Key Differences Between Conservative and Operative Management Rehabilitation Protocols

While rehabilitation protocols for both conservative and surgical management after Achilles emphasize early functional weight-bearing and motion, notable differences exist between the two protocols (Table 12.3). Importantly, it is imperative for those undergoing nonoperative management to begin the rehabilitation process with immobilization in maximal plantarflexion as soon after injury as possible.

In terms of weight-bearing, the nonoperative protocol progresses through weight-bearing to reach full weight-bearing by 6 weeks after injury. On the other hand, postoperative patients are permitted full weight-bearing. Patients undergoing surgery begin weaning from the boot at week 6 postoperatively, while those who did not undergo surgery begin the transition out of heel lifts after week 6. Range of motion is permitted to full at

Table 12.2 Functional rehabilitation protocol after the surgical repair of an Achilles rupture

Time from surgery (week)	Weight-bearing	Immobilization	ROM	Strengthening/activity	Rehabilitation adjuncts
0–2	Full WB	Immobilized in cast, splint, or orthosis at 30° plantarflexion	None	Four-way hip exercises; hamstring curls; knee extensions; toe curls.	Cryotherapy; soft tissue mobilization
3–6	Full WB	Immobilized in splint/orthosis: weekly reduction in plantarflexion by 10° each week until foot is at 0°	Active mobilization of ankle from 0° dorsiflexion, with free AROM in plantarflexion	Isometrics: DF, PF, inversion, eversion; towel scrunches; resistance band exercises: PF, inversion, eversion—exclude DF; seated heel raises; weight shifts when 0° DF is achieved; maintain hip/glut strengthening.	Cryotherapy; soft tissue mobilization; scar mobilization/ massage; blood flow restriction training; stationary bicycle; aquatic therapy (when wounds are healed)
7–12	Full WB	No orthosis; wean from boot	Full progressive ROM in all planes	Single-leg balance/ proprioception; gait training; progressive calf/ ankle strengthening in all planes; maintain general LE CKC/OKC strength.	Cryotherapy; soft tissue mobilization; scar mobilization/ massage; stationary bicycle; blood flow restriction training; aquatic therapy; Alter-G® treadmill

Table 12.2 (continued)

Time from surgery (week)	Weight-bearing	Immobilization	ROM	Strengthening/activity	Rehabilitation adjuncts
12+	Full WB	None	Full	Eccentric calf strengthening; maintain general LE CKC/OKC strength; continue balance/dynamic stability.	Aquatic therapy; return-to-run progression; power; agility; plyometrics
24+	Full WB	None	Full	Continue calf/LE strengthening.	Return to sport

ROM range of motion, *DF* dorsiflexion, *PF* plantarflexion, *WB* weight-bearing, *LE* lower extremity, *CKC* closed kinetic chain, *OKC* open kinetic chain
Alter-G® (AlterG, Inc., Fremont, CA, USA)

Table 12.3 Key differences between conservative and operative management rehabilitation protocols

Domain	Conservative treatment	Surgical Achilles repair
Initiation of protocol	Ideally within 2–3 days of injury	Time to perform surgery ideally sooner than later, though with more leeway than nonoperative management
Weight-bearing	Progression through weight-bearing to weight-bearing as tolerated by week 6	Immediate weight-bearing permitted in plantarflexion immobilization
Immobilization	Longer immobilization in plantarflexion degrees	Wean out of boot at week 7
ROM	Full ROM permitted at week 12	Full ROM permitted at week 7
Strengthening/activity	Slower progressions through strengthening, balance, and functional activities	Quicker progressions through strengthening, balance, and functional activities
Rehabilitation adjuncts	No true limitations beyond weight-bearing, immobilization, and range of motion; less frequently used in the first 2 weeks	May be limited by wound healing and may emphasize scar massage and mobilization

ROM range of motion

week 7 for surgical patients but not allowed full for nonoperative patients until week 12. Furthermore, the progression in strengthening moves more rapidly for those who undergo surgery. On the other hand, because patients managed conservatively do not need to wait for surgical wound healing, the use of certain adjuncts, such as aquatic therapy, may be utilized earlier, while some of the rehabilitation adjuncts for postoperative patients will focus on scar massage and mobilization.

Outcomes for Rehabilitation Protocols

Rehabilitation protocols continue to be a topic of debate and study. As discussed previously, much literature has been dedicated to evaluating reha-

bilitation protocols in terms of the timing of weight-bearing and motion after open repairs or conservatively managed ruptures. Early functional rehabilitation protocols have lacked a standardized definition in the literature, but they are generally accepted to include weight-bearing and exercise-based motion within the first 2 weeks after Achilles rupture or repair, although even the exercises described have been inconsistent [15, 29]. However, randomized controlled trials and meta-analyses support the use of early functional rehabilitation over traditional prolonged immobilization [5, 6, 20, 30–33]. Many studies have demonstrated no differences in rerupture rates, functional outcomes, isokinetic strength, and patient-reported outcomes [31, 33], with some noting higher patient satisfaction with the early rehabilitative protocol [5, 20]. One randomized controlled trial evaluated the hypothesis that immobilization with permitted limited motion would limit tendon elongation [34]. Seventy-five patients undergoing Achilles repair were randomized into three groups: (1) no weight-bearing until week 7, (2) no weight-bearing until week 7 but allowed ankle joint mobilization exercises, and (3) partial weight-bearing until week 5, after which full weight-bearing began. There were no differences in groups in tendon elongation as measured on radiographs, muscle plantarflexion strength, or muscle size [34]. Ultimately, current data supports the safety of early functional mobilization and weight-bearing.

For those undergoing a surgical repair of the Achilles tendon, various surgical approaches have been used. In general, techniques may be classified as open versus percutaneous or minimally invasive techniques for repair. A number of studies have examined outcomes after open relative to minimally invasive approaches. No differences appear to exist based on the meta-analyses of trials comparing these techniques in terms of reruptures, return to activities, or range of motion [35, 36]. Furthermore, minimally invasive surgery has been associated with lower rates of postoperative wound infections and necrosis [36]. However, it is important to note that despite the use of minimally invasive surgery, the risks of wound healing and infection are still higher than those treated conservatively who do not have those same operative risks. In terms of rehabilitation, while many studies have evaluated open repairs, protocols after minimally invasive repair also have demonstrated success with immediate weight-bearing in functional braces with early mobilization [37, 38]. The randomized controlled trial by Groetelaers et al. divided 60 patients into either a cast immobilization group or a functional rehabilitation group for 6 weeks postoperatively [38]. The authors found no significant differences at 1 year between the functional rehabilitation group and the cast immobilization group in terms of Achilles Rupture Performance Scores (96% versus 83% scoring good or excellent, $P > 0.3$), strength (102% versus 96% relative to the uninjured leg, $P > 0.4$), quality of life scores on the Short Form-12 survey ($P > 0.05$), and complaints, including pain and stiffness ($P > 0.1$) [38].

Ultimately, early functional rehabilitation is safe and instrumental in recovery, regardless of the surgical technique.

In the revision surgical setting, additional concerns exist, including the attenuation of grafts that may be used to augment repair, poorer healing response, and additional scar formation. Limited data exist on the optimal protocols for revision surgery or for chronic Achilles ruptures.

Case Study

A 33-year-old male presents to the clinic 2 days after feeling a "pop" in his left ankle while playing basketball. The patient reports that he exercises minimally during the week but will often play basketball for 2 h on the weekends with his friends. After the popping sensation, he was unable to ambulate and return to play. He had initially presented to the emergency room where he was told that radiographs were normal. On physical examination, a palpable defect is noted in his left Achilles tendon proximal to the insertion on the calcaneus.

The ultrasound and MRI findings are demonstrated in Figs. 12.11 and 12.12.

The risks and benefits of surgical and nonoperative care were discussed, and the patient elected nonsurgical management. The patient was placed into a plantarflexed cast for 1 1/2 weeks. At that time, the patient was transitioned into a walking boot with heel lifts in a maximally plantarflexed position with progressive weight-bearing over time. By week 4, he was bearing full weight, and at week 6, the heel lifts were gradually removed to decrease his plantarflexion angle. He progressed through the remainder of the phys-

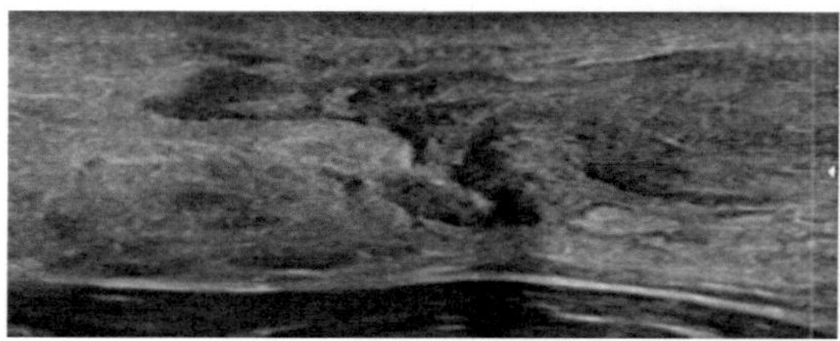

Fig. 12.11 Ultrasound findings demonstrating a midsubstance Achilles tendon rupture

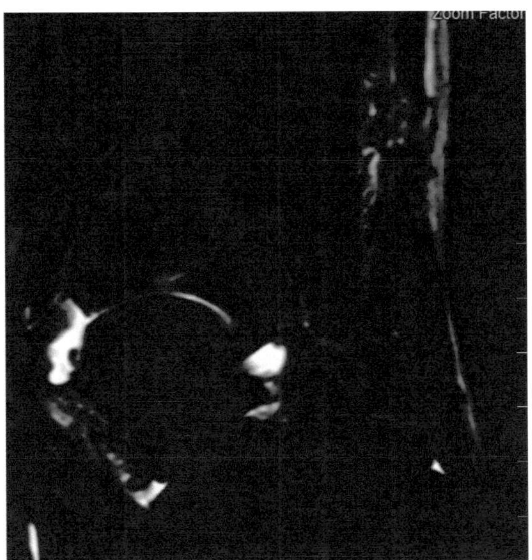

Fig. 12.12 Sagittal T2-weight magnetic resonance image demonstrating a midsubstance Achilles tendon rupture

ical therapy protocol, as described above. At approximately 11 months after the injury, the patient was permitted to return to sport, given the equivalent strength to his contralateral side. He was able to return to recreational basketball play without perceived consequences.

Conclusions

Rehabilitation protocols after Achilles tendon rupture managed conservatively or after repair are critical in progressing patients to return to appropriate function and activity. Early functional rehabilitation protocols with early weight-bearing and range of motion are safe and do not increase risks of rerupture. Furthermore, strength and patient-reported outcome measures tend to be similar between early functional protocols and prolonged immobilization, with some studies favoring patient satisfaction with early functional mobilization. Early functional rehabilitation has been proven beneficial in nonoperative settings in addition to operative repair, whether through open or minimally invasive techniques.

References

1. Gillies H, Chalmers J. The management of fresh ruptures of the Tendo Achillis. J Bone Joint Surg. 1970;52(2):337–43.
2. Keller J, Rasmussen TB. Closed treatment of Achilles tendon rupture. Acta Orthop Scand. 1984;55(5):548–50.
3. Maxwell LC, Enwemeka CS. Immobilization-induced muscle atrophy is not reversed by lengthening the muscle. Anat Rec. 1992;234(1):55–61.
4. Rantanen J, Hurme T, Kalimo H. Calf muscle atrophy and Achilles tendon healing following experimental tendon division and surgery in rats. Comparison of postoperative immobilization of the muscle-tendon complex in relaxed and tensioned positions. Scand J Med Sci Sports. 1999;9(1):57–61.
5. Suchak AA, Bostick GP, Beaupré LA, Durand DC, Jomha NM. The influence of early weight-bearing compared with non-weight-bearing after surgical repair of the Achilles tendon. J Bone Joint Surg Am. 2008;90(9):1876–83.
6. Khan RJK, Fick D, Keogh A, Crawford J, Brammar T, Parker M. Treatment of acute achilles tendon ruptures. A meta-analysis of randomized, controlled trials. J Bone Joint Surg Am. 2005;87(10):2202–10.
7. Barfod KW, Nielsen EG, Olsen BH, Vinicoff PG, Troelsen A, Holmich P. Risk of deep vein thrombosis after acute Achilles tendon rupture: a secondary analysis of a randomized controlled trial comparing early controlled motion of the ankle versus immobilization. Orthop J Sports Med. 2020;8(4):2325967120915900.
8. Matsumoto F, Trudel G, Uhthoff HK, Backman DS. Mechanical effects of immobilization on the Achilles' tendon. Arch Phys Med Rehabil. 2003;84(5):662–7.
9. Yamamoto E, Hayashi K, Yamamoto N. Mechanical properties of collagen fascicles from stress-shielded patellar tendons in the rabbit. Clin Biomech (Bristol, Avon). 1999;14(6):418–25.
10. Speck M, Klaue K. Early full weightbearing and functional treatment after surgical repair of acute achilles tendon rupture. Am J Sports Med. 1998;26(6):789–93.
11. Booth FW. Physiologic and biochemical effects of immobilization on muscle. Clin Orthop Relat Res. 1987;219:15–20.
12. Qin L, Appell HJ, Chan KM, Maffulli N. Electrical stimulation prevents immobilization atrophy in skeletal muscle of rabbits. Arch Phys Med Rehabil. 1997;78(5):512–7.
13. Bring D, Reno C, Renstrom P, Salo P, Hart D, Ackermann P. Prolonged immobilization compromises up-regulation of repair genes after tendon rupture in a rat model: immobilization post-injury impact mRNA levels. Scand J Med Sci Sports. 2009;20(3):411–7.
14. Willits K, Amendola A, Bryant D, Mohtadi NG, Giffin JR, Fowler P, Kean CO, Kirkley A. Operative versus nonoperative treatment of acute Achilles tendon rup-

tures: a multicenter randomized trial using accelerated functional rehabilitation. J Bone Joint Surg Am. 2010;92(17):2767–75.

15. Zellers JA, Christensen M, Kjær IL, Rathleff MS, Silbernagel KG. Defining components of early functional rehabilitation for acute Achilles tendon rupture: a systematic review. Orthop J Sports Med. 2019;7(11):232596711988407.

16. Zellers JA, Carmont MR, Grävare SK. Return to play post-Achilles tendon rupture: a systematic review and meta-analysis of rate and measures of return to play. Br J Sports Med. 2016;50(21):1325–32.

17. Twaddle BC, Poon P. Early motion for Achilles tendon ruptures: is surgery important? A randomized, prospective study. Am J Sports Med. 2007;35(12):2033–8.

18. Nilsson-Helander K, Silbernagel KG, Thomeé R, Faxén E, Olsson N, Eriksson BI, Karlsson J. Acute achilles tendon rupture: a randomized, controlled study comparing surgical and nonsurgical treatments using validated outcome measures. Am J Sports Med. 2010;38(11):2186–93.

19. Lawrence JE, Nasr P, Fountain DM, Berman L, Robinson AHN. Functional outcomes of conservatively managed acute ruptures of the Achilles tendon. Bone Joint J. 2017;99-B(1):87–93.

20. McCormack R, Bovard J. Early functional rehabilitation or cast immobilisation for the postoperative management of acute Achilles tendon rupture? A systematic review and meta-analysis of randomised controlled trials. Br J Sports Med. 2015;49(20):1329–35.

21. Kauwe M. Acute Achilles tendon rupture: clinical evaluation, conservative management, and early active rehabilitation. Clin Podiatr Med Surg. 2017;34(2):229–43.

22. Soroceanu A, Sidhwa F, Aarabi S, Kaufman A, Glazebrook M. Surgical versus nonsurgical treatment of acute Achilles tendon rupture: a meta-analysis of randomized trials. J Bone Joint Surg Am. 2012;94(23):2136–43.

23. Brumann M, Baumbach SF, Mutschler W, Polzer H. Accelerated rehabilitation following Achilles tendon repair after acute rupture—development of an evidence-based treatment protocol. Injury. 2014;45(11):1782–90.

24. Glazebrook M, Rubinger D. Functional rehabilitation for nonsurgical treatment of acute Achilles tendon rupture. Foot Ankle Clin. 2019;24(3):387–98.

25. Hutchison AM, Topliss C, Beard D, Evans RM, Williams P. The treatment of a rupture of the Achilles tendon using a dedicated management programme. Bone Joint J. 2015;97-B(4):510–5.

26. Barfod KW, Bencke J, Lauridsen HB, Ban I, Ebskov L, Troelsen A. Nonoperative dynamic treatment of acute achilles tendon rupture: the influence of early weight-bearing on clinical outcome: a blinded, randomized controlled trial. J Bone Joint Surg Am. 2014;96(18):1497–503.

27. Revak A, Diers K, Kernozek TW, Gheidi N, Olbrantz C. Achilles tendon loading during heel-raising and -lowering exercises. J Athl Train. 2017;52(2):89–96.

28. Saxena A, Ewen B, Maffulli N. Rehabilitation of the operated achilles tendon: parameters for predicting return to activity. J Foot Ankle Surg. 2011;50(1):37–40.

29. Christensen M, Zellers JA, Kjær IL, Silbernagel KG, Rathleff MS. Resistance exercises in early functional rehabilitation for Achilles tendon ruptures are poorly described: a scoping review. J Orthop Sports Phys Ther. 2020;23:1–41.

30. Zhao J-G, Meng X-H, Liu L, Zeng X-T, Kan S-L. Early functional rehabilitation versus traditional immobilization for surgical Achilles tendon repair after acute rupture: a systematic review of overlapping meta-analyses. Sci Rep. 2017;7(1):39871.

31. Lantto I, Heikkinen J, Flinkkila T, Ohtonen P, Siira P, Laine V, Leppilahti J. A prospective randomized trial comparing surgical and nonsurgical treatments of acute Achilles tendon ruptures. Am J Sports Med. 2016;44(9):2406–14.

32. Huang J, Wang C, Ma X, Wang X, Zhang C, Chen L. Rehabilitation regimen after surgical treatment of acute Achilles tendon ruptures: a systematic review with meta-analysis. Am J Sports Med. 2015;43(4):1008–16.

33. Mark-Christensen T, Troelsen A, Kallemose T, Barfod KW. Functional rehabilitation of patients with acute Achilles tendon rupture: a meta-analysis of current evidence. Knee Surg Sports Traumatol Arthrosc. 2016;24(6):1852–9.

34. Eliasson P, Agergaard A-S, Couppé C, Svensson R, Hoeffner R, Warming S, Warming N, Holm C, Jensen MH, Krogsgaard M, Kjaer M, Magnusson SP. The ruptured Achilles tendon elongates for 6 months after surgical repair regardless of early or late weightbearing in combination with ankle mobilization: a randomized clinical trial. Am J Sports Med. 2018;46(10):2492–502.

35. Grassi A, Amendola A, Samuelsson K, Svantesson E, Romagnoli M, Bondi A, Mosca M, Zaffagnini S. Minimally invasive versus open repair for acute Achilles tendon rupture: meta-analysis showing reduced complications, with similar outcomes, after minimally invasive surgery. J Bone Joint Surg Am. 2018;100(22):1969–81.

36. Gatz M, Driessen A, Eschweiler J, Tingart M, Migliorini F. Open versus minimally-invasive surgery for Achilles tendon rupture: a meta-analysis study. Arch Orthop Trauma Surg. 2020;

37. Braunstein M, Baumbach SF, Boecker W, Carmont MR, Polzer H. Development of an accelerated functional rehabilitation protocol following minimal invasive Achilles tendon repair. Knee Surg Sports Traumatol Arthrosc. 2018;26(3):846–53.

38. Groetelaers RPTGC, Janssen L, van der Velden J, Wieland AWJ, Amendt AGFM, Geelen PHJ, Janzing HMJ. Functional treatment or cast immobilization after minimally invasive repair of an acute Achilles tendon rupture: prospective, randomized trial. Foot Ankle Int. 2014;35(8):771–8.

Chronic Tendinopathy of the Achilles Tendon

Nonoperative Management of Insertional and Noninsertional Achilles Tendinopathy

Justin Paoloni and George A. C. Murrell

Anatomy

The soleus and gastrocnemius muscles combine in the calf to form the Achilles tendon, which inserts onto the posterior process of the calcaneus. The Achilles musculotendinous unit is the primary ankle plantar flexor. The Achilles tendon is the largest and strongest tendon in the body and is able to accept weight-bearing forces of ten times the body weight [1].

The Achilles tendon has a spiral configuration, internally rotating prior to inserting inferiorly onto the posterior calcaneus. The retrocalcaneal bursa lies anterior to the Achilles tendon, is located between the tendon and the calcaneus immediately proximal to its insertion, and provides lubrication for the tendon passing over the bone. The retro-Achilles bursa is posterior to the Achilles tendon at its insertion and functions to lubricate motion between the Achilles tendon and the overlying skin. In insertional Achilles tendinopathy, both the retrocalcaneal bursa and calcaneal tuberosity, and also the retro-Achilles bursa, are potentially involved in the pathologic process [2].

J. Paoloni (✉)
Premier Orthopaedics and Sports Medicine, Sydney, NSW, Australia

G. A. C. Murrell
Department of Orthopaedic Surgery, Orthopaedic Research Institute, University of New South Wales, St. George Hospital Campus, Sydney, NSW, Australia
e-mail: murrell.g@ori.org.au

Biomechanics

During the stance phase of walking, the ankle plantar flexor muscles are dominant, and large forces act on the Achilles. Running surfaces such as hills or cambers, changes in training intensity or mileage, and inadequate footwear are proposed causes of Achilles tendinopathy [3–5].

As the Achilles tendon inserts into the calcaneus, talocalcaneal (subtalar) motion causes tendon-shearing forces, and thus functional subtalar hyperpronation may be an etiologic factor in Achilles tendinopathy [6, 7]. Subtalar pronation causes tibial internal rotation, while knee extension causes tibial external rotation, and this tendon "whipping action" may compromise tendon vascularity and lead to collagen fiber degeneration.

Pathophysiology

Achilles tendinopathy is a degenerative tendinopathy [8, 9] that has an incidence in runners of 6.5–18% [1, 3, 5], and it is suggested that a combination of anatomic and biomechanical factors cause tendon substance degeneration [3–7, 10, 11].

In Achilles tendon injury, metabolic changes in the paratenon result in increased catabolism, decreased oxygenation, and the impairment of the paratenon gliding function [8, 9, 12]. The early paratenon injury probably leads to subsequent tendon substance degeneration and tendinopathy. Tendon substance degeneration may also occur as a result of tenocyte apoptosis due to repetitive loading [13].

Histopathologically, the features of degenerative tendinopathy include collagen fiber disorganization and disruption, mucoid degeneration, neovascularization, and an absence of inflammatory cells [8, 9, 14].

Animal tendon metabolism is relatively sluggish, as evidenced by its having only 13% of the oxygen uptake of muscle, and requires more than 100 days to synthesize structurally and biomechanically mature collagen [15]. Normally, it takes 12–16 weeks for the development of the collagen fibers with effective cross-bonding to provide a strong elastic scar [16]. This 3–4-month time frame of animal tendon healing has implications for treating human tendinopathy, and this may be the reason that tendinopathies, such as Achilles tendinopathy, have a tendency to chronicity.

Classification

Achilles tendinopathy is classified as insertional or noninsertional. Noninsertional tendinopathy is tendon substance degeneration in the relatively hypovascular region of the Achilles tendon that is 2–6 cm proximal to the calcaneal insertion [17]. Insertional tendinopathy involves the tendon–bone interface and may be associated with a prominent posterosuperior calcaneal tuberosity (Haglund's deformity) [2]. Haglund's deformity contributes to the development of insertional tendinopathy through mechanical abrasion and chemical erosion of the retrocalcaneal bursa and overlying tendon. The retro-Achilles bursa may also be involved in the pathologic process, often as a result of friction from footwear.

Clinical Features

The dominant symptom of Achilles tendinopathy is tendon pain. The location of the Achilles tendon pain and tenderness differentiates between

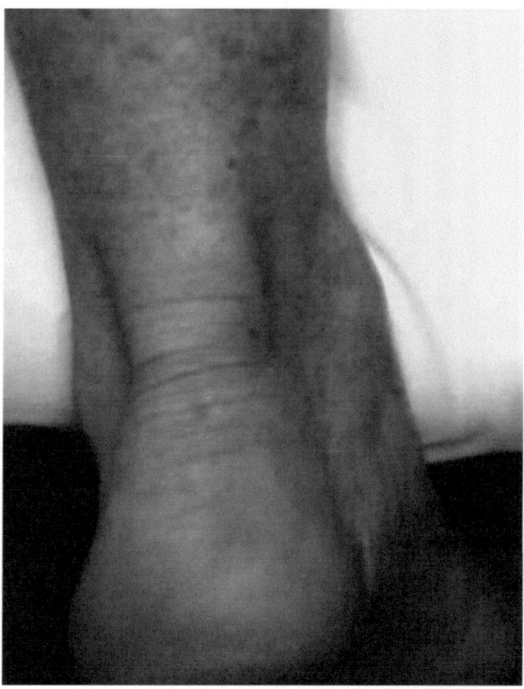

Fig. 13.1 The site of pain, swelling, and tenderness in noninsertional Achilles tendinopathy, commonly 2 to 6 cm from the Achilles tendon insertion

insertional and noninsertional Achilles tendinopathy. With noninsertional tendinopathy, pain, swelling, and tenderness are localized 2–6 cm proximal to the calcaneal insertion (Fig. 13.1), whereas in insertional tendinopathy, the site of pain and tenderness is localized to the tendon insertion onto the calcaneus. The pain is usually worse in the morning and may be associated with morning tendon stiffness, is initially reduced with exercising the tendon, and then may recur after exercise (see sect "Case Study", below). With disease progression, the pain may become constant, even during light exercise such as walking.

A clinical examination reveals localized tendon tenderness and often tendon thickening and crepitus on palpation. Achilles tenderness may be reduced by passive ankle dorsiflexion (London test). In insertional Achilles tendinopathy, an obvious retro-Achilles bursitis may be noted. Subtalar hyperpronation (Fig. 13.2) or pes planus may be present.

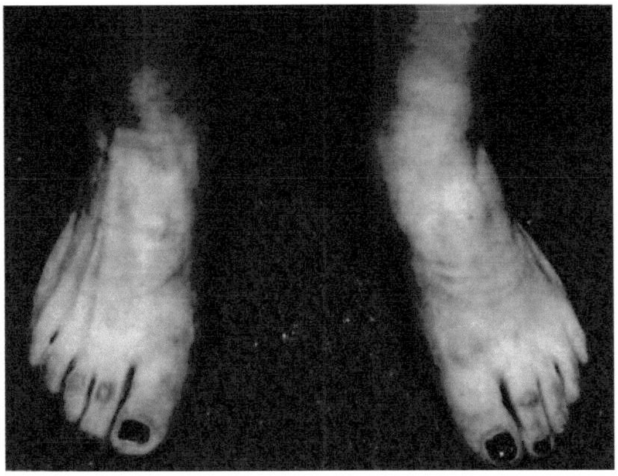

Fig. 13.2 Subtalar hyperpronation in the stance phase, most prominent in the left foot with some collapse of the medial longitudinal arch of the foot. Excessive subtalar hyperpronation may increase torsional forces on the Achilles tendon and its vasculature and contribute to the development of Achilles tendinopathy

Restricted ankle range of movement and clinical decreases in ankle plantarflexion strength are uncommon.

Case Study

A 42-year-old man presented with an insidious onset of 4 months of left posterior heel pain during and after running. Over the past 7 months, he had increased his running distance in an effort to lose weight and had progressed from running on a treadmill twice a week to road running four times a week. He said that he had morning pain and stiffness in the Achilles and Achilles tendon stiffness after inactivity.

On examination, it was noted that he had pes planus and subtalar hyperpronation while standing, and there was posterior heel pain with weight-bearing ankle inversion and eversion. Tenderness was present 3–5 cm proximal to the Achilles tendon insertion, and there was decreased tenderness in this region when the tendon was placed under passive stretch (London test).

The ankle X-ray was normal, but ultrasound demonstrated a fusiform thickening in the Achilles tendon with hypoechoic regions and collagen fiber disorganization and disruption.

Clinically and radiologically, the patient had noninsertional Achilles tendinopathy, and treatment included regular ice application, paracetamol/acetaminophen as required for pain, avoidance of aggravating activities in the short term, regular Achilles stretching, and an eccentric Achilles strengthening program. Other measures, such as foot control through supportive shoes and orthotics, were emphasized.

The patient presented 4 weeks later with moderate improvement in his Achilles pain, but he still had morning pain and stiffness as well as stiffness after inactivity. Walking was pain free. Tenderness persisted in the Achilles tendon on examination. Orthotics were prescribed, and he was directed to wear them and his supportive footwear at all times. He was encouraged to continue the stretching and exercise program, and 1.25-mg/24-h topical glyceryl trinitrate patches were commenced.

On review 4 weeks later, he had been compliant with all of his nonoperative treatment measures. The Achilles was virtually asymptomatic, except for mild morning stiffness. Mild Achilles tenderness persisted on examination. Again, he was encouraged to continue the exercise program, wear his supportive shoes and orthotics, and use the topical glyceryl trinitrate patches.

At a further review 4 weeks later, a total of 12 weeks after commencing therapy, he had been asymptomatic for the past 2–3 weeks. A graded return to running was implemented, which entailed gradually reintroducing running, having rest days from activity, and wearing supportive shoes when running. He was told to continue his stretches and exercises for a further 6–8 weeks.

At the 16-week review, he was asymptomatic and had returned to running 2–3 km three times a week without symptoms. He was advised to slowly increase his running and to continue maintenance stretching and exercise.

Investigations

Achilles tendinopathy is a clinical diagnosis. Weight-bearing ankle X-rays can be used to exclude bony pathology. Ultrasound (Fig. 13.3)

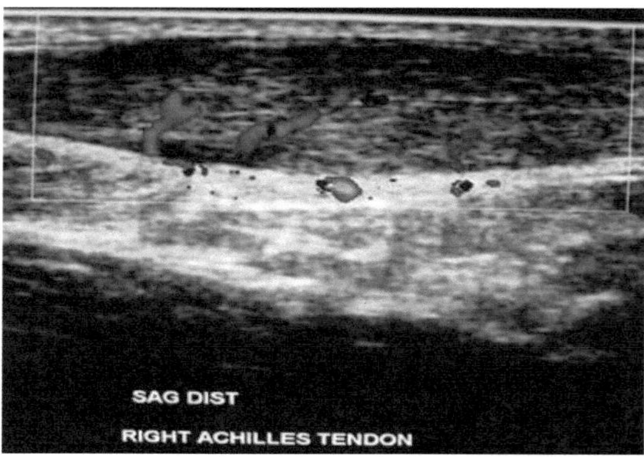

Fig. 13.3 Doppler ultrasound scan demonstrating noninsertional Achilles tendinopathy, with fusiform tendon thickening, hypoechoic regions, and increased tendon blood flow suggestive of neovascularization on Doppler mode

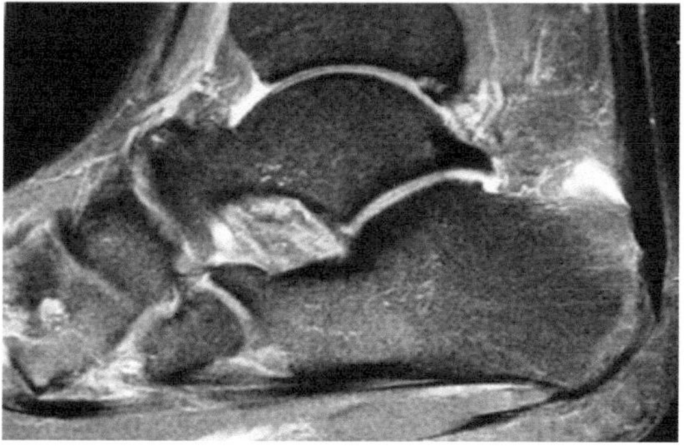

Fig. 13.4 Magnetic resonance imaging (MRI) demonstrating insertional Achilles tendinopathy with retrocalcaneal bursitis and Haglund's bony deformity of the posterior calcaneal process

and magnetic resonance imaging (MRI) (Fig. 13.4) demonstrate pathology but are generally unnecessary. There is a high incidence of asymptomatic Achilles tendon degeneration seen with both ultrasound and MRI scans that may confound the diagnosis [18–20].

Treatment

Exercise rehabilitation is the mainstay of treatment for Achilles tendinopathy [4, 10, 11, 21, 22]. There are many other suggested treatment approaches, but exercise rehabilitation has the best evidence of efficacy and should be at the core of any treatment program.

Resting from aggravating activities (relative rest or activity modification) is logical but lacks evidence of clinical efficacy. However, given that it is generally accepted that Achilles tendon degeneration results from overuse or overload and that the time frame for tendon healing is probably 3–4 months, it is reasonable to instruct the patient to avoid aggravating activities in the short term. If the patient is unable to rest or has severe pain, a plaster boot with a rocker-bottom sole is advocated for 6 weeks to enforce relative rest [4].

Analgesics may be required for the pain of Achilles tendinopathy, and initially, regular ice application should be encouraged as a simple measure for controlling tendon pain and swelling. Paracetamol/acetaminophen/Tylenol is as effective as nonsteroidal anti-inflammatory drugs (NSAIDs) for analgesia in soft tissue injury [23, 24], and NSAIDs have not demonstrated clinical efficacy in treating Achilles tendinopathy [25–27]. Thus, if analgesia is required in Achilles tendinopathy, paracetamol/acetaminophen is probably the best choice. In bursitis associated with insertional Achilles tendinopathy, NSAIDs may be appropriate for analgesia.

Heel lift devices reduce Achilles tendon plantarflexion stresses during walking [28] and are an inexpensive treatment modality. It is suggested that these 1.5-cm heel lifts be used bilaterally in all shoes [4]. Orthotic devices can control subtalar motion in patients with subtalar hyperpronation and have been advocated to reduce Achilles tendon stress during weight-bearing activities such as walking or running [4, 6, 7, 29–32].

Stretching the Achilles tendon restores tendon length and stimulates tendon healing along the lines of normal force loading [33, 34]. While stretching has limited evidence of clinical efficacy in treating Achilles tendinopathy, basic science research suggests that stretching assists in the restoration of the normal biomechanical properties of an injured tendon. Prolonged static stretching of both the gastrocnemius and soleus muscles (with straight knee and bent knee stretches, respectively) is therefore advocated as part of the treatment program.

Eccentric Achilles tendon exercises such as heel-drop exercises off a step (Fig. 13.5) decrease pain and hasten the return-to-normal activity in patients with chronic noninsertional Achilles tendinopathy when performed at high repetitions for 12 weeks (Alfredson protocol) [35]. Concentric heel raises to return to the neutral ankle position are not performed on the affected leg with this exercise regime as they decrease efficacy [36]. Eccentric exercise used in the treatment of insertional Achilles tendinopathy appears to be less effective [37], and early in the course of treatment, stretching or exercise may increase Achilles tendon pain. It may be advisable to avoid these activities in the initial stages of treating insertional Achilles tendinopathy and to concentrate on decreasing mechanical trauma to the tendon

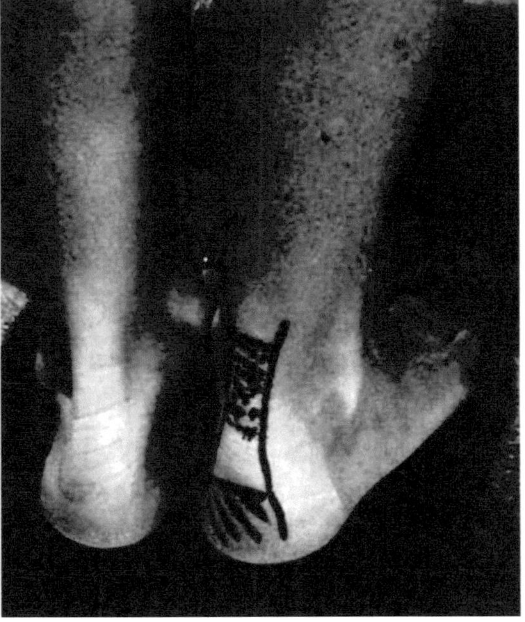

Fig. 13.5 Eccentric Achilles tendon strengthening exercises as per the Alfredson protocol. These exercises are often described as "heel-drop" exercises and are performed with the forefoot on the step and the hindfoot hanging off the edge of the step in order to lower the heel below the level of the step. This lowering of the heel causes Achilles tendon lengthening under load, and this eccentric exercise stimulates tendon healing. Note that there is no concentric component to the exercises

and inflammation, such as with concomitant bursitis [10, 24, 38].

Corticosteroid injections have a demonstrated lack of efficacy in Achilles tendinopathy and peritendinitis [39], have a risk of tendon rupture with intratendinous injection, and generally should not be used to treat noninsertional Achilles tendinopathy [40–42]. Corticosteroid injection may be used in insertional Achilles tendinopathy where concomitant bursitis is present and symptomatic [24, 41, 43].

Extracorporeal shock wave therapy (ESWT) has shown efficacy in treating recalcitrant insertional Achilles tendinopathy [44] and recently has shown treatment benefits in treating noninsertional Achilles tendinopathy that are similar to those of eccentric exercise [45]. Currently, ESWT is probably best reserved for treating recalcitrant Achilles tendinopathy.

Continuous topical glyceryl trinitrate treatment at a dosage of 1.25 mg/24 h has demonstrated efficacy in improving asymptomatic patient outcomes in chronic noninsertional Achilles tendinopathy when combined with exercise rehabilitation [46], and these effects persist at the 3-year follow-up [47](Fig. 13.6). This therapy is best used in chronic noninsertional Achilles tendinopathy if the initial treatment is ineffective, and it should be recognized that this drug has not been approved for this purpose by the Food and Drug Administration (FDA) at the time of publication. Side effects include headache and rash in 5–10% of patients. The efficacy in treating insertional Achilles tendinopathy is not established.

Aprotinin, a metalloprotease and collagenase inhibitor, has limited evidence of efficacy in decreasing tendon pain and improving functional outcomes in Achilles tendinopathy [48], with recent research suggesting it is no more effective than a placebo [49].

The most common side effect is a mild allergic reaction in 3% of patients, although anaphylactic reactions can occur. Aprotinin injections are probably best reserved for recalcitrant tendinopathy due to the risk of anaphylaxis, and it should be recognized that this drug had not been approved for this purpose by the FDA at the time of publication.

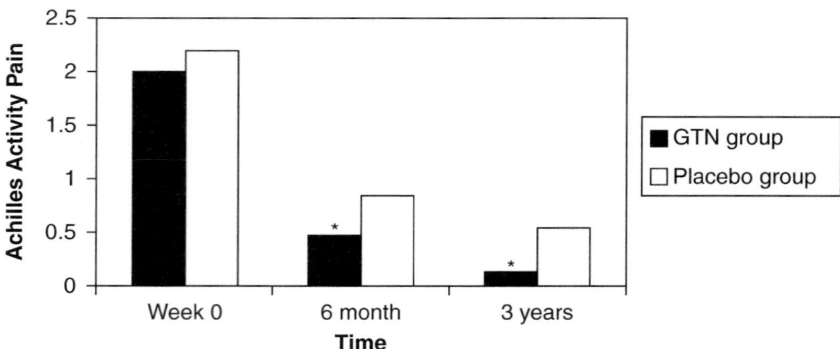

Fig. 13.6 Graph illustrating the effects of continuous topical glyceryl trinitrate (GTN) treatment on Achilles tendon pain with activity in patients with chronic noninsertional Achilles tendinopathy. Significant differences at the $p < 0.05$ level are denoted by an asterisk

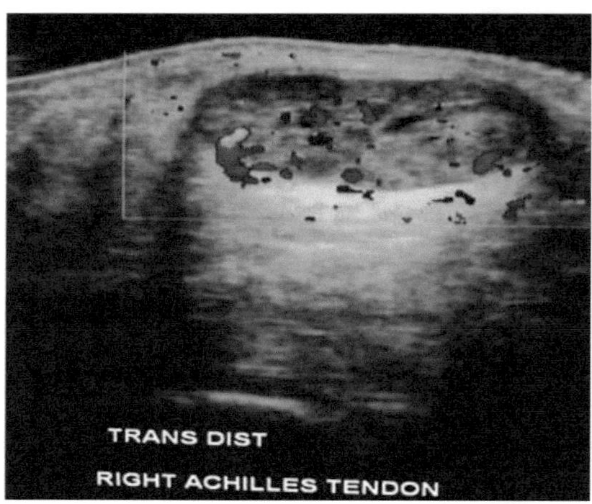

Fig. 13.7 Cross-sectional view of the Achilles tendon with Doppler ultrasound demonstrating increased blood flow within the tendon substance, suggestive of neovascularization in tendinopathy. Note that the majority of increased blood flow is in the deep aspect of the tendon. This neovascularization can be obliterated using polidocanol sclerosant injections, similar to the process of treating varicose veins, and provides 80% pain reduction in 80% of people over 4–6 months.</FL>

Doppler ultrasound-guided polidocanol injections, a sclerosant agent used to obliterate regions of neovascularization in tendinopathy (Fig. 13.7), has evidence of efficacy in decreasing pain and improving patient outcomes in Achilles tendinopathy [50, 51], and this effect persists at 2-year follow-up [52]. This therapy has no side effects, but it is relatively new, and therefore availability is currently limited to specialized centers.

Another treatment that has been advocated for use in musculoskeletal injury such as Achilles tendinopathy is prolotherapy—the use of proliferative agents such as high-strength glucose—although there is no evidence of its efficacy in treating any tendon injury [53, 54]. The use of prolotherapy in Achilles tendinopathy would generally be considered a last resort.

With any tendinopathy, including Achilles tendinopathy, failure of symptom resolution within 6–12 months of nonoperative treatment may indicate the necessity for surgical intervention. The presence of unacceptable pain or disability from the patient's perspective should prompt an orthopedic surgical referral.

Return to Sports

In Achilles tendinopathy, return to full sports activity is variable but may take as long as 6–12 months. Cross-training to maintain fitness and to control body weight should be encouraged and will generally involve pain-free, non-weight-bearing activities such as cycling, swimming, or rowing. Once the patient is asymptomatic with daily activities such as walking, then a graded return to more vigorous weight-bearing activities, such as walking for exercise or running, may be instituted. This return to heavy weight-bearing activity should always be performed gradually with an emphasis on wearing supportive footwear to control excessive foot motion, ensuring rest days to allow for tendon adaptation to increased stress, and monitoring Achilles symptoms to prevent overload and injury recurrence.

Prognosis

One of the few studies of the natural course of Achilles tendinopathy was an 8-year follow-up study to determine the long-term outcome of patients initially treated nonoperatively for acute or subacute Achilles tendinopathy [54]. This study demonstrated that the long-term prognosis of patients with Achilles tendinopathy was generally good, with 94% of people being asymptomatic or experiencing only mild Achilles tendon pain on strenuous exercise and 84% of people returning to full levels of physical activity. Despite these encouraging outcomes, there was a clear side-to-side difference between the involved and the uninvolved Achilles tendon in the performance tests, clinical examination, and ultrasonography, and 29% of patients with Achilles tendinopathy failed to respond to nonoperative treatment and required surgical treatment.

References

1. Clain M, Baxter DE. Achilles tendinitis. Foot Ankle Int. 1992;13(8):482–7.
2. Merkel K, Hess H, Kunz M. Insertional tendinopathy in athletes: a light microscope, histochemical and electron microscope examination. Pathol Res Pract. 1982;173:303–9.
3. Clement D, Taunton JE, Smart GW. A survey of overuse running injuries. Phys Sports Med. 1981;9(5):47–58.
4. Brukner P, Khan K. Clinical sports medicine. 3rd ed. Sydney: Blackwell Scientific; 2005.
5. Krissoff W, Ferris WD. Runner's injuries. Phys Sports Med. 1979;7(12):55–64.
6. Burdett R. Forces predicted at the ankle during running. Med Sci Sports. 1982;14:308–16.
7. Scott S, Winter DA. Internal forces at chronic running injury sites. Med Sci Sports Exerc. 1990;22(3):357–69.
8. Khan K, Cook JL, Bonar F, et al. Histopathology of common tendinopathies. Sports Med. 1999;27(6):393–408.
9. Astrom M, Rausing A. Chronic Achilles tendinopathy: a survey of surgical and histopathological findings. Clin Orthop. 1995;316:151–64.
10. Alfredson R, Lorentzon H. Chronic Achilles tendinosis. Recommendations for treatment and prevention. Sports Med. 2000;29(2):135–46.
11. Renstrom AFH. An introduction to chronic overuse injuries. In: Harris M, Williams C, Stanish WD, et al., editors. Oxford textbook of sports medicine. New York: Oxford University Press; 1994. p. 531–45.
12. Kvist M, Jozsa L, Jarvinen M. Chronic Achilles paratenonitis in athletes: a histological and histochemical study. Pathology. 1987;19:1–11.
13. Arnoczky S, Tian T, Lavagnino M, et al. Activation of stress-activated protein kinases (SAPK) in tendon cells following cyclic strain: the effects of strain frequency, strain magnitude, and cytosolic calcium. J Orthop Res. 2002;20:947–52.
14. Puddu G, Ippolito E, Postacchini F. A classification of Achilles tendon disease. Am J Sports Med. 1976;4:145–50.
15. Murrell G, Jang D, Deng XH, et al. Effects of exercise on Achilles tendon healing in a rat model. Foot Ankle Int. 1998;19(9):598–603.
16. Vailas A, Tipton CM, Laughlin HL, et al. Physical activity and hypophysectomy on the aerobic capacity of ligaments and tendons. J Appl Physiol. 1978;44(4):542–6.
17. Lagergen C. Vascular distribution in Achilles tendon—an angiographic and microangiographic study. Acta Chir Scand. 1958;116:491–5.
18. Harris CA, Peduto AJ. Achilles tendon imaging. Australas Radiol. 2006;50(6):513–25.
19. Cook JL, Khan KM, Purdam C. Achilles tendinopathy. Manual Ther. 2002;7(3):121–30.
20. Kainberger F, Mittermaier F, Seidl G, et al. Imaging of tendons-adaptation, degeneration, rupture. Eur J Radiol. 1997;25(3):209–22.
21. Werd MB. Achilles tendon sports injuries: a review of classification and treatment. J Am Podiatr Med Assoc. 2007;97(1):37–48.
22. McLauchlan GJ, Handoll HH. Interventions for treating acute and chronic Achilles tendinitis. Cochrane Database Syst Rev. 2001;(2):CD000232.
23. DeGara C, Taylor M, Hedges A. Assessment of analgesic drugs in soft tissue injuries presenting to an accident and emergency department—a comparison of antrafenine, paracetamol, and placebo. Postgrad Med J. 1982;58:489–92.
24. Paoloni JA, Orchard J. The use of therapeutic medications in soft tissue injuries. Med J Aust. 2005;183(7):384–8.
25. McLauchlan G, Handoll HHG. Interventions for treating acute and chronic Achilles tendinitis. Cochrane Database Syst Rev. 2004;2:4.
26. Astrom M, Westlin N. No effect of piroxicam on Achilles tendinopathy. A randomized study of 70 patients. Acta Orthop Scand. 1992;63(6):631–4.
27. Auclair J, Georges M, Grapton X, et al. A double-blind controlled multicenter study of percutaneous niflumic acid gel and placebo in the treatment of Achilles heel tendinitis. Curr Ther Res Clin Exp. 1989;46(4):782–8.
28. Akizuki KH, Gartman EJ, Nisonson B, et al. The relative stress on the Achilles tendon during ambulation in an ankle immobiliser: implications for rehabilitation after Achilles tendon repair. Br J Sports Med. 2001;35(5):329.

29. Wilson JJ, Best TM. Common overuse tendon problems: a review and recommendations for treatment. Am Fam Phys. 2005;72(5):811–8.
30. Wallace RG, Traynor IE, Kernohan WG, et al. Combined conservative and orthotic management of acute ruptures of the Achilles tendon. J Bone Joint Surg. 2004;86(6):1198–202.
31. Mazzone MF, McCue T. Common conditions of the Achilles tendon. Am Fam Phys. 2002;65(9):1805–10.
32. Sobel E, Levitz SJ, Caselli MA. Orthoses in the treatment of rear foot problems. J Am Podiatr Med Assoc. 1999;89(5):220–33.
33. Iwuagwu F, McGrouther DA. Early cellular response in tendon injury: the effect of loading. Plast Recon Surg. 1998;102(6):2064–71.
34. Kvist M, Jarvinen M. Clinical, histochemical and biomechanical features in repair of muscle and tendon injuries. Int J Sports Med. 1982;3:12–4.
35. Alfredson H, Pietila T, Jonsson P, et al. Heavy-load eccentric calf muscle training for the treatment of chronic Achilles tendinosis. Am J Sports Med. 1998;26(3):360–6.
36. Niesen-Vertommen S, Taunton JE, Clement DB. The effect of eccentric versus concentric exercise in the management of Achilles tendonitis. Clin J Sports Med. 1992;2:109–13.
37. Fahlstrom M, Jonsson P, Lorentzon R, et al. Chronic Achilles tendon pain treated with eccentric calf-muscle training. Knee Surg Sports Traumatol Arth. 2003;11(5):327–33.
38. Krishna Sayana M, Maffulli N. Insertional Achilles tendinopathy. Foot Ankle Clin. 2005;10(2):309–20.
39. DaCruz DJ, Geeson M, Allen MJ, et al. Achilles paratendonitis: an evaluation of steroid injection. Br J Sports Med. 1988;22(2):64–5.
40. Kennedy J, Willis RB. The effects of local steroid injections on tendons: a biomechanical and microscopic correlative study. Am J Sports Med. 1976;4:11–21.
41. Hayes DW Jr, Gilbertson EK, Mandracchia VJ, et al. Tendon pathology in the foot. The use of corticosteroid injection therapy. Clin Podiatr Med Surg. 2000;17(4):723–35.
42. Shrier I, Matheson GO, Kohl HW. Achilles tendonitis: are corticosteroid injections useful or harmful? Clin J Sport Med. 1996;6(4):245–50.3rd.
43. Speed CA. Fortnightly review: corticosteroid injections in tendon lesions. Br Med J. 2001;323(7309):382–6.
44. Furia JP. High-energy extracorporeal shock wave therapy as a treatment for insertional Achilles tendinopathy. Am J Sports Med. 2006;34(5):733–40.
45. Rompe JD, Nafe B, Furia JP, et al. Eccentric loading, shock-wave treatment, or a wait-and-see policy for tendinopathy of the main body of tendo Achillis: a randomized controlled trial. Am J Sports Med. 2007;35(3):374–83.
46. Paoloni JA, Appleyard RC, Nelson J, et al. Topical glyceryl trinitrate application in the treatment of non-insertional Achilles tendinopathy: a randomized, double-blind, placebo controlled clinical trial. J Bone Joint Surg. 2004;86A(5):916–22.
47. Paoloni J, Murrell GAC. Three-year prospective comparison study of topical glyceryl trinitrate treatment in chronic noninsertional Achilles tendinopathy. Foot Ankle Int. 2007;28:1064–8.
48. Capasso G, Maffulli N, Testa V. Preliminary results with peritendinous protease inhibitor injections in the management of Achilles tendinitis. J Sports Traumatol Rel Res. 1993;15:37–40.
49. Brown R, Orchard J, Kinchington M, et al. Aprotinin in the management of Achilles tendinopathy: a randomised controlled trial. Br J Sports Med. 2006;40(3):275–9.
50. Alfredson H, Ohberg L. Sclerosing injections to areas of neo-vascularisation reduce pain in chronic Achilles tendinopathy: a double-blind randomised controlled trial. Knee Surg Sports Traumatol Arth. 2005;13(4):338–44e.
51. Alfredson H, Lorentzon R. Sclerosing polidocanol injections of small vessels to treat the chronic painful tendon. Cardiovasc Hematol Agents Med Chem. 2007;5(2):97–100.
52. Lind B, Ohberg L, Alfredson H. Sclerosing polidocanol injections in mid-portion Achilles tendinosis: remaining good clinical results and decreased tendon thickness at 2–year follow-up. Knee Surg Sports Traumatol Arth. 2006;14(12):1327–32.
53. Rabago D, Best TM, Beamsley M, et al. A systematic review of prolotherapy for chronic musculoskeletal pain. Clin J Sport Med. 2005;15(5):376–80.
54. Paavola M, Kannus P, Paakkala T, et al. Long-term prognosis of patients with Achilles tendinopathy: an observational 8-year follow-up study. Am J Sports Med. 2000;28(5):634–42.

Tendoscopy of Noninsertional Achilles Tendinopathy

14

Christopher C. Cychosz and Phinit Phisitkul

Introduction

Noninsertional Achilles tendinopathy, or midportion tendinopathy, is an overuse injury resulting in pain and swelling located approximately 2–7 cm proximal to the insertion of the Achilles tendon on the calcaneus [1]. Conservative treatment modalities such as eccentric strengthening, activity modification, extracorporeal shock wave therapy (ECSWT), platelet-rich plasma (PRP) injections, and orthoses are often the first-line treatment options; however, up to one quarter of patients ultimately fail conservative management and go on to require surgery [2].

The etiology of pain associated with this condition remains poorly understood. Some studies have suggested that the occurrence of neovascularization in the areas of tendon degenerative changes may be associated with the pain experienced in patients with chronic noninsertional Achilles tendinopathy [3]. It has also been hypothesized that vascular ingrowth is also accompanied by the ingrowth of nerve endings, which may also be responsible for the generation of pain [4]. However, it is still not clear which is the predominant factor in symptoms associated with chronic tendinopathy. Recent studies have shown a relationship between gastrocnemius contracture and Achilles tendinopathy indicated by good outcomes after gastrocnemius recessions.

Traditionally, surgical procedures involving the Achilles tendon were performed through an open approach. However, more recently, less invasive procedures have been gaining popularity, given the high complication rate associated with incisions in this area, including skin necrosis, superficial or deep infections, hematoma, scarring, and sural nerve injury [5, 6]. While the first description of tendoscopy in the literature was by Wertheimer et al. in a 1995 case report to treat tenosynovitis of the tibialis posterior, it was not until 2 years later, in 1997, that Achilles tendoscopy was described in a series by van Dijk [7, 8]. Since that time, tendoscopy of the Achilles tendon has been proposed to serve a variety of diagnostic and therapeutic indications, such as assisting with percutaneous Achilles tendon repairs, Haglund excision, retrocalcaneal bursitis, tendinopathy, and paratendinopathy [9]. In this chapter, we will focus on the use of tendoscopy for the treatment of noninsertional Achilles tendinopathy.

C. C. Cychosz (✉)
Department of Orthopaedics and Rehabilitation, University of Iowa, Iowa City, IA, USA
e-mail: christopher-cychosz@uiowa.edu

P. Phisitkul
Department of Orthopaedics, Tri-State Specialists, LLP, Sioux City, IA, USA

Principles of Tendoscopy

Tendoscopy is typically performed while using fluid irrigation (e.g., normal saline) to aid in the distention of the tendon sheath as well as to decrease visual interference from bleeding. However, dry tendoscopy can be used in certain circumstances using a slotted cannula with the scope for procedures such as gastrocnemius recession [10]. In our experience, low-pressure flow up to 40 mmHg or gravity flow is enough to provide adequate insufflation of the area of interest while minimizing fluid extravasation from the surgical site.

The advancement of endoscopic instrumentation, including a smaller camera size, has been crucial to tendoscopic technique development. Typically for larger tendons such as the Achilles and proximal flexor hallucis longus (FHL), a 4 mm, 30-degree camera is best suited for most indications. Sometimes a smaller 2.7 mm, 30-degree camera may be used as well; however, this is often better suited for smaller structures such as the distal FHL and other tendons of the foot and ankle besides the Achilles. We recommend using the largest camera that can comfortably fit in the tendon sheath or peritendinous space.

Portal placement is typically in line with the tendon guided by direct palpation. It is helpful to keep at least 1 cm of soft tissue between the skin incision and tendon pathology if possible to prevent the camera from dislodging. An endoscopic trocar or a hemostat is frequently used in cases where adhesions are present to aid in stripping the tendon from surrounding scar tissue prior to camera insertion. Furthermore, the camera is often helpful as a retractor if strategically placed while performing the tendoscopy. Familiarity with the use of percutaneous incisions for minimally invasive longitudinal tenotomies can help address cases with extreme tendon enlargement or cystic changes. Of course, the surgeon should always anticipate the possibility of needing to convert to an open approach if needed.

Indications

Patients with noninsertional Achilles tendinopathy may be noted to have diffuse thickening of the tendon, local degenerative changes within the tendon but structurally intact, or tendon insufficiency with partial rupture [11]. Those with chronic paratendinopathy may complain of pain along the medial aspect of the tendon, and only the paratenon will be involved upon magnetic resonance imaging (MRI) [12]. The soleus and plantaris tendons are separated by the paratenon medially, and the plantaris tendon is allowed to glide freely in relation to the Achilles in unaffected patients. However, in those with paratendinopathy, adhesions may develop between the Achilles and plantaris, causing them to become fixed [13].

Achilles tendoscopy has been described in the literature as being used in the evaluation or treatment of central tendinopathy or tendinosis, paratendinopathy or tendinosis, chronic partial tears of the Achilles tendon through lysis of adhesions, excision of degenerative tissues/scar tissue, and excision of the plantaris tendon and also to guide percutaneous tenotomy to stimulate a healing response.

Surgical Technique

The patient is placed in a prone position with a pneumatic tourniquet over the thigh. A bump may be placed under the hip to keep the operative limb in neutral rotation. It is important that the patient be placed distal enough on the table to allow the surgeon to manipulate the ankle into full dorsiflexion and plantarflexion throughout the procedure.

The area of tendon enlargement is palpated, and a proximal medial portal is created approximately 2 cm proximal to this area, while the distal lateral portal is created 2 cm distally and 1 cm anterior to the lateral margin of the Achilles (Fig. 14.1). A hemostat is inserted through each

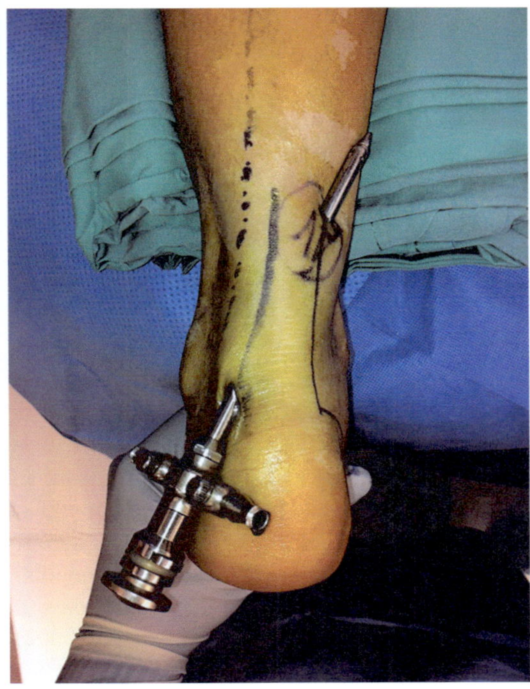

Fig. 14.1 Left leg is positioned over a bump in a prone position. Arthroscopic cannula is inserted from the distal lateral portal through the proximal medial portal

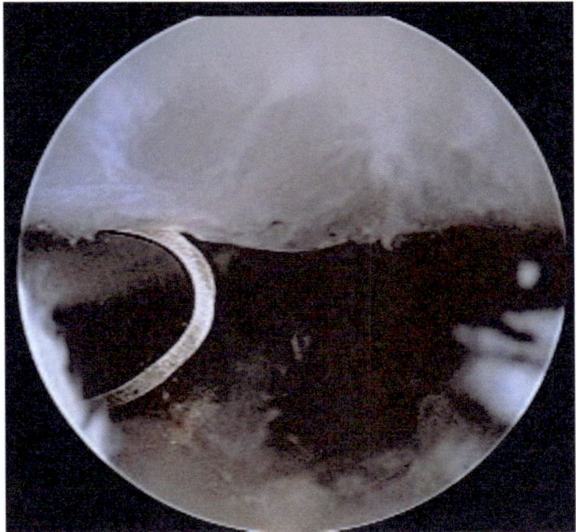

Fig. 14.2 With the camera inserted from the distal lateral portal, the debridement of adhesion ventral to the Achilles tendon is performed using a 4.5 mm shaver from the proximal medial portal

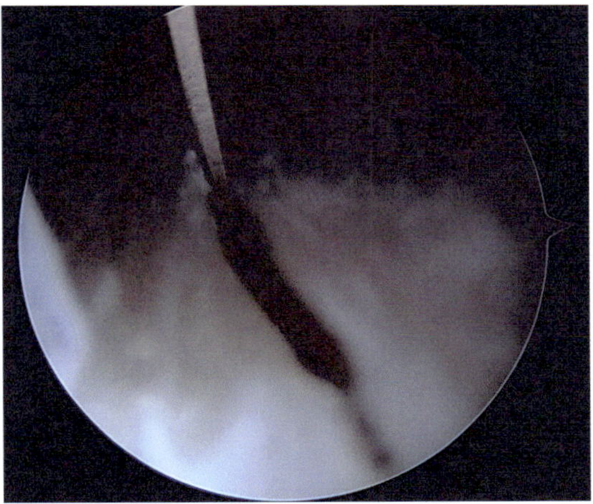

Fig. 14.3 Longitudinal tenotomy of the Achilles tendon is performed percutaneously under arthroscopic guidance

portal to create a space around the Achilles tendon using a "nick and spread" technique. Care must be taken to avoid injuring the sural nerve. Significant adhesions are frequently encountered, especially anteriorly. Next, a 4 mm, 30-degree camera is inserted into the distal medial portal along the anterior aspect of the tendon. A 4.5 mm shaver is introduced from the other portal for debridement of scar tissue or adhesions (Fig. 14.2). Pressure over the Achilles tendon toward the arthroscopic shaving device may be useful to facilitate debridement of the anterior surface of the tendon [14]. Longitudinal tenotomies of the ventral tendon surface may be performed using a retrograde knife or number 11 scalpel percutaneously under direct visualization if significant intratendinous lesions are noted (Fig. 14.3). If mass occupying lesions are present, such as ganglion cysts, an accessory muscle belly, low-lying soleus muscle, or enlarged degenerated tendon substance, they may be excised as well (Fig. 14.4). At the end of

the procedure, portals are closed with 3-0 nylon sutures and dressings of the surgeon's choice. Patients with an associated gastrocnemius contracture may also benefit from a gastrocnemius recession using either open or endoscopic technique in the prone position. The patient is placed into a walking boot and can start progressive weight-bearing immediately. Patients will typically begin to wean out of the boot by approximately 4–6 weeks.

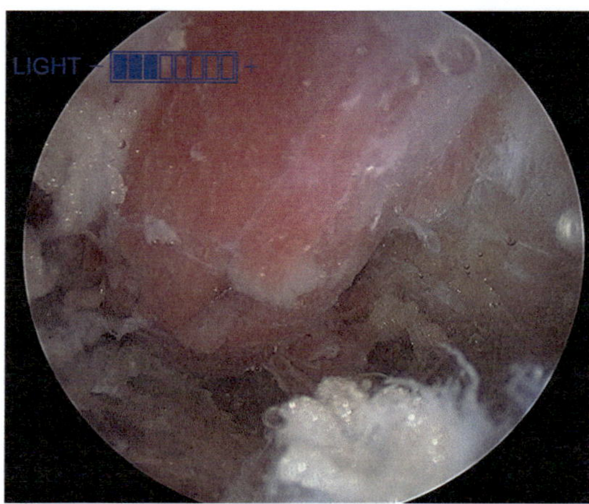

Fig. 14.4 Low-lying soleus muscle is observed from the distal lateral portal

Outcomes of Tendoscopy for Noninsertional Achilles Tendinopathy

Current evidence supporting the use of tendoscopy for noninsertional Achilles tendinopathy consists mainly of small case series and expert opinions. Steenstra and van Dijk reported the outcome of endoscopic paratenon release with the release of the plantaris tendon in 20 patients diagnosed with combined paratendinopathy and intratendinous lesions [13]. At a mean of 6 years postoperatively, 16 patients were available for follow-up, and most reported that they were able to resume their sporting activities within 4–8 weeks after surgery. No complications were reported in this series.

Two years later, in 2008, Vega et al. reported a retrospective series of eight patients with chronic Achilles tendinopathy treated using an endoscopic technique where degenerative or pathologic tissue of the Achilles tendon was resected while performing multiple longitudinal tenotomies with a retrograde knife [15]. All eight patients reported excellent results at a mean follow-up of 27.1 months (range: 18–40 months), and all patients were pain free. On physical examination, all nodules had disappeared except in two cases. MRI obtained 6 months after surgery showed normal signals in five out of eight

(63%) patients, and the remaining three showed minimal signs of local deterioration.

The first prospectively designed study was published by Thermann et al. in 2009, in which eight consecutive patients suffering from chronic midportion Achilles tendinopathy underwent endoscopic debridement of the ventral, neovascularized portion of the Achilles tendon as well as the paratenon [6]. The authors reported that all patients experienced immediate postoperative pain relief with a mean VAS improvement from 40 preoperatively to 97.5 at a 6-month follow-up. No complications occurred.

Pearce et al. published a retrospective case series of 11 patients with noninsertional Achilles tendinopathy who had failed at least 6 months of conservative treatment measures [16]. At a minimum follow-up of 2 years (range: 24–39 months), the mean AOFAS scores improved from 68 preoperatively to 92 postoperatively ($p < 0.0002$). The Ankle Osteoarthritis Scale (AOS) scores improved for pain (28–8%, $P = 0.0004$) and disability (38–10%, $p = 0.0005$). SF-36 scores also improved in this consecutive series from 76 preop to 87 postoperatively but did not reach a level of statistical significance ($p = 0.059$). No complications occurred. At final follow-up, 8/11 (73%) of patients were satisfied with the results of the procedure. The authors of this study reported that the plantaris tendon was released and divided in all patients included in this study given it's suspected role in symptomatology with this condition [16]

Maquirriain et al. demonstrated promising long-term results in a series of 27 patients undergoing endoscopic debridement with longitudinal tenotomies for midportion Achilles tendinopathy [17]. At a minimum follow-up of 5 years, the Victorian Institute Sports Assessment-Achilles questionnaire score improved from 37.0 to 97.5 ($p = 0.0006$), and the Achilles Tendon Scoring System (ATSS) improved from 32.6 to 97.2 ($p = 0.000006$). Two complications were reported in this group, including a keloid lesion and a seroma with chronic fistula formation.

The largest series to date was published by Opdam et al. in 2018 [18]. The authors reported the results of 59 patients who underwent endoscopic treatment of patients with chronic midportion Achilles tendinopathy including release of the paratenon with resection of the plantaris tendon between 2000 and 2013. The median satisfaction score for treatment was 9 out of 10 for those treated unilaterally and 9.5 out of 10 for those treated bilaterally. The median numeric rating scale pain scores during running and sport were 1 for the unilateral group and 0 for the bilaterally treated group. One reoperation for the recurrence of symptoms was necessary. The authors found high patient satisfaction with EuroQol 5D scores and good functional outcomes in this cohort.

Recently, Wagner et al. reported on a retrospective case series consisting of 11 patients who underwent Achilles tendoscopy with excision and debridement of all ventral paratenon adhesions and debridement of Kager's fat pad in addition to the retrocalcaneal bursa adhesions on the deep tendon surface [19]. No tenotomy of the plantaris tendon was performed in this group. Ten of the 11 patients (91%) were satisfied, and all patients returned to the same sporting level compared to their preoperative level at a median time of 4 months (range: 2–12 months). No complications were reported other than one patient who developed tarsal tunnel syndrome, which was operated on 8 months after the index procedure.

Tendoscopic augmentation with the flexor hallucis longus has also been reported in a series of five patients with chronic noninsertional tendinopathy by T.H. Lui in 2012 [14]. An accessory plantar portal with a bone tunnel through the posterior calcaneal tubercle was used for the FHL portion of this procedure. Five patients had greater than 50% tendon involvement on preoperative MRI evaluation and a mean symptom duration of 37 months (range: 6–132 months). At a mean follow-up of 19.8 months (range: 13–29 months), the Achilles Tendinopathy Scoring System (ATSS) scores improved from 29.4 to 89. No complications occurred.

Equinus contracture leading to mechanical overload of the Achilles tendon has been described as an underlying factor in the development of noninsertional Achilles tendinopathy [20]. Several authors have published case series using isolated gastrocnemius recession as a treatment for Achilles tendinopathy with promising results [20–23]. The largest series consisting of 320 patients who underwent endoscopic gastrocnemius recession demonstrated a mean VAS improvement from 7 to 3 ($p < 0.01$) with significant improvements in both SF-36 physical and mental components ($p < 0.01$ for both). In this series, 11/320 (3.4%) patients reported plantarflexion weakness, and sural nerve dysesthesia was reported in 10/320 patients (3.1%).

Conclusions

The treatment of noninsertional Achilles tendinopathy has evolved substantially in the last decade. The use of arthroscopy allows orthopedic surgeons to evaluate the condition of the tendon and peritendinous tissue, remove scar tissue or space-occupying lesions, and alter the mechanics of the tendon with a gastrocnemius recession. The promising results are based on the preservation of soft tissue envelope and minimized postoperative complications.

References

1. Baltes TPA, Zwiers R, Wiegerinck JI, van Dijk CN. Surgical treatment for midportion Achilles tendinopathy: a systematic review. Knee Surg Sports Traumatol Arthrosc. 2017;25(6):1817–38.
2. Kvist M. Achilles tendon injuries in athletes. Sports Med. 1994;18(3):173–201.
3. Ohberg L, Lorentzon R, Alfredson H. Neovascularisation in Achilles tendons with painful tendinosis but not in normal tendons: an ultrasonographic investigation. Knee Surg Sports Traumatol Arthrosc. 2001;9(4):233–8.
4. Andersson G, Danielson P, Alfredson H, Forsgren S. Nerve-related characteristics of ventral paratendinous tissue in chronic Achilles tendinosis. Knee Surg Sports Traumatol Arthrosc. 2007;15(10):1272–9.
5. Maffulli N, Oliva F, Maffulli GD, Giai Via A, Gougoulias N. Minimally invasive Achilles tendon stripping for the management of tendinopathy of the main body of the Achilles tendon. J Foot Ankle Surg. 2017;56(5):938–42.
6. Thermann H, Benetos IS, Panelli C, Gavriilidis I, Feil S. Endoscopic treatment of chronic mid-portion

Achilles tendinopathy: novel technique with short-term results. Knee Surg Sports Traumatol Arthrosc. 2009;17(10):1264–9.

7. Wertheimer SJ, Weber CA, Loder BG, Calderone DR, Frascone ST. The role of endoscopy in treatment of stenosing posterior tibial tenosynovitis. J Foot Ankle Surg. 1995;34(1):15–22.

8. Niek van Dijk C, Scholten PE, Kort NP. Tendoscopy (tendon sheath endoscopy) for overuse tendon injuries. Oper Tech Sports Med. 1997;5(3):170–8.

9. Cychosz CC, Phisitkul P, Barg A, Nickisch F, van Dijk CN, Glazebrook MA. Foot and ankle tendoscopy: evidence-based recommendations. Arthroscopy. 2014;30(6):755–65.

10. Phisitkul P, Barg A, Amendola A. Endoscopic recession of the gastrocnemius tendon. Foot Ankle Int. 2017;38(4):457–64.

11. Carreira D, Ballard A. Achilles tendoscopy. Foot Ankle Clin. 2015;20(1):27–40.

12. Segesser B, Goesele A, Renggli P. The Achilles tendon in sports. Orthopade. 1995;24(3):252–67.

13. Steenstra F, van Dijk CN. Achilles tendoscopy. Foot Ankle Clin. 2006;11(2):429–38. viii

14. Lui TH. Treatment of chronic noninsertional Achilles tendinopathy with endoscopic Achilles tendon debridement and flexor hallucis longus transfer. Foot Ankle Spec. 2012;5(3):195–200.

15. Vega J, Cabestany JM, Golanó P, Pérez-Carro L. Endoscopic treatment for chronic Achilles tendinopathy. Foot Ankle Surg. 2008;14(4):204–10.

16. Pearce CJ, Carmichael J, Calder JD. Achilles tendinoscopy and plantaris tendon release and division in the treatment of non-insertional Achilles tendinopathy. Foot Ankle Surg. 2012;18(2):124–7.

17. Maquirriain J. Surgical treatment of chronic achilles tendinopathy: long-term results of the endoscopic technique. J Foot Ankle Surg. 2013;52(4):451–5.

18. Opdam KTM, Baltes TPA, Zwiers R, Wiegerinck JI, van Dijk CN. Endoscopic treatment of mid-portion Achilles tendinopathy: a retrospective case series of patient satisfaction and functional outcome at a 2- to 8-year follow-up. Arthroscopy. 2018;34(1):264–9.

19. Wagner P, Wagner E, Ortiz C, Zanolli D, Keller A, Maffulli N. Achilles tendoscopy for non insertional Achilles tendinopathy. A case series study. Foot Ankle Surg. 2020;26(4):421–4.

20. Duthon VB, Lübbeke A, Duc SR, Stern R, Assal M. Noninsertional Achilles tendinopathy treated with gastrocnemius lengthening. Foot Ankle Int. 2011;32(4):375–9.

21. Kiewiet NJ, Holthusen SM, Bohay DR, Anderson JG. Gastrocnemius recession for chronic noninsertional Achilles tendinopathy. Foot Ankle Int. 2013;34(4):481–5.

22. Gurdezi S, Kohls-Gatzoulis J, Solan MC. Results of proximal medial gastrocnemius release for Achilles tendinopathy. Foot Ankle Int. 2013;34(10):1364–9.

23. Tallerico VK, Greenhagen RM, Lowery C. Isolated gastrocnemius recession for treatment of insertional Achilles tendinopathy: a pilot study. Foot Ankle Spec. 2015;8(4):260–5.

24. Lysholm J, Wiklander J. Injuries in runners. Am J Sports Med. 1987;15(2):168–71.

Open Debridement of Noninsertional Achilles Tendinopathy

15

Mark E. Easley and Ian L. D. Le

Although symptomatic Achilles tendinopathy can be managed nonoperatively [1, 2], histologic analysis of tissue obtained at the time of surgery demonstrates degenerative fibrous tissue, no inflammatory cells, and no healing response [3, 4]. Surgical management of noninsertional Achilles tendinopathy is indicated when nonoperative management fails. Surgical options for noninsertional Achilles tendinopathy include the following:

1. Percutaneous tenotomy
2. Tenosynovectomy
3. Open Achilles debridement with repair of the residual Achilles tendon
4. Open Achilles debridement with reconstruction of the residual Achilles tendon

Percutaneous tenotomy can be applied to any case of Achilles tendinopathy but is perhaps best reserved for mild-to-moderate Achilles tendinopathy [5–7]. Open debridement affords a comprehensive evaluation and debridement of the diseased Achilles tendon, with the option for augmentation of the repair or reconstruction, and includes tenosynovectomy in virtually all cases.

Following debridement, Achilles tendon repair is generally recommended when 50% or more of the cross-sectional volume of the diseased tendon segment comprises healthy tendon fibers. In contrast, reconstruction or augmentation is typically warranted when the majority of the segment in question is diseased. In approximately 19–23% of the cases, a partial rupture of the Achilles tendon will be identified at the segment of the tendon in question [3, 8]. In a majority of cases, the partial rupture is associated with degenerated/unhealthy tissue. The repair of the partial rupture should be performed in conjunction with the excision of the degenerated portion of the tendon.

Preoperative Evaluation

The patient generally reports pain in the posterior calf. There is a fusiform thickening within the Achilles tendon substance, located proximal to the Achilles' calcaneal insertion, and the nodule usually limits activities that require push-off during gait. On clinical exam, this tender fusiform mass is located approximately 4–6 cm proximal to the Achilles insertion—the site that is also commonly associated with an acute Achilles tendon rupture. The tendon is noted to be in continuity, and the patient has a negative Thompson test. The painful arc sign may distinguish between paratendonitis and Achilles tendinopathy [9]. The sign occurs with an ankle range

M. E. Easley (✉)
Division of Orthopaedic Surgery, Duke University
Medical Center, Morrisville, NC, USA
e-mail: mark.e.easley@duke.edu

I. L. D. Le
Division of Orthopaedics 2675 36st NE, University of
Calgary, Calgary, AB, Canada

of motion, where the tender mass remains localized in paratenonitis but moves up and down with the Achilles tendon in tendinopathy. While not always present, hyperdorsiflexion of the ankle may be observed in patients with nodular Achilles tendinopathy. Radiographs are of little value but may reveal calcification within the diseased portion of the tendon. Magnetic resonance imaging (MRI) is not a prerequisite to surgical intervention but does offer guidance as to the presence and extent of disease, with potentially some prognostic value and reasonable clinical correlation [10–13].

Isolated paratendonitis [3, 14] is not associated with intrasubstance tendon signal change viewed via MRI. However, noninsertional Achilles tendon disorders may exist on a continuum, and therefore pantendonitis may be present, with fluid in the paratenon (paratenonitis) and intrasubstance tendon signal change (tendinopathy) occurring simultaneously. The axial MRI view suggests the extent of tendon disease in the cross-section, and the sagittal view demonstrates the extent of tendon disease over the course of the tendon. Likewise, ultrasound has proven effective in determining the extent of tendon disease and may provide some prognostic value and reasonable clinical correlation [10, 15, 16]. Both MRI and ultrasound may identify a partial rupture at the site of tendon degeneration [10, 15]. More recently, MRI has proven effective in monitoring the response to both nonoperative and operative treatments of Achilles tendinopathy [13, 17].

Longitudinal Percutaneous Tenotomy

Background

While not an open technique, percutaneous longitudinal tenotomy bears mentioning in the oper-

ative management of noninsertional Achilles tendinopathy. Like nitroglycerine and extracorporeal shock wave therapy, percutaneous tenotomy induces low-grade trauma to the degenerated portion of the tendon to stimulate a healing response [5–7]. As it is a minimally invasive technique, percutaneous longitudinal tenotomy may be combined with brisement [14] (see Chap. 13) to address stenosing tenosynovitis and tendinopathy. Intraoperative ultrasound is applied by some surgeons to identify the exact location of tendon disease when performing percutaneous tenotomy [6]. The minimally invasive nature of this procedure may reduce soft tissue complications associated with open debridement.

Surgical Technique [5–7]

Proponents of percutaneous longitudinal tenotomy recommend prone positioning, with the patient's feet protruding beyond the operating table and the ankles supported by a bump (Fig. 15.1a, b). Tourniquet use is unnecessary, and only local anesthesia is required. Via palpation or ultrasound guidance, the diseased tendon segment is identified. In the configuration of the number 5 on a game die, five separate stab incisions are performed in sequence into the diseased tendon using a size 11 surgical scalpel blade. With each introduction of the knife, the blade is held stationary, while the ankle is passively dorsiflexed and plantarflexed, and for each incision, the knife blade is introduced twice—the first time with the blade facing distally and the second with the blade directed proximally. The stab incisions are spaced approximately 2 cm from one another. Alternatively, with ultrasound guidance, a single, central stab incision can serve to create multiple tenotomies by angling the blade with each introduction [6]. The wounds are covered with Steri-Strips, and a mildly compressive dressing and a protective bandage are applied (Fig. 15.1c, d).

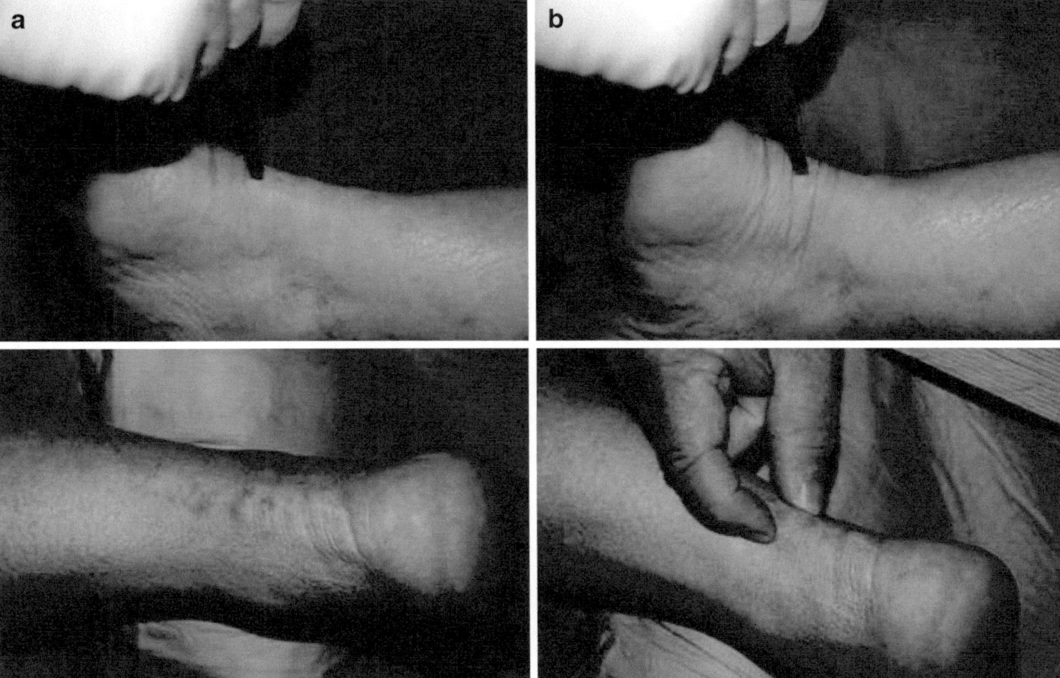

Fig. 15.1 (**a**, **b**) Percutaneous longitudinal tenotomies performed into thickened, fusiform portion of Achilles tendon. (**a**) Scalpel inserted percutaneously through the Achilles, directed proximally, and the ankle is dorsiflexed. (**b**) Same position with the ankle plantarflexed. This procedure is repeated in the same location with the scalpel redirected distally and the dorsiflexion/plantarflexion repeated. Then the technique is repeated in four more locations within the thickened fusiform portion of the tendon. (**c**) Appearance of the tendon 8 months following percutaneous longitudinal tenotomy. (**d**) Some residual thickening is evident, but tenderness is resolved

Open Achilles Tendon Debridement with Repair

Positioning/Tourniquet Use/Anesthesia

The patient may be positioned either prone or supine with a bump under the opposite hip. A tourniquet is optional. If a tourniquet is utilized, a thigh tourniquet offers the advantage over a calf tourniquet of preserving unrestricted gastrocnemius-soleus mobility during surgery. Anesthesia ranges from regional to general and is dictated by surgeon preference and tourniquet use. We prefer to place the patient in the prone position, use a thigh tourniquet, and have the anesthesiologist administer a lumbar plexus/sciatic/femoral regional block. Typically, we exsanguinate the operative extremity with the patient supine on the stretcher and inflate the tourniquet prior to prepping/draping and positioning the patient in the prone position. While this sequence consumes a few extra minutes of tourniquet time, it is safer for the patient's lumbar spine, which otherwise would need to be hyperextended to exsanguinate the extremity.

Surgical Approach

A longitudinal incision is made immediately posteromedial to the diseased portion of the Achilles tendon, extending approximately 2 cm proximal and distal to the fusiform tendon mass (Fig. 15.2). Careful soft tissue handling is important as the blood supply to the skin in this area is not robust. At no point is forceful traction applied to the skin edges, and forceps are only used on tissues deep into the epidermis. Delamination of the dermal layer from the paratenon overlying the Achilles

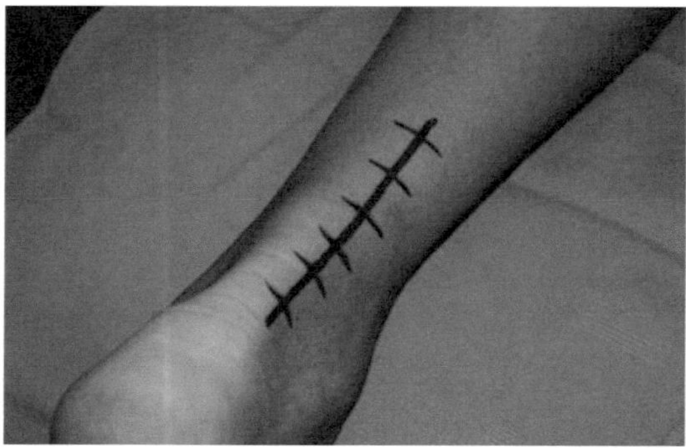

Fig. 15.2 Medial longitudinal approach adjacent to the fusiform thickening of the Achilles tendon

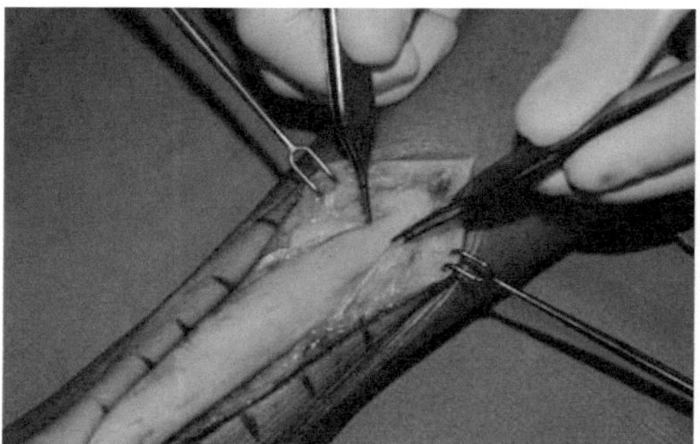

Fig. 15.3 Exposure and reflection of the paratenon

tendon is minimized. The paratenon is exposed and longitudinally divided directly over the fusiform mass within the tendon (Fig. 15.3). With long-standing paratenonitis, the paratenon may be adherent to the underlying tendon; separation of the paratenon and tendon usually is still possible but may be difficult. Several small-diameter tagging sutures may be placed in the paratenon to facilitate the closure of the paratenon at the completion of the surgery (Fig. 15.4). The following adjacent structures are at risk and must be protected: the sural nerve, the tibial nerve, and the posterior tibial artery. We do not recommend routinely identifying these structures as it requires greater dissection, but the surgeon must maintain awareness of the close proximity of these structures at risk.

Achilles Tendon Debridement and Repair

The Achilles tendon is incised longitudinally over the segment of the tendon in question to expose the diseased tissue. The unhealthy tendon is generally easily distinguished from the healthy tendon fibers (Fig. 15.5). Unhealthy, degenerated tissue has a "crabmeat" appearance without distinct orientation in contrast to the healthy, longitudinally organized, collagen fibers of a normal tendon. Although the temptation is great to avoid excessive debridement to preserve adequate tendon substance, leaving a diseased tendon most likely results in persistent symptoms. All of the unhealthy fibers must be removed, even if augmentation is thereby necessitated. Often, the unhealthy tissue is enucleated, leaving a rim of healthy fibers at the diseased segment (Fig. 15.6). Should a partial tear of the Achilles tendon be identified, a repair is indicated but only after the degenerated/unhealthy tissue is fully debrided.

Repair of the residual healthy Achilles tendon without augmentation is an intraoperative decision. Generally, when at least 50% of the diseased tendon segment is occupied by healthy

Fig. 15.4 Several small-diameter tagging sutures may be placed in the paratenon to facilitate the closure of the paratenon at the completion of the surgery

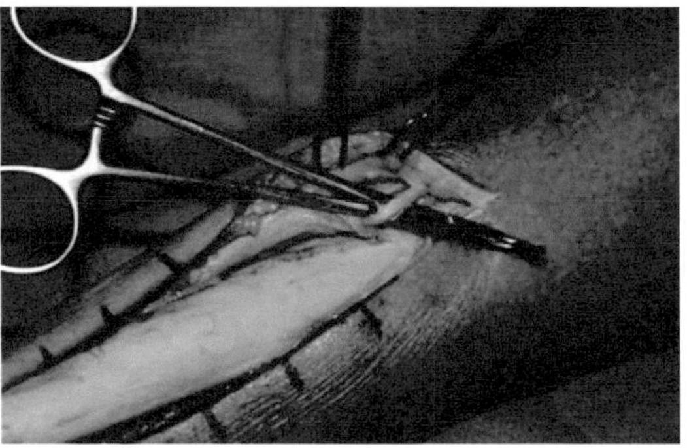

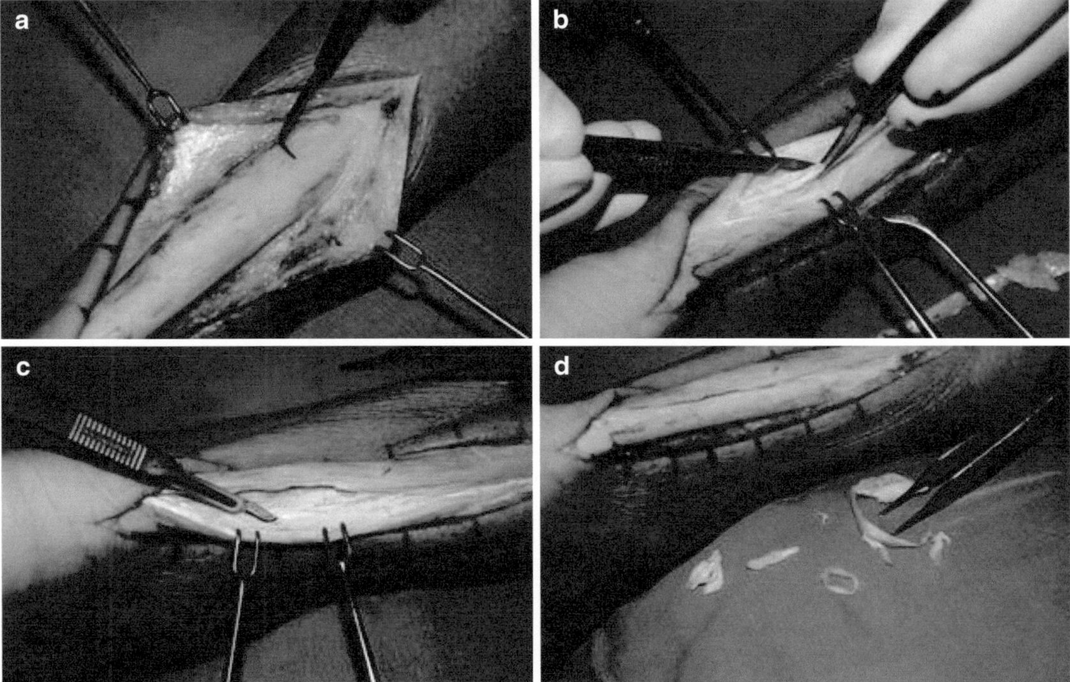

Fig. 15.5 (a) Longitudinal incision directly into the focus of the Achilles tendinopathy. (b) Debridement of the diseased portion of the tendon, leaving only healthy Achilles tendon fibers. Note that diseased fibers are typically centrally located. (c) Repair of the remaining healthy Achilles tendon. (d) "Hollow" Achilles tendon. "Tubularized" tendon

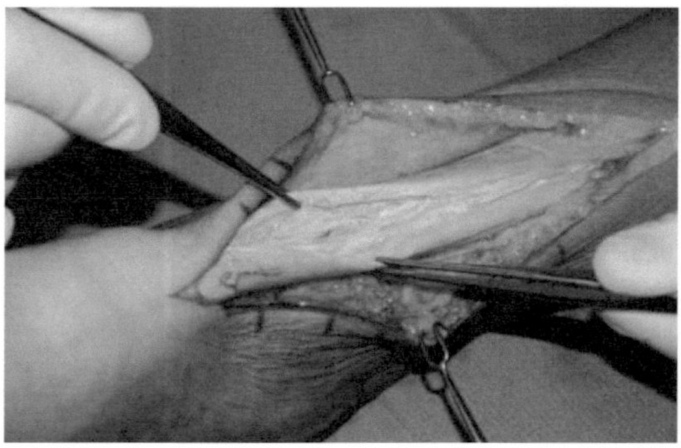

Fig. 15.6 Repair with nonabsorbable suture. Note the reestablishment of the near-physiologic dimension of the Achilles tendon

fibers, a repair is recommended. We perform a common tendon repair technique known as "tubularization" (Fig. 15.7). The healthy tendon fibers are imbricated to create a tubular appearance to the tendon, thereby reinforcing and contouring the tendon at the site of previous pathology. The nonabsorbable suture is recommended, and attempts may be made to bury the knots of these tendons within the imbrication. However, burying these knots is not always possible.

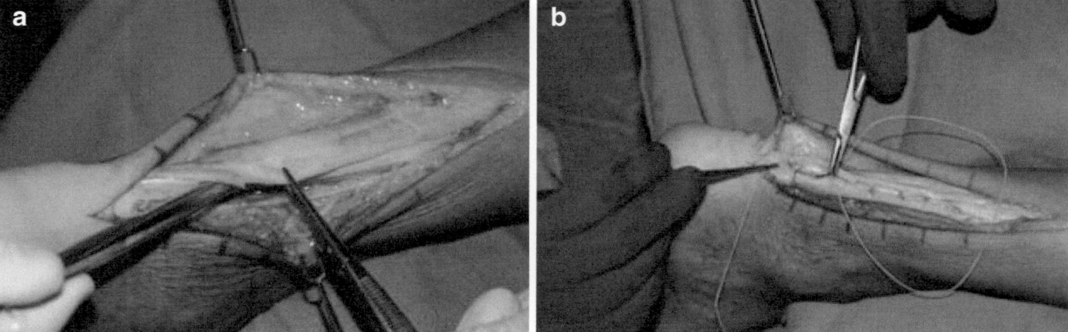

Fig. 15.7 (**a**) Repair of the paratenon. Proximal reapproximation of the paratenon. (**b**) Sural nerve identified and protected. Distal reapproximation of the paratenon

Achilles Tendon Debridement and Reconstruction

Should less than 50% of healthy tendon remain following the debridement of the diseased segment, reconstruction/augmentation must be considered. We prefer to augment the repair with a flexor hallucis longus (FHL) tendon, a technique introduced by Wapner et al. [18] for the management of chronic Achilles tendon ruptures. The FHL tendon is in close proximity and represents the second strongest flexor of the ankle. The harvest of the FHL requires a deep compartment fasciotomy, directly anterior to the Achilles tendon. The FHL muscle is visible through the deep fascia, and the longitudinal fasciotomy can be safely performed directly over this muscle. The posteromedial neurovascular bundle lies directly medial to the FHL tendon and must be protected.

With the tibial nerve and posterior tibial artery identified and protected, the FHL is harvested. Surgeon preference dictates whether a short or long FHL harvest is performed. A long harvest requires a separate plantar foot incision, places the medial plantar nerve at risk, and offers approximately 3 cm more tendon than a short harvest. A long harvest may prove beneficial if the majority of the diseased Achilles tendon segment has to be removed due to extensive disease, thereby potentially affording two strands of augmentation to the defect site. Based on a cadaveric study, a long FHL harvest affords approximately 8 cm of FHL tendon versus 5 cm for a short FHL harvest [19]. Alternatively or additionally, a V-Y advancement or turndown procedure, as described for chronic, neglected Achilles tendon ruptures, may be employed (see Chaps. 10 and 12).

With a short FHL harvest, the ankle and toes are maximally plantarflexed, the posteromedial neurovascular bundle is protected, and the FHL is transected as far distally as possible within its fibro-osseous tunnel in the posteromedial ankle/foot. The FHL tendon is then secured distally, either directly to the distal Achilles tendon or anchored to the calcaneus, just anterior to the distal Achilles tendon. We prefer to anchor the FHL to the calcaneus using a bioabsorbable interference screw technique. With the posteromedial

neurovascular bundle protected, a tunnel is created in the calcaneus from dorsal to plantar with increasingly larger diameter drill bits/reamers. The proper position for the tunnel is determined on intraoperative fluoroscopy with the initial small diameter drill bit. The final tunnel diameter is dictated by the size of the FHL tendon and the desired interference screw. A nonabsorbable suture is placed in the end of the FHL tendon and passed through the tunnel to the plantar heel using a long needle. With the desired tension (usually with the ankle slightly plantarflexed), the interference screw is placed in the calcaneal tunnel. Several additional nonabsorbable sutures are passed side to side from the FHL tendon to the distal Achilles tendon and to the surrounding calcaneal periosteum. The suture protruding from the heel is tensioned, cut flush with the skin, and allowed to retract.

A long FHL harvest allows for the tendon augmentation to be passed through a calcaneal tunnel so that two portions of the FHL tendon can be used to augment the previous site of tendon disease. This FHL tendon can then be sewn side to side to the residual Achilles tendon and to itself; alternatively, it can be woven through the residual Achilles tendon.

Closure

After irrigation, the paratenon is closed over the repair, usually with a running locked absorbable suture (Fig. 15.8). The previously placed tag sutures facilitate the identification

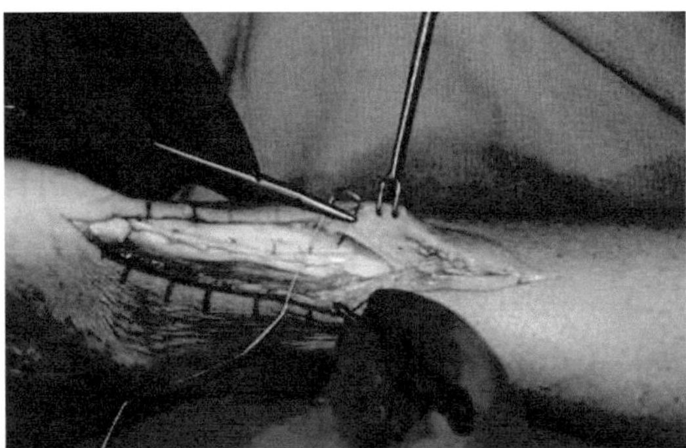

Fig. 15.8 Repair reinforced with absorbable suture

of the paratenon and its proper alignment during closure. The tourniquet should be released prior to wound closure to ensure meticulous hemostasis and avoid hematoma formation, which may induce wound complications. With careful soft tissue handling, the subcutaneous layer is closed, avoiding excessive skin traction or trapping the sural nerve. The skin can be reapproximated with a monofilament suture or staples. The use of a drain is according to the surgeon's preference. Sterile dressings, adequate padding, and a posterior splint are applied with the patient's ankle at its resting tension.

Aftercare

The postoperative course is dictated by (1) wound healing, (2) strength of the repair/reconstruction, and (3) patient compliance. Ideally, range of motion should be initiated as early as possible, but it should not compromise skin healing and the repair/fixation.

Percutaneous Tenotomy [5, 7].

Postoperative day 1: elevation, nonsteroidal anti-inflammatory drugs (NSAIDs), protected weight-bearing (WB), isometric strength training with active dorsiflexion and plantarflexion.

Postoperative day 2: weight-bearing as tolerated (WBAT) with crutches; continue isometric strength training.

Week 1: full weight-bearing (FWB); continue isometric strength training.

Week 2: swimming, water running.

Week 4: stationary bike; gentle running; isometric, concentric, eccentric calf muscle strengthening.

Weeks 10 to 12: unrestricted return to sports.

Open Debridement and Repair

Weeks 1 and 2: elevation, non-weight-bearing (NWB) splinting in slight plantarflexion (resting tension).

Weeks 3 and 4: if wound healed, touch-down weight bearing (TDWB) gentle range-of-motion exercises without resistance.

Weeks 5 and 6: TDWB, isometric, concentric, eccentric calf muscle strengthening.

Weeks 7–12: progressive WB, stationary bike, water running; continue calf strengthening.

Weeks 13–16: gentle running; increase resistance exercises.

Weeks 17–20: unrestricted return to sports.

Open Debridement and Reconstruction

The following schedule must be tempered by the quality of the reconstruction/fixation of augmentation:

Weeks 1 and 2: elevation, NWB splinting in slight plantarflexion (resting tension).

Weeks 3–6: if wound healed, TDWB gentle range-of-motion exercises without resistance.

Weeks 7–12: gradual progression of partial weight-bearing to FWB; stationary bike; water running; isometric, concentric, eccentric calf muscle strengthening.

Weeks 13–20: FWB, gentle running; increase resistance exercises.

Weeks 21–24: unrestricted return to sports.

Complications

Wound Complications

Drawing from the literature reporting the open management of Achilles tendon disorders, including acute Achilles tendon repair, the wound complication rate is approximately 10%. Wound complications include wound edge necrosis, hematoma formation, associated superficial wound infections, and symptomatic fibrosis/scar formation. In the majority of cases, these wound complications can be effectively managed with local wound care, wound healing agents, and extending the period of immobilization. When there is no response to local wound care, plastic surgery consultation is indicated. There should be little delay in plastic surgery consultation since, physiologically, there is very little soft tissue coverage over the repaired/reconstructed Achilles tendon. If the paratenon was effectively reapproximated, a wound vacuum-assisted closure (VAC) can prove effective in avoiding tissue transfer procedures.

Infection

The reported prevalence of superficial wound infections following open Achilles tendon surgery ranges from less than 1% to almost 20%; for deep wound infections, the prevalence has been reported to be 2.2% [20–23]. These estimates combine reports of surgical management of Achilles tendon disorders, including acute rupture, neglected ruptures, and tendinopathy. Superficial wound infections can often be managed with topical antibiotic ointments and oral antibiotics. As for wound complications, if in close follow-up the response to local wound care is ineffective, the threshold for surgical management should be low. Irrigation and debridement, followed by local wound care or wound VAC management, may prove effective for infections not violating the paratenon.

Deep infections necessitate the takedown of the repair/reconstruction and the removal of nonabsorbable sutures. Although unfortunate, the removal of all foreign bodies is essential. Within the paratenon, an inadequately treated infection could readily spread to infect the entire gastrocnemius/soleus complex.

Rupture

As previously noted, occasionally the degenerated portion of the Achilles tendon develops a partial rupture. In fact, there is histologic evidence that suggests that degenerated tendons are predisposed to rupture. Therefore, it is essential to excise all of the degenerated tendon at the index procedure even if that necessitates creating an intercalary defect within the tendon. Martin et al. [24] completely excised the involved segment of a tendon in all cases and bridged the defect with a long FHL transfer (double strand) without reestablishing the continuity of the two ends of the Achilles tendon. Although their conclusions rely on follow-up by questionnaire in some of their patients, the authors report no cases of reconstruction FHL rupture. Their finding of no FHL ruptures is supported by Wilcox et al. [25].

Persistent Pain

Reported persistent pain following these procedures ranges from 0% to 15%. Not all Achilles tendinopathy is symptomatic, so the exact cause of pain prior to the index procedure is perhaps not fully understood. However, it is generally accepted that symptoms are secondary to the patient having to rely on unhealthy, degenerated tissue over a segment of the Achilles tendon during push-off. Accordingly, persistent pain is generally attributed to the incomplete resection of a diseased tendon. To ensure the satisfactory removal of a diseased tendon, some surgeons routinely create an intercalary defect in the area of tendon degeneration and then bridge the defect with Achilles tendon advancement or tendon transfer [24].

Occasionally, sural neuralgia is experienced postoperatively. Since most surgeons use a medial approach to the diseased portion of the tendon and elevate the paratenon, direct injury to the sural nerve is relatively uncommon. More likely, scar formation postoperatively results in an adhesive neuralgia. While direct trauma to the sural nerve can be diagnosed clinically within the first few weeks after surgery, adhesive neuralgia may not become apparent for several months. Proper soft tissue handling with deep retraction may lead to traction neuralgia of the sural nerve, a phenomenon that typically resolves over several weeks to months postoperatively.

Loss of Toe Push-off Strength (Following Flexor Hallucis Longus Transfer)

The transfer of the FHL tendon to augment/reconstruct the Achilles tendon should result in the loss of great toe push-off strength. Coull et al. [26]. studied the effects of FHL transfer for Achilles tendinopathy and chronic Achilles tendon ruptures in 16 patients. Despite pedobarographic evaluation suggesting a trend toward a reduction in peak pressure loading on the distal phalanx, AOFAS hallux metatarsophalangeal-interphalangeal (MTP-IP) scores and Short Form (SF)-36 questionnaire data failed to demonstrate functional deficits of the hallux in this limited group of patients.

Results

Overview

Reported results of the operative management of nodular Achilles tendinopathy are supported almost exclusively by no more than level IV evidence (case series) and are frequently clouded by the fact that several studies include results for the treatment of both insertional and noninsertional Achilles tendinopathy. However, our review of the following studies provides some indication of anticipated results in the surgical management of noninsertional Achilles tendinopathy.

Meta-Analysis

In an analysis of 26 studies that report the results of the surgical management of Achilles tendinopathy, Tallon et al. [27] identified a negative correlation between success rate and overall method scores. To reach this conclusion, the authors created a highly reproducible methodology score. Important is their observation that although study methods continue to improve, evidence-based guidelines for this area of research are required to provide accurate outcome data for the surgical management of Achilles tendinopathy.

Comparative Analysis

In a case-controlled study, Maffulli et al. [28] suggested that athletic patients respond better to operative management than nonathletic patients. In their investigation, 80% of athletes and 52% of nonathletes had good to excellent results, respectively. The nonathletic population had a higher complication rate, and 19% of the nonathletic population required reoperations.

Benazzo et al. [29] noted that younger age and a relatively short duration of Achilles tendon symptoms were associated, with a more favorable outcome, with operative intervention in the management of Achilles tendinopathy. The authors concluded that the shorter duration of symptoms correlated with less Achilles tendon pathology.

Open Debridement and Repair

Maffulli et al. [30] reported results in 14 athletes undergoing surgical excision of central core degenerative lesions after failing an exhaustive regimen of nonoperative measures. At a mean follow-up of 35 months, only five patients had an excellent or good result. Even reoperation in six patients failed to improve the outcome. Based on this limited patient population, the authors suggested that a long-standing disease—an average of 87 months from the onset of the symptoms of surgical management in this cohort—may have a negative impact on the outcome. In fact, they extrapolated to recommend that perhaps earlier surgical intervention should be indicated.

Johnston et al. [14] reported the management of 41 patients with Achilles tendinopathy and an average duration of symptoms of 14 weeks. Approximately 50% responded to nonsurgical management over an 18-week period, and an additional three patients recovered satisfactory function following a brisement procedure. The remaining 17 patients failing nonoperative management underwent tenosynovectomy and limited tendon debridement for tendinosis; all patients managed surgically returned to full function at an average of 31 weeks. Patients responding to nonoperative management tended to be younger (average age 33 years) than those managed surgically (average age 48 years).

Ohberg et al. [31] studied the recovery of calf muscle strength following surgically managed noninsertional Achilles tendinopathy in 24 patients. Using concentric and eccentric peak torque measures, the authors noted that calf strength deficits in the affected extremity, compared to the uninvolved extremity observed preoperatively, persisted at an average follow-up of 5 years despite a rigorous calf-strengthening rehabilitation protocol. The authors concluded that the deficits may be clinically insignificant since 92% of the patients reported no functional deficits at final follow-up.

Leach et al. [32] noted successful long-term outcomes in nine competitive runners undergoing surgical debridement and repair for noninsertional Achilles tendinopathy. Although all patients returned to their desired high level of function, two required reoperation to achieve that status.

Saxena and Cheung [33, 34] reported that athletic patients, particularly male runners, tended to return to their desired level of activity more rapidly than nonathletic patients. Two retrospective reviews comprised a variety of diagnoses accounting for achillodynia, including noninsertional tendinopathy, insertional tendinopathy, and tenosynovitis. Patients undergoing surgical management requiring bony procedures (insertional) necessitated the greatest time to return to full activity (average 18.6 weeks). Patients with noninsertional Achilles tendinopathy (undergoing excision/repair procedures) returned to full activity by an average of 13.2 weeks for mucoid degeneration and 14.4 weeks for calcific tendinosis. Reconstructive procedures for chronic Achilles tendon ruptures returned at an average of 34.0 weeks. In contrast, patients without tendinopathy and only paratenonitis and those undergoing only tenolysis/tenosynovectomy returned to the desired level of function, on average, by 7.7 weeks.

Schepsis et al. [35] reviewed a wide variety of Achilles tendon pathology managed surgically and noted that the surgical management of tendinopathy yielded the lowest percentage of satisfactory outcomes. The cohort of 79 patients comprised a relatively active patient population, with an average age of 33 years (range: 17–59 years) with diagnoses of paratenonitis ($n = 23$), noninsertional tendinopathy ($n = 15$), retrocalcaneal bursitis ($n = 24$), insertional tendinopathy ($n = 7$), and combined findings ($n = 10$). Good to excellent outcomes were as follows: paratenonitis (87%), insertional tendinopathy (8%), retrocalcaneal bursitis (75%), and noninsertional tendinopathy (67%). Furthermore, the noninsertional tendinopathy group also required the highest number of reoperations.

In a prospective study, Paavola et al. [36] demonstrated a more favorable outcome for the surgical management of peritendinous adhesions than peritendinous adhesions associated with tendinopathy. At relatively short-term follow-up (7 months), of the 42 patients evaluated preoperatively and at 7 months or later, satisfactory results were 88% for the group with peritendinous adhesions and 54% for the groups with peritendinous adhesions and tendinosis. Likewise, the incidence of complications was 6% for the peritendinous adhesion group and 27% for the group with peritendinous adhesions and tendinosis.

In two separate prospective studies of surgical management of Achilles tendinopathy, Alfredson et al. [37, 38] observed that the recovery of plantarflexion muscle strength to equal that of the unaffected side typically takes 6 -12 months. The evaluation focused on concentric and eccentric peak torque measures. The investigators could not identify any differences in outcome if the surgically managed tendon was immobilized for

2 weeks or 6 weeks in the immediate postoperative period.

The surgical management of isolated tenosynovitis, or tenosynovitis without associated tendinopathy, almost uniformly yields a favorable outcome with a relatively rapid return to the desired functional level. Gould and Korson [39] reported successful outcomes with a return to full function within only a few months in eight of nine patients undergoing excision of a pseudosheath of degenerative tissue that was creating a stenosing tenosynovitis.

The results of reconstruction using an FHL augmentation for inadequate residual healthy tendons have been favorable [24, 25]. At an average follow-up of 14 months, Wilcox et al. [25] reported that 90% of their 20 patients undergoing debridement and FHL augmentation for noninsertional Achilles tendinopathy scored 70 points or higher on the AOFAS hindfoot-ankle score. No wound complications, ruptures, or recurrences of tendinopathy were reported. Although the SF-36 outcome measure for physical function was lower than that for United States norms, the authors suggested that FHL reconstruction is a reasonable option for the reconstruction of Achilles tendinopathy.

Martin et al. [24] reported the results of 56 surgically managed Achilles tendinopathies in 44 patients. In all cases, a complete excision of the diseased portion of the tendon was performed, and the defect was spanned via an FHL tendon transfer. Although over half of the patients responded only by questionnaire and only 19 were examined at final follow-up, the authors concluded that the SF-36 scores of their surgically managed patients were not statistically significantly different from the scores for the general United States population. This conclusion was made even though the plantarflexion range of motion and plantarflexion strength were significantly less than the unaffected side in the 19 patients tested. In these 19 patients, the average AOFAS score was 91 points. Pain was decreased in 96% ($n = 42$), and satisfaction was 86% ($n = 38$).

Percutaneous Longitudinal Tenotomy

In three separate investigations of athletic patients with Achilles tendinopathy with an average follow-up ranging from 16 to 36 months, Testa and Maffulli and coauthors [5–7] reported satisfactory results of percutaneous longitudinal tenotomy, with or without ultrasound guidance, in a majority of patients. Maffulli et al. [5] noted good to excellent results in 77% of middle- to long-distance runners, and Testa et al. [7] observed good to excellent results in 86% of track-and-field athletes. In a separate study, 75% of athletes evaluated after ultrasound-guided percutaneous tenotomy returned to preinjury levels of activity [6]. These authors conclude that percutaneous tenotomy is a reasonably safe outpatient procedure for noninsertional Achilles tendinopathy when nonoperative measures fail. They caution that diffuse or multinodular tendinopathy or pantendinopathy may be better managed with open paratenon stripping and multiple longitudinal tenotomies.

References

1. Ohberg L, Alfredson H. Effects on neovascularisation behind the good results with eccentric training in chronic mid-portion Achilles tendinosis? Knee Surg Sports Traumatol Arthrosc. 2004;12(5):465–70.
2. Ohberg L, Lorentzon R, Alfredson H. Eccentric training in patients with chronic Achilles tendinosis: normalised tendon structure and decreased thickness at follow up. Br J Sports Med. 2004;38(1):8–11.
3. Astrom M, Rausing A. Chronic Achilles tendinopathy. A survey of surgical and histopathologic findings. Clin Orthop Rel Res. 1995;316:151–64.
4. Maffulli N, Kader D. Tendinopathy of tendo achillis. J Bone Joint Surg (Br). 2002;84(1):1–8.
5. Maffulli N, Testa V, Capasso G, et al. Results of percutaneous longitudinal tenotomy for Achilles tendinopathy in middle- and long-distance runners. Am J Sports Med. 1997;25(6):835–40.
6. Testa V, Capasso G, Benazzo F, et al. Management of Achilles tendinopathy by ultrasound-guided percutaneous tenotomy. Med Sci Sports Exerc. 2002;34:(4)573–80:573.
7. Testa V, Maffulli N, Capasso G, et al. Percutaneous longitudinal tenotomy in chronic Achilles tendonitis. Bull Hosp Joint Dis. 1996;54(4):241–4.

8. Astrom M. Partial rupture in chronic Achilles tendinopathy. A retrospective analysis of 342 cases. Acta Orthop Scand. 1998;69(4):404–7.

9. Maffulli N, Wong J, Almekinders LC. Types and epidemiology of tendinopathy. Clin Sports Med. 2003;22(4):675–92.

10. Astrom M, Gentz CF, Nilsson P, et al. Imaging in chronic Achilles tendinopathy: a comparison of ultrasonography, magnetic resonance imaging and surgical findings in 27 histologically verified cases. Skelet Radiol. 1996;25(7):615–20.

11. Karjalainen PT, Soila K, Aronen HJ, et al. MR imaging of overuse injuries of the Achilles tendon. AJR Am J Roentgenol. 2000;175(1):251–60.

12. Gardin A, Bruno J, Movin T, et al. Magnetic resonance signal, rather than tendon volume, correlates to pain and functional impairment in chronic Achilles tendinopathy. Acta Radiol. 2006;47(7):718–24.

13. Shalabi A, Kristoffersen-Wilberg M, Svensson L, et al. Eccentric training of the gastrocnemius-soleus complex in chronic Achilles tendinopathy results in decreased tendon volume and intratendinous signal as evaluated by MRI. Am J Sports Med. 2004;32(5):1286–96.

14. Johnston E, Scranton P Jr, Pfeffer GB. Chronic disorders of the Achilles tendon: results of conservative and surgical treatments. Foot Ankle Int. 1997;18(9):570–4.

15. Lehtinen A, Peltokallio P, Taavitsainen M. Sonography of Achilles tendon correlated to operative findings. Ann Chir Gynaecol. 1994;83(4):322–7.

16. Paavola M, Paakkala T, Kannus P, et al. Ultrasonography in the differential diagnosis of Achilles tendon injuries and related disorders. A comparison between pre-operative ultrasonography and surgical findings. Acta Radiol. 1998;39(6):612–9.

17. Shalabi A, Kristoffersen-Wiberg M, Papadogiannakis N, et al. Dynamic contrast-enhanced MR imaging and histopathology in chronic Achilles tendinosis. A longitudinal MR study of 15 patients. Acta Radiol. 2002;43(2):198–206.

18. Wapner KL, Pavlock GS, Hecht PJ, et al. Repair of chronic Achilles tendon rupture with flexor hallucis longus tendon transfer. Foot Ankle. 1993;14(8):443–9.

19. Tashjian RZ, Hur J, Sullivan RJ, et al. Flexor hallucis longus transfer for repair of chronic Achilles tendinopathy. Foot Ankle Int. 2003;24(9):673–6.

20. Khan RJ, Fick D, Keogh A, et al. Treatment of acute Achilles tendon ruptures. A meta-analysis of randomized, controlled trials. J Bone Joint Surg Am. 2005;87(10):2202–10.

21. Paavola M, Orava S, Leppilahti J, et al. Chronic Achilles tendon overuse injury: complications after surgical treatment. An analysis of 432 consecutive patients. Am J Sports Med. 2000;28(1):77–82.

22. Pajala A, Kangas J, Ohtonen P, et al. Rerupture and deep infection following treatment of total Achilles tendon rupture. Bone Joint Surg. 2002;84:2016.

23. Chiodo CP, Wilson MG. Current concepts review: acute ruptures of the Achilles tendon. Foot Ankle Int. 2006;27(4):305–13.

24. Martin RL, Manning CM, Carcia CR, et al. An outcome study of chronic Achilles tendinosis after excision of the Achilles tendon and flexor hallucis longus tendon transfer. Foot Ankle Int. 2005;26(9):691–7.

25. Wilcox DK, Bohay DR, Anderson JG. Treatment of chronic Achilles tendon disorders with flexor hallucis longus tendon transfer/augmentation. Foot Ankle Int. 2000;21(12):1004–10.

26. Coull R, Flavin R, Stephens MM. Flexor hallucis longus tendon transfer: evaluation of postoperative morbidity. Foot Ankle Int. 2003;24(12):931–4.

27. Tallon C, Coleman BD, Khan KM, et al. Outcome of surgery for chronic Achilles tendinopathy. A critical review. Am J Sports Med. 2001;29(3):315–20.

28. Maffulli N, Testa V, Capasso G, et al. Surgery for chronic Achilles tendinopathy yields worse results in nonathletic patients. Clin J Sport Med. 2006;16(2):123–8.

29. Benazzo F, Stennardo G, Valli M. Achilles and patellar tendinopathies in athletes: pathogenesis and surgical treatment. Bull Hosp Joint Dis. 1996;54(4):236–40.

30. Maffulli N, Binfield PM, Moore D, et al. Surgical decompression of chronic central core lesions of the Achilles tendon. Am J Sports Med. 1999;27(6):747–52.

31. Ohberg L, Lorentzon R, Alfredson H. Good clinical results but persisting side-to-side differences in calf muscle strength after surgical treatment of chronic Achilles tendinosis: a 5-year follow-up. Scand J Med Sci Sports. 2001;11(4):207–12.

32. Leach RE, Schepsis AA, Takai H. Long-term results of surgical management of Achilles tendinitis in runners. Clin Orthop Relat Res. 1992;282:208–12.

33. Saxena A, Cheung S. Surgery for chronic Achilles tendinopathy. Review of 91 procedures over 10 years. J Am Podiatr Med Assoc. 2003;93(4):283–91.

34. Saxena A. Results of chronic Achilles tendinopathy surgery on elite and nonelite track athletes. Foot Ankle Int. 2003;24(9):712–20.

35. Schepsis AA, Jones H, Haas AL. Achilles tendon disorders in athletes. Am J Sports Med. 2002;30(2):287–305.

36. Paavola M, Kannus P, Orava S, et al. Surgical treatment for chronic Achilles tendinopathy: a prospective seven month follow up study. Br J Sports Med. 2002;36(3):178–82.

37. Alfredson H, Pietila T, Lorentzon R. Chronic Achilles tendinitis and calf muscle strength. Am J Sports Med. 1996;24(6):829–33.

38. Alfredson H, Pietila T, Ohberg L, et al. Achilles tendinosis and calf muscle strength. The effect of short-term immobilization after surgical treatment. Am J Sports Med. 1998;26(2):166–71.

39. Gould N, Korson R. Stenosing tenosynovitis of the pseudosheath of the tendo Achilles. Foot Ankle Int. 2002;23(7):595–9.

Operative Management of Insertional Achilles Tendinopathy

Amanda N. Fletcher, Albert T. Anastasio, and James A. Nunley

Insertional Achilles Tendinopathy: Introduction/Definition

Insertional Achilles tendinopathy is a disorder of the distal Achilles tendon located at the tendinous insertion onto the calcaneus. It comprises a spectrum of acute and chronic pathology involving the Achilles tendon insertion and its surrounding tissues. As the term tendinopathy implies, degenerative changes within the tendon occur and result in a constellation of histopathologic, radiographic, and clinical signs and symptoms presenting as posterior heel pain. The posterior heel is a complex anatomic region, and insertional Achilles tendinopathy often encompasses multifactorial pathology involving the Achilles tendon proper, retrocalcaneal bursa, and superior calcaneal process.

Anatomy

Achilles Tendon

The Achilles tendon is the thickest and strongest tendon in the body and is subjected to high tensile loads of up to ten times body weight during running, jumping, hopping, and skipping [1]. It originates from the aponeuroses of the gastrocnemius, soleus, and, variably, plantaris muscle. The tendon internally rotates 90 degrees as it courses distally before inserting onto the posterosuperior aspect of the calcaneal tuberosity. Given this rotation, the soleus contribution inserts anteromedially, and the gastrocnemius fibers insert posterolaterally. The plantaris tendon variably joins the anteromedial side of the Achilles. The tendon inserts at the enthesis located 2 cm distal on the posterosuperior calcaneal prominence via Sharpey's fibers. The Achilles tendon insertion is broad and measures 19.8 mm in height with a width of 23.8 mm proximally and 31.2 mm distally [2].

Retrocalcaneal Bursa

There are two bursae located at the posterior heel: one located posterior or superficial to the Achilles tendon between the Achilles tendon and the skin (termed superficial, subcutaneous, or Achilles bursa) and one between the Achilles tendon and the posterosuperior aspect of the calcaneus (retrocalcaneal bursa). The retrocalcaneal bursa is a horse-shoe-shaped structure located between the anterior Achilles tendon and posterior calcaneus. The bursae function to lubricate and protect the Achilles tendon by reducing friction between the tendon and adjacent tissues [3]. Inflammation of these bursae can cause pain at the posterior heel, termed Achilles tendon bursi-

A. N. Fletcher (✉) · A. T. Anastasio · J. A. Nunley
Department of Orthopaedic Surgery, Duke University
Medical Center, Durham, NC, USA
e-mail: amanda.fletcher@duke.edu;
albert.anastasio@duke.edu; james.nunley@duke.edu

tis. More specifically, either retrocalcaneal bursitis and/or subcutaneous Achilles bursitis can result. These conditions can occur in isolation or in conjunction with insertional Achilles tendinopathy, which can be clinically challenging to differentiate.

Superior Calcaneal Process

An enlargement of the posterosuperior calcaneal process was first described by Haglund in 1928 and was termed Haglund's deformity [4]. An isolated Haglund's deformity may be asymptomatic or may lead to adjacent soft tissue impingement and posterior heel pain. A symptomatic Haglund's deformity, presenting as pain and tenderness at the posterolateral calcaneal prominence, is termed Haglund's disease. While this can occur in isolation, patients may also present with a combination of Haglund's deformity, insertional Achilles tendinopathy, retrocalcaneal bursitis, and retrocalcaneal exostosis, collectively termed Haglund's syndrome. Posterior heel pain can result from any disease process that affects one or all of these components. While there are inconsistencies with Achilles nomenclature in the literature, it is important to understand the anatomy to diagnose correctly and treat patients who present with posterior heel pain.

Pathophysiology

Insertional Achilles tendinopathy is a combined process of inflammation and degeneration with the insertion of the Achilles tendon. Lyman et al. studied the strain behavior of the distal Achilles and noted that insertional Achilles tendinopathy tends to involve the anterior part of the tendon, although the highest strain on biomechanical testing is actually posterior [5]. Given the anterior tendon involvement, it was initially postulated that a prominent superior posterolateral calcaneal tuberosity caused friction at the anterior Achilles insertion, resulting in local damage to the tendon and longitudinal tears at the inser-

tion. However, Kang et al. reported no difference in radiographic parameters of Haglund's deformity between patients with insertional Achilles tendinopathy and control patients [6]. Additionally, Lu et al. found no correlation between the size of the Haglund process and the development of symptoms or the outcome of treatment [7].

Another theory is that repetitive microtrauma causes micro tears within the tendon itself. The subsequent inflammatory response leads to attritional changes within the tendon, including collagen degeneration and the loss of parallel structure, fatty infiltration, fibrosis, and capillary proliferation [8]. Tendon degeneration is manifested by increased tendon thickness and, ultimately, calcification and ossification within the Achilles tendon. The bony metaplasia can result in enthesophytes at the tendinous insertion and intratendinous calcification of the Achilles tendon proper. The calcifications may continue to enlarge and irritate the Achilles tendon, causing further degeneration and necrosis. Cystic changes within the bone along the posterior calcaneal tuberosity may also be present. Contributing factors to the disease process include a gastrocnemius contracture, a cavus foot that results in a more vertical calcaneus, a prominent posterosuperior angle of the calcaneus, and an excessively long calcaneus; these features are proposed to cause impingement of the Achilles tendon and retrocalcaneal bursa on the posterior aspect of the calcaneus, resulting in bursitis, tenosynovitis, and chronic tendinopathy [9].

With all of these concomitant processes, insertional Achilles tendinopathy is thought to begin as an acute process (tendonitis) but is often not treated until its chronic stages (tendinosis or calcific tendinosis) [10]. The semantics of Achilles terminology is often inconsistent, and improper terms are used interchangeably. The term "tendinopathy" should be utilized for clinical diagnosis, whereas the terms "tendinitis" and "tendinosis" should only be applied when a histologic confirmation of tendon pathology is made.

Epidemiology

The incidence of insertional Achilles tendinopathy has been reported to be around 4% in the general population [11] and 14% in the athletic population [12]. The highest prevalence rates have been reported in runners with up to 21% of running athletes affected [13]. There are two distinct groups of patients who present with this condition: younger, athletic individuals and older, more comorbid individuals. In general, the younger patients represent an overuse, inflammatory phenomenon and are treated successfully nonoperatively. The older patients are often more sedentary and comorbid, and their symptoms are typically caused by degenerative changes rather than overuse. These patients are typically older than 45 years of age and more frequently female. An association between systemic diseases such as hypertension and diabetes with Achilles tendinopathy has also been demonstrated [14]. This older patient population typically does not respond well to conservative treatment.

History and Physical Exam

The diagnosis of insertional Achilles tendinopathy is primarily established from the history and physical examination. Patients most commonly present with the chief complaint of posterior heel pain. They may also report swelling, stiffness, or weakness. The pain is typically exacerbated by activity or pressure from closed-back shoes. Similar to most tendinopathies, the pain begins intermittently and gradually becomes constant as the disease progresses. Routine physical examination should begin with observation of gait and overall foot alignment. Particular attention should be paid to hindfoot alignment as a cavovarus foot can be a contributing factor. Inspection may reveal visible erythema, fullness, and swelling at the posterior heel secondary to thickening of the pathologic tendon or concomitant bursitis. A Haglund's deformity can present as a prominence of the lateral calcaneal ridge, termed a "pump bump," referring to the irritation caused by certain shoe wear. Further physical examination often reveals pain with palpation along the distal aspect of the tendon and posterior calcaneus. The pain is often localized more lateral at the heel. Routine range of motion and strength testing should be performed. Depending on the severity and chronicity of the disease process, weakness with push-off, an equinus contracture, or calf atrophy may be present. Special tests should include the Silfverskiold test to evaluate for an isolated gastrocnemius contracture. A Thompson should be performed if there is concern for an acute Achilles tendon rupture, which occurs more commonly in patients with preexisting tendon pathology. A double- and single-leg heel raise can help assess the degree of push-off weakness.

Imaging

While insertional Achilles tendinopathy is primarily a clinical diagnosis, imaging is routinely obtained to help confirm the diagnosis, examine associated pathophysiology, rule out other conditions on the differential diagnosis, determine the extent of tendon involvement, and aid with preoperative planning when indicated. Radiographs should include a weight-bearing anterior-posterior, mortise, lateral, and Harris heel or Saltzman view to allow the evaluation of hindfoot alignment, Haglund deformity, enthesophyte, and intratendinous calcification (Fig. 16.1).

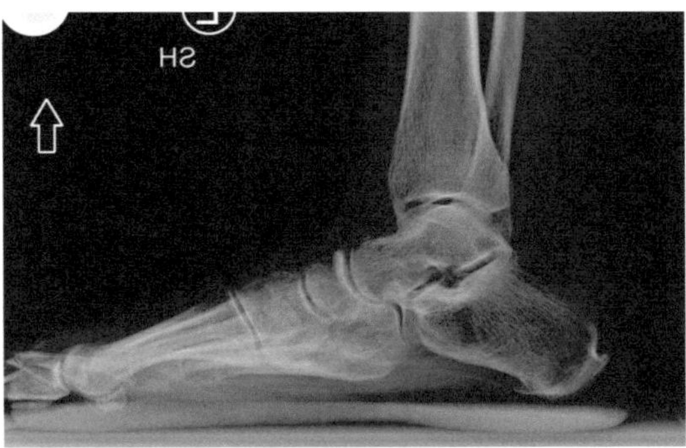

Fig. 16.1 Lateral weight-bearing radiograph of the foot and ankle demonstrating an enthesophyte at the distal Achilles insertion, ossification within the Achilles tendon, and a prominence of the posterosuperior calcaneus (Haglund's deformity)

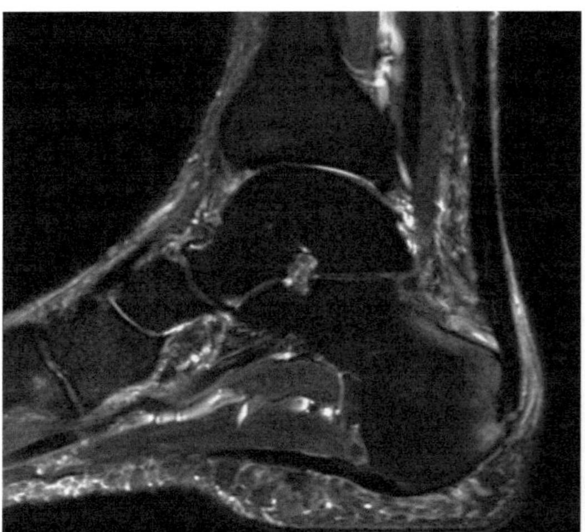

Fig. 16.2 Sagittal T2 fat-suppressed magnetic resonance imaging (MRI) demonstrating Achilles tendinosis and peritenonitis. There is a mild signal and a thickening of the distal Achilles tendon and peritenon. There is a small amount of fluid in the retrocalcaneal bursa and a signal within Kager's fat pad. There are also reactive bony changes in the posterosuperior calcaneus at the tendon insertion

Advanced imaging modalities, including sonography and magnetic resonance imaging (MRI), can be used to examine for soft tissue (tendon degeneration, neovascularization, bursitis, paratendinitis) as well as bony changes (bone marrow edema or cystic changes at the insertion) (Fig. 16.2). Sonography offers the benefits of being inexpensive and has a distinct advantage of facilitating dynamic assessment.

Operative Indications

Posterior heel pain is multifactorial and includes paratendinopathy, retrocalcaneal bursitis, subcutaneous Achilles bursitis, and insertional tendinopathy with or without partial tears. Each of these entities is distinct, but they often occur concomitantly. Regardless of the pathology present, nonoperative management should be considered first. This includes rest, ice, elevation, activity modification, shoe wear modification, orthotics, nonsteroidal anti-inflammatories, and physical therapy. Therapy should focus on heel cord stretching and eccentric calf-muscle training.

Ultrasound modalities, including dexamethasone iontophoresis, high-energy extracorporeal shock wave therapy, dry needling, and treatments with biologics such as platelet-rich plasma, may also be considered. Symptoms recalcitrant to conservative therapies after 3 to 6 months warrant consideration of operative management.

Multiple authors have tried to identify clinical or image-based risk factors for the success or failure of nonoperative management. Nicholson and colleagues described a system to predict the potential success of the nonoperative treatment of insertional Achilles tendinosis dependent on the degree of involvement of the tendon based on MRI [15]. Type I involvement (tendon thickening <8 mm with nonuniform intramural splits) had the greatest chance of success (87.5%), while greater tendon involvement with confluent areas of intrasubstance signal changes indicative of intramural degeneration (types II and III) responded more poorly to conservative management with failure rates up to 90%. Stenson et al. identified four clinical factors that correlated with failing nonoperative treatment: worse visual analog scale scores, limited ankle range of motion, previous corticosteroid injection, and the presence of Achilles tendon enthesophyte [16]. As the number of these risk factors increased, so did the chance of failing nonoperative treatment. The early identification of these patients and appropriate anticipatory guidance, including an earlier discussion of surgical interventions, may result in improved satisfaction and functional outcomes. In regard to tendon ossification or a Haglund's deformity, these do not necessarily produce pain and may be identified incidentally [6, 7].

In general, the indications for the surgical treatment of insertional Achilles tendinopathy are persisting pain and limitations in daily activities and/or sports activities despite exhausting conservative measures. In elderly patients who present with chronic symptoms, patients with significant tendon involvement, patients with the aforementioned risk factors, and those with partial or impending tears, operative intervention may be considered earlier in the treatment course. Contraindications to surgical intervention include arterial insufficiency; poor skin and soft tissues, with an active heel wound considered a strict contraindication; poorly controlled comorbidities, particularly diabetes; and inability to comply with a postoperative protocol. Preoperative education and optimization in patients with diabetes or tobacco dependence should include glycemic control and smoking cessation.

Operative Techniques

Approaches and Techniques

The surgical technique must address all pathology that is producing the pain, and one should consider the degree and severity of tendon involvement, the presence and extent of calcification, and the presence of a prominent posterosuperior calcaneus, retrocalcaneal bursitis, or equinus deformity. Multiple surgical approaches have been described, and the posterior midline transtendinous approach has become the most commonly utilized [17, 18]. Some historical and less common approaches include a lateral incision, medial J-shaped or vertical incision, dual medial and lateral incisions, and a transverse (Cincinnati) incision. Additionally, endoscopic and percutaneous techniques are becoming increasingly common.

Recent literature has suggested that the transtendinous approach allows for adequate exposure of the most commonly diseased area of the tendon and the calcaneal exostosis, with excellent postoperative pain and functional results [19–27]. This transtendinous approach also allows optimal visualization and debridement of the intrasubstance tendinosis and calcification. It is suggested that this approach is the safest in terms of blood supply and healing potential. A review of the angiosomes of the hindfoot by Attinger et al. demonstrates that the midline transtendinous approach divides the peroneal angiosome from the posterior tibial angiosome, thereby preventing injury to the distal angiosome boundaries [28]. Additionally, the concern with scar formation and shoe irritation using the central approach

is offset by the decompression of the posterior heel that occurs with this approach [10].

Irrespective of surgical approach, the operative strategy for insertional Achilles tendinopathy is the removal of the degenerative tendon and decompression of the posterior heel via excision of the inflamed retrocalcaneal bursa and resection of the prominent posterior calcaneal prominence. While tendon-sparing techniques have been described, adequate debridement of the Achilles tendon typically requires splitting the tendon and some amount of detachment from the calcaneal insertion; anywhere from partial to complete detachment has been described. The number of tendons that can be safely detached and debrided has been debated. Kolodziej et al. performed a biomechanical study releasing the tendon in different directions and increments and subsequently performed repeated cyclic loading of three times body weight [2]. After performing 75% superior-to-inferior resection, 88.9% ($n = 8$ of 9) of the specimen remained intact after the cyclic loading. Wagner et al. demonstrated that a complete detachment and reconstruction of the Achilles tendon with a proximal V-Y lengthening and suture anchor reattachment does not decrease the working capacity of the gastric-soleus muscle and plantarflexion strength is maintained [29]. Thus, both clinical and biomechanical studies support the safety of tendon detachment from its insertion when required.

When greater than 50% of the Achilles tendon is detached from the calcaneus, a repair of the reflected tendon with suture anchors is recommended [30, 31]. There are various techniques to repair the tendon back to its insertion on the calcaneus. Anywhere from one to four anchors have been described, utilizing single- or double-row repair, and a variety of anchor and suture types. Recent clinical and biomechanical evidence supports the benefits of a double-row repair. In a retrospective review of 40 patients who underwent surgery for insertional Achilles tendinopathy, Ettinger et al. reported that patients treated with two suture anchors or the double-row fixation technique have significantly improved American Orthopaedic Foot and

Ankle Society (AOFAS) and Foot and Ankle Outcome Score (FAOS) scores compared to those with single anchor fixation [32]. Recent biomechanical evidence demonstrated that a double-row repair results in a significantly larger contact area and leads to a significantly higher peak load to failure compared to a single-row repair [31]. Given this evidence, the increased footprint area of the tendon on the calcaneal tuberosity afforded by the double-row construct confers the theoretical benefit of improved fixation and may allow for earlier weight-bearing and rehabilitation [19]. The postoperative protocols also vary significantly between providers, from immobilization and non-weight-bearing to early range of motion and weight-bearing. There is limited level 1 evidence to support the superiority of any surgical techniques or postoperative protocol.

Posterior Midline Transtendinous Approach and Repair Technique

The most established surgical treatment utilizes a posterior midline transtendinous approach; partial or complete tendon detachment from the insertion; debridement of the diseased tendon, including all pathologic calcification; resection of the retrocalcaneal bursa; calcaneal exostectomy of the prominent posterosuperior process; and repair of the healthy residual Achilles tendon to the calcaneus. A deep tendon transfer, most commonly with the flexor hallucis longus (FHL), may also be performed in more severe or revision cases. If this is necessary, another advantage of the transtendinous approach is easy access to the FHL tendon through this same incision.

The patient undergoes appropriate anesthesia, commonly regional blocks with sedation or general anesthesia. A more proximal block, such as a sciatic nerve block, allows for the preferred thigh tourniquet. Additionally, general anesthesia with a popliteal block for postoperative pain control may also be considered. A popliteal block alone with sedation would necessitate a calf tourniquet and may interfere with the mobilization of the

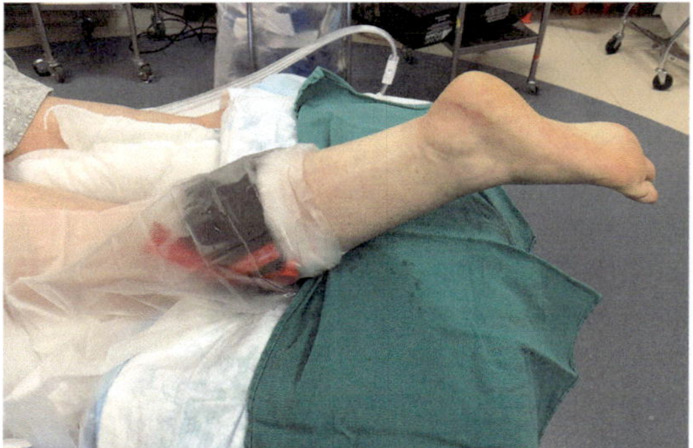

Fig. 16.3 Patient positioning. The patient is positioned prone, and a calf tourniquet is utilized

gastrocnemius/soleus complex. Preoperative intravenous antibiotics are recommended. A thigh tourniquet is placed with the patient supine prior to positioning. The patient is positioned prone, and bony prominences are well padded. The patient should be distal enough on the table so the surgeon can comfortably operate from the foot of the bed with the foot suspended freely (Fig. 16.3). The operative leg is exsanguinated with an elastic bandage and the tourniquet inflated to 250–300 mmHg. Ensure to minimize excessive leg manipulation and putting undue stress on the patient's lumbar spine'. A towel or foam bump may be placed under the foot to slightly flex the knee.

The Achilles tendon is palpated, and a 5–10 cm posterior longitudinal incision is marked at the midline of the Achilles tendon and calcaneus. The incision should extend distally to where the nonglabrous tissue meets the glabrous plantar skin. This allows safe distal exposure for Haglund's resection and anchor placement (Fig. 16.4).

The skin and subcutaneous tissue are incised with a 15-blade scalpel, and full-thickness flaps are maintained. The paratenon is split at the midline of the Achilles tendon, in line with the skin incision. Full-thickness paratenon flaps are raised medially and laterally with the scalpel and preserved to allow for later closure (Fig. 16.5). A longitudinal, full-thickness split is then made in the midline of the Achilles tendon with a horizontal "T" at the distal-most aspect of the insertion to

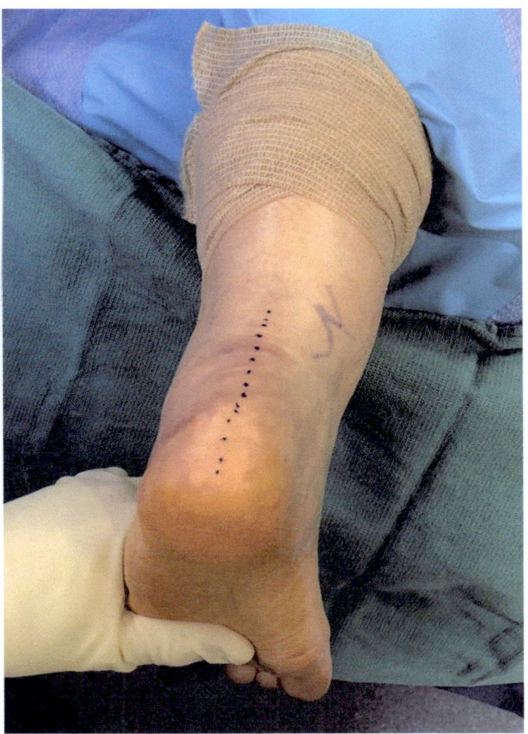

Fig. 16.4 The planned surgical incision for a posterior midline transtendinous approach. The incision must extend distal enough to the glabrous plantar skin to allow access to the calcaneus

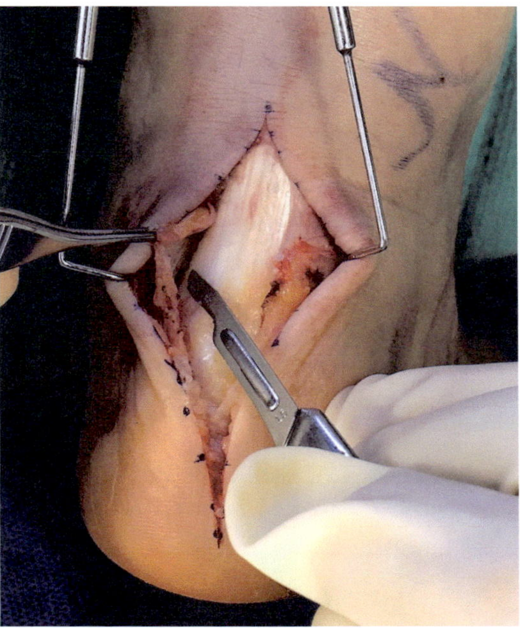

Fig. 16.5 The paratenon is longitudinally incised and carefully dissected from the Achilles tendon. This creates full-thickness medial and lateral paratenon flaps to allow proper repair upon closure

accommodate lifting medial and lateral distal limbs (Fig. 16.6). This allows for adequate exposure to the degenerative tendon, ectopic calcification, retrocalcaneal bursitis, and Haglund's deformity. During exposure, it is imperative to avoid undue tension on the skin edges to prevent wound complications. We recommend double-prong skin hooks, a spring retractor, or a Gelpi retractor for deep soft tissue retraction without direct pressure on the skin edges.

The inflamed retrocalcaneal bursa is then excised given its contribution to the disease process and for improved visualization (Fig. 16.7). To facilitate adequate bony decompression and the debridement of the diseased tendon, a proportion of the Achilles tendon is partially detached. Beginning centrally at the horizontal "T" created, the insertion is released laterally and medially by sharply elevating the Sharpey's fibers directly from the calcaneus using a 15-blade scalpel

(Fig. 16.8). Biomechanical and clinical studies demonstrate that 50% of the Achilles insertion may be elevated without compromising insertional strength or the risk of avulsion [2, 33]. It has become a routine practice to detach about 50–75% of the tendon with subsequent suture anchor repair back to the insertion on the calcaneus. Using sharp subperiosteal dissection, the insertional fibers of the Achilles tendon are detached from their insertion to better expose the calcaneus and anterior tendon fibers.

If present, the enthesophyte should be removed using a rongeur, rasp, or saw (Fig. 16.9). The exostectomy is then performed to remove Haglund's deformity. Then the prominent posterolateral bone on the superior calcaneus ridge is located. At this stage, deep gelpie retractors or Hohmann retractors placed between the remaining Achilles attachments and the calcaneus medially and laterally help to facilitate exposure without compromising the skin. Using an oscillating saw, chisel, or osteotome, exostectomy is performed from posterior-inferior to anterior-

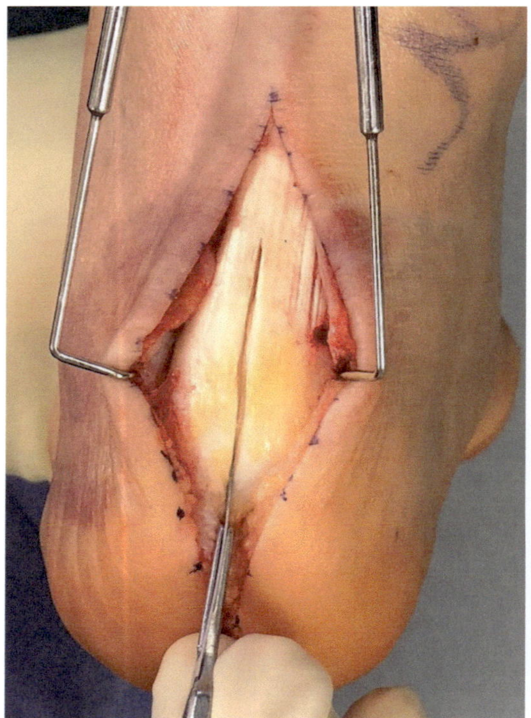

Fig. 16.6 A longitudinal, full-thickness split is made in the midline of the Achilles tendon

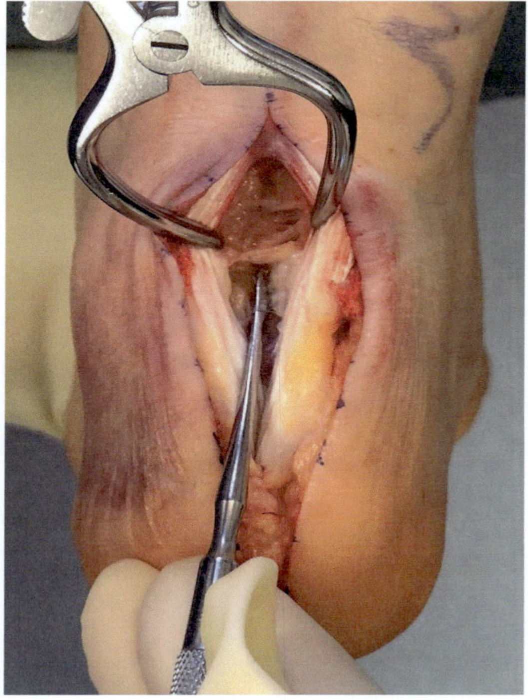

Fig. 16.7 The inflamed retrocalcaneal bursa is visualized anterior to the Achilles tendon and excised

superior, exiting the superior aspect of the calcaneus (Fig. 16.10). The medial and lateral aspect of the posterior calcaneus should also be resected in a "chamfer" fashion, further decompressing the space. After adequate bony resection, the cut distal edges of the calcaneus are then smoothed with a rasp or feathered with a saw blade. The adequacy of the bony resection is confirmed by both direct visualization and fluoroscopic lateral heel imaging (Fig. 16.11).

The tendon is then inspected and palpated. All areas of intratendinous degeneration and calcification are sharply excised until only a healthy tendon remains (Fig. 16.12). The distal portion of the Achilles tendon is then reattached to the calcaneus with suture anchors. Given the earlier bony resection, the posterior calcaneus is now a smooth surface of the cancellous bone, which helps facilitate the healing of the tendon back to the calcaneus. Anywhere from two to four suture

anchors with nonabsorbable suture can be utilized for reattachment (Fig. 16.13). Irrespective of the anchor type used, satisfactory fixation may be confirmed by the ability to lift the lower leg by the anchors' sutures.

With the foot held in neutral to slight plantarflexion, the medial and lateral sutures are then passed through the Achilles tendon (Fig. 16.14). The two suture limbs from the medial anchor are passed through the far medial aspect of the medial limb of the detached tendon. Similarly, the two suture limbs from the lateral anchor are passed through the far lateral aspect of the lateral limb of the detached tendon. The two suture limbs from each anchor are tied to one another, securing the tendon back to the calcaneus. Care should be taken to repair the tendon in a neutral ankle position with a tension-free repair. To achieve a tension-free repair, drape the detached limbs of the Achilles tendon over the suture anchors prior to repair; the sutures should exit the Achilles ten-

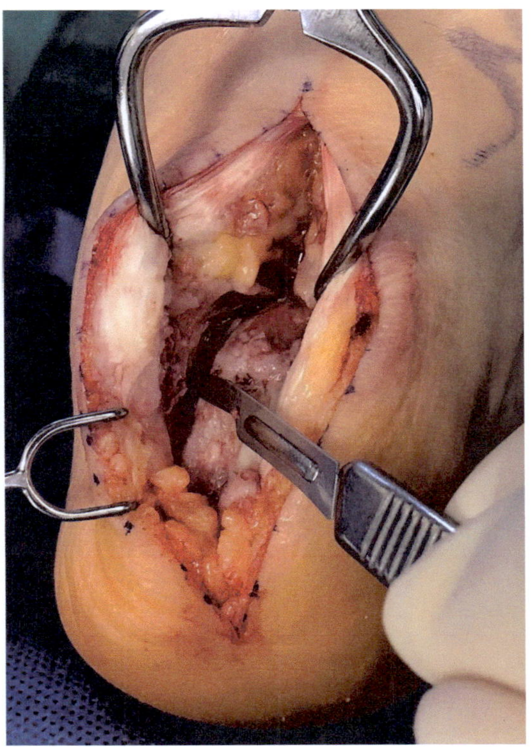

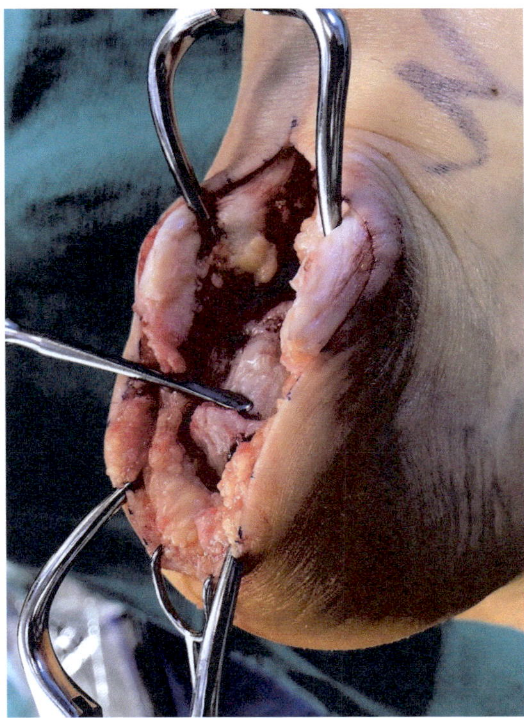

Fig. 16.8 The Achilles tendon insertion is partially detached from the calcaneus using sharp subperiosteal dissection, creating medial and lateral limbs

Fig. 16.9 The freer elevator is localizing an enthesophyte at the distal Achilles insertion, which was subsequently resected with a rongeur

don from anterior to posterior at the level of the anchor. Suturing the tendon too proximally would overtension the tendon, while suturing the tendon too distally would result in a loose repair. Additionally, passing the sutures out of the far lateral and far medial aspects of the tendon prevents prominent suture knots under the incision.

The wound is thoroughly irrigated prior to closure. The longitudinally split Achilles's fibers are then loosely reapproximated with buried absorbable sutures in an interrupted or running fashion. Care should be taken to avoid any prominent suture knots. The paratenon is then reapproximated with an absorbable suture. The subcutaneous tissue and skin are then closed. Again, gentle manipulation of the skin with judicial use of forceps should be a priority to prevent wound-healing issues.

Postoperatively, the patient is immobilized in a well-padded short-leg splint or controlled ankle

motion (CAM) boot with the ankle in 10° of plantarflexion to minimize tension on the repair. The splint is removed at 2 weeks postoperatively for wound inspection and suture removal. The postoperative protocol varies depending on the treating physician's preference and the extent of repair. The leg is again reimmobilized in a splint, cast, or CAM boot for an additional 2–4 weeks. Some surgeons may allow protected weight-bearing in a plantarflexed CAM boot or cast at 3 or 4 weeks; however, others maintain non-weight-bearing for a total of 6 weeks. Gentle range of motion may begin 4–6 weeks postoperatively. The patient may begin weight-bearing as tolerated around 4–6 weeks postoperatively in a removable CAM boot with a heel lift. Heel lifts are recommended for the first 4–8 weeks of weight-bearing to minimize the tension on the repair. It is recommended to start with a larger heel lift and gradually decrease the height of the lift every 1–2 weeks. Unrestricted weight-bearing

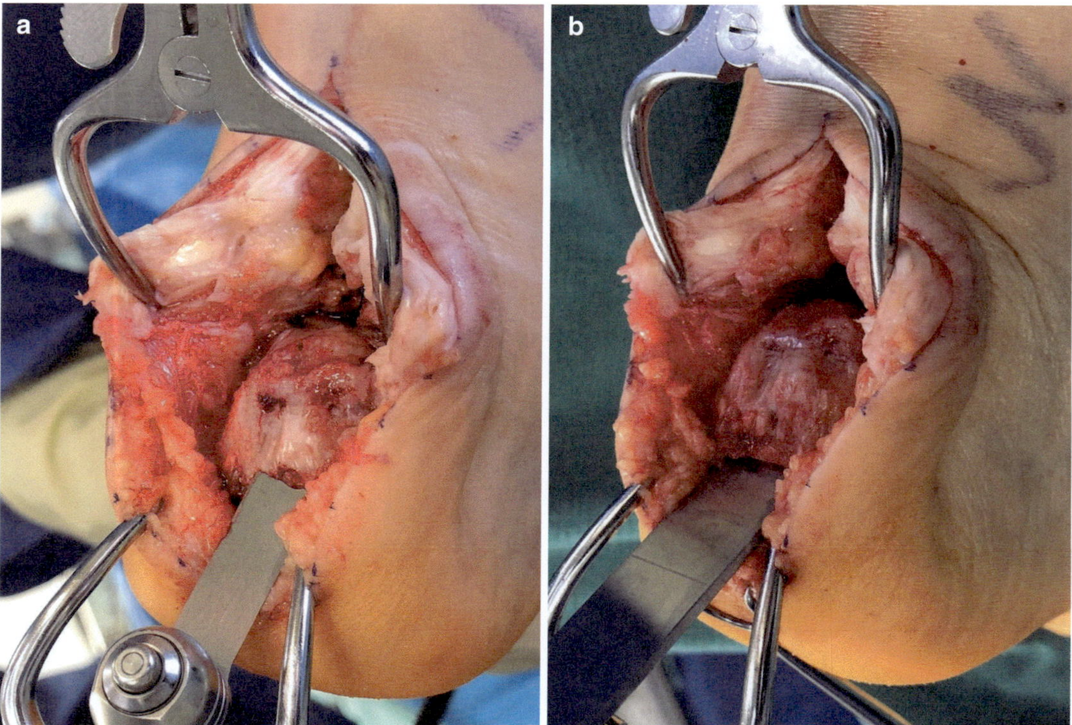

Fig. 16.10 (**a**) Haglund's deformity exostectomy is performed using an oscillating saw from posterior-inferior to anterior-superior, exiting the superior aspect of the calcaneus. (**b**). Haglund's deformity exostectomy is completed with a straight osteotome

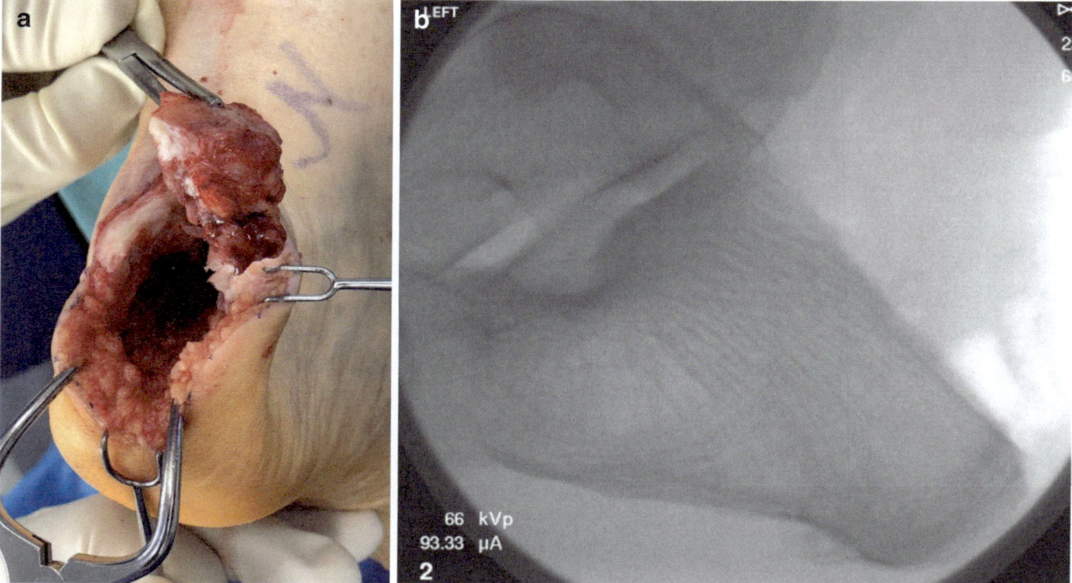

Fig. 16.11 (**a**) The resected Haglund's deformity removed from the posterosuperior calcaneus. (**b**) Intraoperative lateral heel fluoroscopic imaging confirming adequate resection of Haglund's deformity

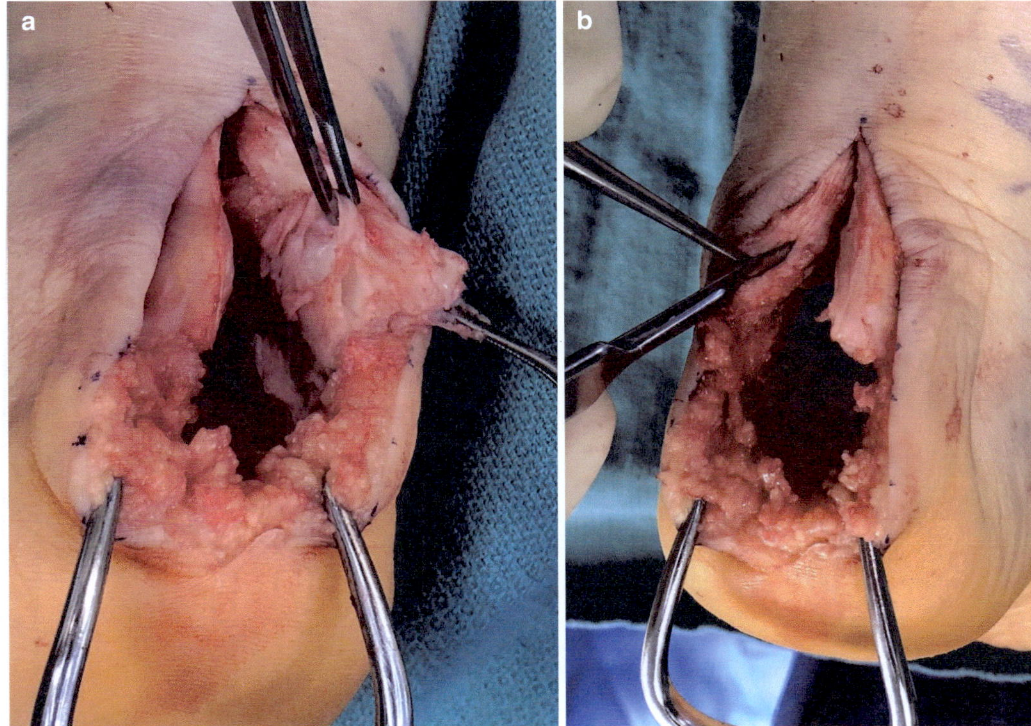

Fig. 16.12 (**a**) Degenerative changes of the anterior Achilles tendon evidenced by tendon fraying, a loss of uniform parallel tendon structure, and intratendinous cal-cification. (**b**). Sharp excision of all degenerative tendon and intratendinous calcification is performed

should not ensue until a minimum of 6–8 weeks after surgery. Plantarflexion strengthening begins around 10–12 weeks postoperatively. Athletic activity should be restricted until about 4–6 months. Physical therapy may be recommended postoperatively for gait training, gentle ankle range of motion exercise, an eccentric stretching protocol, and a graduated gastrocnemius-soleus strengthening program. Patients should be counseled preoperatively that this surgery necessitates a prolonged recovery of 6–12 months.

When to Augment with an FHL Transfer

The FHL tendon has been described as an effective transfer to augment a deficient Achilles tendon. The FHL transfer was first described in 1993 by Wapner et al. for the repair of chronic Achilles tendon rupture [34]. This technique has been advocated for use in patients with insertional Achilles tendinopathy in the setting of more severe tendinosis, in patients older than 50 years old, and in patients with a high body mass index (BMI) [23, 35–37]. The FHL tendon is recruited because of its close proximity to the Achilles tendon, its large size, its strong vascular supply, its function as a secondary plantarflexor, and the fact that it is in-phase with the gastrocnemius-soleus muscle to provide a synergistic effect to the Achilles tendon [38]. The theoretical benefit of FHL augmentation is mechanical support to protect the reattached Achilles tendon, with the addition of a muscle with significant volume and strength. It is also believed that the low-laying muscle belly may optimize the healing response by perfusing the healing Achilles tendon [39]. FHL can be harvested through the posterior trans-

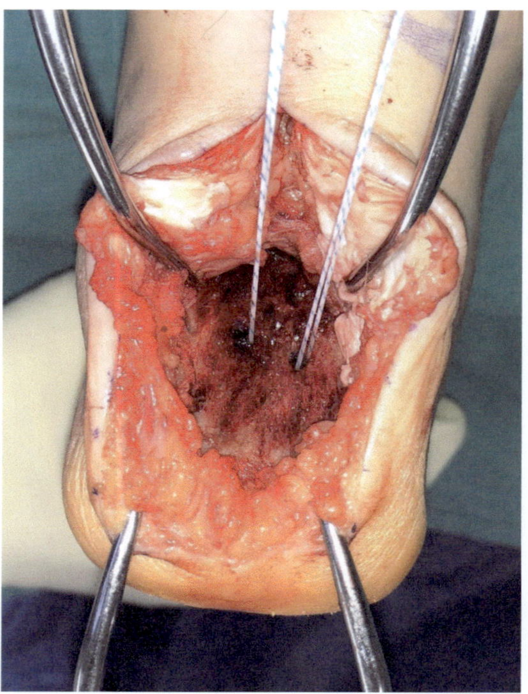

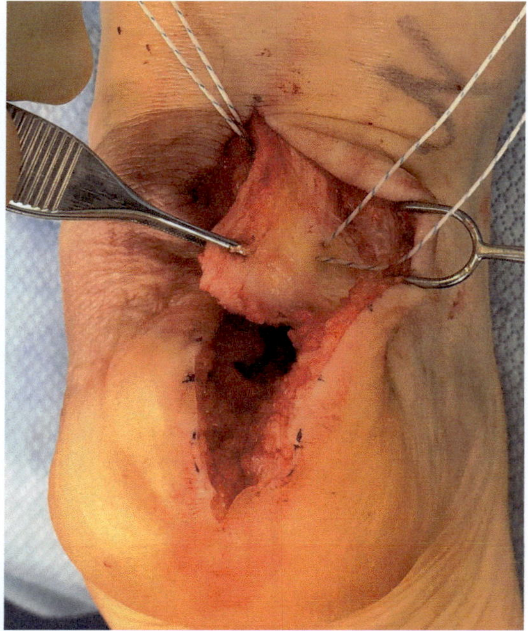

Fig. 16.14 The foot is placed in neutral ankle dorsiflexion to slight plantarflexion. The two suture limbs from the medial anchor are passed through the far medial aspect of the medial limb of the detached tendon. The two medial suture anchor limbs are tied together. This is repeated for the lateral anchor and lateral limb of the detached tendon

Fig. 16.13 Two suture anchors are utilized for a single-row repair. The anchors are drilled and then placed in the bed of the bleeding cancellous bone created by Haglund's deformity resection at the posterior calcaneus

tendinous incision; however, harvesting through a separate more plantar and distal incision yields an FHL greater than 4 cm in length [40]. Augmentation with FHL became increasingly common for older or overweight patients with extensive insertional Achilles tendon disease and in the setting of revision surgery. Good results have been presented in the case of a series of patients treated with FHL augmentation [35–37, 41]. Additionally, while there was initial concern for the loss of hallux flexion strength, Hunt et al. and Schon et al. found that FHL transfer does not affect hallux strength or balance [27, 37].

An FHL tendon transfer was routinely recommended if debridement of greater than 50–75% was performed for either insertional or noninsertional Achilles tendinopathy. Schmidtberg et al. performed a biomechanical study demonstrating that an FHL transfer significantly increased the load to failure of the Achilles tendon with a noninsertional defect involving 25%, 50%, and 75%

of the tendon width. The mechanism of failure was usually through the defect in the specimens with a 50% or 75% defect, supporting the use of FHL augmentation with debridement of greater than 50% [42]. This technique has commonly been extrapolated to insertional disease as well.

This common practice was later challenged by a prospective randomized controlled trial performed by Hunt et al. to determine if FHL augmentation was associated with superior clinical outcome scores and greater ankle plantarflexion strength compared with Achilles debridement alone [27]. This investigation studied pain (visual analog scale (VAS)), functional outcome (AOFAS), patient satisfaction, plantarflexion strength, and complications of patients with and without FHL transfer. They reported that there was greater ankle plantarflexion strength in the FHL group at 6 months and 1 year compared with the control group; however, pain, functional outcome, satisfaction, and complications were similar between the two groups. Thus, while ankle plantarflexion strength appeared to be improved with FHL transfer, the strength may not translate to a meaningful clinical difference or benefit, and FHL transfer may not be necessary for primary cases. Following these findings, it is becoming increasingly recognized that FHL transfer is not indicated as a primary procedure but should be considered for failed treatment.

Endoscopic Bursectomy and Calcaneoplasty

With the advent of improved endoscopy techniques and an increased focus on minimally invasive techniques, endoscopic techniques have been described for the treatment of insertional Achilles tendinopathy. Endoscopic intervention is typically recommended in younger patients who do not have calcification or evidence of substantial intratendinous changes on MRI. In general, endoscopic debridement should be avoided in patients with bone formation within the distal Achilles tendon insertion, and rather open debridement is indicated. However, there are authors who describe and advocate for combined endoscopic and minimally invasive approaches that address all facets of insertional Achilles tendinosis: endoscopic calcaneoplasty; percutaneous dorsal closing wedge calcaneal osteotomy; endoscopic debridement of the ventral surface of the Achilles tendon; endoscopic debridement of the Achilles insertion; endoscopic gastrocnemius with or without soleus aponeurotic recession; endoscopic-assisted FHL transfer; endoscopic subcutaneous adventitial Achilles bursa resection; and resection of diseased tendon segment, minimally invasive gastrocnemius-soleus aponeurotic recession, and reattachment of Achilles tendon [43].

In a level II prospective study comparing endoscopic decompression of the retrocalcaneal space to open techniques in patients with the same diagnostic criteria, Leitze et al. reported that endoscopic decompression produces final results equal to or better than those of an open technique, with a similar recovery time, fewer complications, and a better cosmetic appearance [44]. A systematic review of 35 studies and 1260 ankles summarized endoscopic procedures and demonstrated better final AOFAS, a lower rate of complications and failures, and shorter recovery time when compared to open techniques [45]. However, it is important to recognize the limitations of such conclusions, including heterogeneous patient populations and selection bias for patients undergoing open versus endoscopic procedures. Moreover, despite the limited case series, it may not be possible to entirely remove the enthesophyte, Haglund's prominence, or all diseased tissues in patients with full-thickness intratendinous calcifications via an endoscopic approach. Therefore, for less familiar surgeons, endoscopic techniques may be more appropriate for patients with a disease characterized primarily by the enlargement of the posterior superior calcaneal tuberosity. A further large-scale and comparative prospective study is needed to further evaluate the safety and efficacy of these minimally invasive procedures.

Zadek Osteotomy

A Zadek osteotomy is a dorsal closing wedge osteotomy of the posterior calcaneus. The procedure was first described by Zadek in 1939 [46]. Since this time, multiple authors have reported positive outcomes with both open [47–49] and percutaneous [43, 50] Zadek osteotomy techniques. Tourne et al. recently provided a radiographic analysis to explain the efficacy of the Zadek osteotomy, theorizing that it improves the functional and clinical results in Haglund's syndrome due to the change of the shape and position of the calcaneus [9]. They theorize that the osteotomy reduces the overall length of the calcaneus, elevates the insertion of the Achilles tendon, tilts the heel prominence anteriorly, and decreases the vertical position of the calcaneus. Thus, the lever arm of the Achilles tendon is shortened, leading to a reduction of tension at the Achilles insertion [9].

The Zadek osteotomy has resulted in positive outcomes in patients with calcific insertional pathology [49] as well as athletes [48]. Maffulli et al. studied the outcomes of a modified Zadek osteotomy, without excision of the intratendinous calcification, in patients with calcific insertional Achilles tendinopathy; they reported successful union in all 25 patients at an average of 5 weeks, return to normal activities at 23 weeks, significant improvement in VAS pain scores and the Victorian Institute of Sports Assessment-Achilles (VISA-A) scores up to 2 years, and minimal complications [49]. Georgiannos et al. reported outcomes of the Zadek osteotomy in 52 athletes with painful insertional Achilles pathology; they similarly reported significant improvements in AOFAS and VISA-A scores with a return to previous sports activity at 21 weeks [48]. In one of the largest series of 50 patients with 7-year follow-up, Tourne et al. report excellent clinical and functional outcomes following Zadek calcaneal osteotomy in addition to an exostosectomy for Haglund's syndrome of the heel [9]. Others who challenge these theories and outcomes share a common concern that osteotomy does not address the true pathology, and no direct intervention of the tendon is performed.

Y-V Advancement

Achilles V-Y advancement was originally described by Abraham and Pankovich in 1975 [51] for the repair of neglected Achilles tendon ruptures. In this procedure, the diseased tendon is excised, and a V-shaped incision is made in the tendon aponeurosis, allowing the tendon to lengthen distally and reconnect to the calcaneus. With extensive insertional Achilles degeneration, complete debridement and excision of the distal Achilles tendon may be required, and a V-Y advancement allows for direct repair back to the calcaneus. Investigators popularizing this technique report that this comprehensive approach results in high patient satisfaction and does not compromise the working capacity of the gastric-soleus muscle [29, 52, 53]. In a comparative study of FHL transfer and V-Y advancement for chronic insertional Achilles tendinopathy performed by Staggers et al., the authors reported

similar high satisfaction rates, positive functional outcomes, and low complication rates in both operative groups [52]. An FHL tendon transfer and V-Y advancement may be performed in conjunction in advanced diseased stages; however, both autograft and allograft reconstruction techniques are available as well.

Gastrocnemius Recession

For patients with a gastrocnemius contracture, a gastrocnemius procedure should be performed in combination with open debridement. Conflicting low-level evidence, including a small number of retrospective case series, exist regarding the use of isolated gastrocnemius release for the treatment of insertional Achilles tendinopathy. Proponents report that an isolated gastrocnemius recession for chronic insertional Achilles tendinopathy can provide high satisfaction, pain relief, and a faster recovery period with few or no complications [54, 55]. However, Gurdezi et al. reported that an isolated gastrocnemius recession may be less efficacious in patients with heel spurs [56]. Moreover, a gastrocnemius recession may not be appropriate for athletic patients given the subsequent deficits in plantarflexion power and endurance [55]. Additional investigations are warranted to understand the efficacy of an isolated gastrocnemius recession or as an adjunct to other operative procedures in the treatment of Achilles pathology.

Complications

The complication rate following operative repair ranges widely in the current literature, from a series with no complications reported to others with complication rates up to 30% [57]. In a systematic review by Wiegerinck et al., they reported an overall major complication rate of 3.1% and a minor complication rate of 20%; however, this included multiple different approaches and was not limited to the now more commonly accepted posterior transtendinous approach [58]. Horterer et al. recently reported complications associated with the posterior transtendinous incision in 118 patients with a minimum of 12 months follow-up [20]. Complications included 14% with a minor complication, the majority (75%) of which were surgical site infections. The satisfaction rate was 78%. Shoe conflict, reported in 32% of patients, was the factor identified to negatively affect patient satisfaction. The most commonly reported complications include delayed wound healing, superficial infection, scar hypertrophy or hypersensitivity, sural nerve injury or sural neuritis, the persistence or recurrence of insertional pain, and deep vein thrombosis [59]. Wound-healing issues tend to be one of the most common complications following surgery; therefore, gentle skin and soft tissue handling is fundamental to any surgical technique.

Overall Outcomes

The consistently good postoperative outcomes across a range of level I– IV studies, despite variations in surgical techniques, continue to support the use of operative treatment for insertional Achilles tendinopathy when conservative measures have failed [18, 59]. Postoperative patient-reported outcomes, including patient satisfaction, self-reported function, and pain are generally positive following operative treatment. Postoperative AOFAS ankle-hindfoot scores range from 81 to 96 [57], and an average patient satisfaction of 89% has been reported [58]. Nunley et al. reported the longest follow-up to date with clinical outcomes of 29 ankles following the posterior transtendinous technique at an average of 7 years postoperative [25]. Their cohort resulted in an average recovery time of 5.7 months, an average AOFAS hindfoot score of 96, a 96% satisfaction rate, and no significant difference in plantarflexion strength compared to the nonoperative side. Overall, patients with insertional Achilles tendinopathy refractory to conservative measures experience positive results following operative intervention.

References

1. O'Brien M. The anatomy of the Achilles tendon. Foot Ankle Clin. 2005;10(2):225–38.
2. Kolodziej P, Glisson RR, Nunley JA. Risk of avulsion of the Achilles tendon after partial excision for treatment of insertional tendonitis and Haglund's deformity: a biomechanical study. Foot Ankle Int. 1999;20(7):433–7.
3. Frey C, Rosenberg Z, Shereff MJ, Kim H. The retrocalcaneal bursa: anatomy and bursography. Foot Ankle. 1992;13(4):203–7.
4. 49:49. HP. Beitrag zur Klinik der Achillesssshne. Zeitschr Orthop Chir. 1928;49:49–58.
5. Lyman J, Weinhold PS, Almekinders LC. Strain behavior of the distal achilles tendon: implications for insertional achilles tendinopathy. Am J Sports Med. 2004;32(2):457–61.
6. Kang S, Thordarson DB, Charlton TP. Insertional Achilles tendinitis and Haglund's deformity. Foot Ankle Int. 2012;33(6):487–91.
7. Lu CC, Cheng YM, Fu YC, Tien YC, Chen SK, Huang PJ. Angle analysis of Haglund syndrome and its relationship with osseous variations and Achilles tendon calcification. Foot Ankle Int. 2007;28(2):181–5.
8. Klauser AS, Miyamoto H, Tamegger M, et al. Achilles tendon assessed with sonoelastography: histologic agreement. Radiology. 2013;267(3):837–42.
9. Tourne Y, Baray AL, Barthelemy R, Karhao T, Moroney P. The Zadek calcaneal osteotomy in Haglund's syndrome of the heel: clinical results and a radiographic analysis to explain its efficacy. Foot Ankle Surg. 2021;28:79.
10. DeOrio MJ, Easley ME. Surgical strategies: insertional achilles tendinopathy. Foot Ankle Int. 2008;29(5):542–50.
11. Waldecker U, Hofmann G, Drewitz S. Epidemiologic investigation of 1394 feet: coincidence of hindfoot malalignment and Achilles tendon disorders. Foot Ankle Surg. 2012;18(2):119–23.
12. Kvist M. Achilles tendon injuries in athletes. Ann Chir Gynaecol. 1991;80(2):188–201.
13. Schepsis AA, Jones H, Haas AL. Achilles tendon disorders in athletes. Am J Sports Med. 2002;30(2):287–305.
14. Holmes GB, Lin J. Etiologic factors associated with symptomatic achilles tendinopathy. Foot Ankle Int. 2006;27(11):952–9.
15. Nicholson CW, Berlet GC, Lee TH. Prediction of the success of nonoperative treatment of insertional Achilles tendinosis based on MRI. Foot Ankle Int. 2007;28(4):472–7.
16. Stenson JF, Reb CW, Daniel JN, Saini SS, Albana MF. Predicting failure of nonoperative treatment for insertional Achilles tendinosis. Foot Ankle Spec. 2018;11(3):252–5.
17. Barg A, Ludwig T. Surgical strategies for the treatment of insertional Achilles tendinopathy. Foot Ankle Clin. 2019;24(3):533–59.

18. Moen R, Hagenbucher JR, Shinabarger AB. Surgical treatment of insertional Achilles tendinopathy: a systematic review. J Am Podiatr Med Assoc. 2020;110(5):131.

19. Shakked RJ, Raikin SM. Insertional tendinopathy of the Achilles: debridement, primary repair, and when to augment. Foot Ankle Clin. 2017;22(4):761–80.

20. Hörterer H, Baumbach SF, Oppelt S, et al. Complications associated with midline incision for insertional Achilles tendinopathy. Foot Ankle Int. 2020;41(12):1502–9.

21. Miao XD, Jiang H, Wu YP, Tao HM, Yang DS, Hu H. Treatment of calcified insertional Achilles tendinopathy by the posterior midline approach. J Foot Ankle Surg. 2016;55(3):529–34.

22. McAlister JE, Hyer CF. Safety of achilles detachment and reattachment using a standard midline approach to insertional enthesophytes. J Foot Ankle Surg. 2015;54(2):214–9.

23. McGarvey WC, Palumbo RC, Baxter DE, Leibman BD. Insertional Achilles tendinosis: surgical treatment through a central tendon splitting approach. Foot Ankle Int. 2002;23(1):19–25.

24. Ahn JH, Ahn CY, Byun CH, Kim YC. Operative treatment of Haglund syndrome with central Achilles tendon-splitting approach. J Foot Ankle Surg. 2015;54(6):1053–6.

25. Nunley JA, Ruskin G, Horst F. Long-term clinical outcomes following the central incision technique for insertional Achilles tendinopathy. Foot Ankle Int. 2011;32(9):850–5.

26. Johnson KW, Zalavras C, Thordarson DB. Surgical management of insertional calcific achilles tendinosis with a central tendon splitting approach. Foot Ankle Int. 2006;27(4):245–50.

27. Hunt KJ, Cohen BE, Davis WH, Anderson RB, Jones CP. Surgical treatment of insertional Achilles tendinopathy with or without flexor Hallucis longus tendon transfer: a prospective, randomized study. Foot Ankle Int. 2015;36(9):998–1005.

28. Attinger C, Cooper P, Blume P, Bulan E. The safest surgical incisions and amputations applying the angiosome principles and using the Doppler to assess the arterial-arterial connections of the foot and ankle. Foot Ankle Clin. 2001;6(4):745–99.

29. Wagner E, Gould J, Bilen E, Fleisig GS, Wilk K, Fowler R. Change in plantarflexion strength after complete detachment and reconstruction of the Achilles tendon. Foot Ankle Int. 2004;25(11):800–4.

30. Maffulli N, Testa V, Capasso G, Sullo A. Calcific insertional Achilles tendinopathy: reattachment with bone anchors. Am J Sports Med. 2004;32(1):174–82.

31. Beitzel K, Mazzocca AD, Obopilwe E, et al. Biomechanical properties of double- and single-row suture anchor repair for surgical treatment of insertional Achilles tendinopathy. Am J Sports Med. 2013;41(7):1642–8.

32. Ettinger S, Razzaq R, Waizy H, et al. Operative treatment of the insertional Achilles tendinopathy through a transtendinous approach. Foot Ankle Int. 2016;37(3):288–93.

33. Calder JD, Saxby TS. Surgical treatment of insertional Achilles tendinosis. Foot Ankle Int. 2003;24(2):119–21.

34. Wapner KL, Pavlock GS, Hecht PJ, Naselli F, Walther R. Repair of chronic Achilles tendon rupture with flexor hallucis longus tendon transfer. Foot Ankle. 1993;14(8):443–9.

35. Den Hartog BD. Flexor hallucis longus transfer for chronic Achilles tendonosis. Foot Ankle Int. 2003;24(3):233–7.

36. Elias I, Raikin SM, Besser MP, Nazarian LN. Outcomes of chronic insertional Achilles tendinosis using FHL autograft through single incision. Foot Ankle Int. 2009;30(3):197–204.

37. Schon LC, Shores JL, Faro FD, Vora AM, Camire LM, Guyton GP. Flexor hallucis longus tendon transfer in treatment of Achilles tendinosis. J Bone Joint Surg Am. 2013;95(1):54–60.

38. Gaston TE, Daniel JN. Achilles insertional tendinopathy-is there a gold standard? Arch Bone Jt Surg. 2021;9(1):5–8.

39. Martin RL, Manning CM, Carcia CR, Conti SF. An outcome study of chronic Achilles tendinosis after excision of the Achilles tendon and flexor hallucis longus tendon transfer. Foot Ankle Int. 2005;26(9):691–7.

40. Sakaki MH, Godoy-Santos AL, Ortiz RT, Araújo A, Fernandes TD. Flexor hallux tendon transfer: comparative study through double or single approach. Acta Ortop Bras. 2014;22(3):140–3.

41. Wegrzyn J, Luciani JF, Philippot R, Brunet-Guedj E, Moyen B, Besse JL. Chronic Achilles tendon rupture reconstruction using a modified flexor hallucis longus transfer. Int Orthop. 2010;34(8):1187–92.

42. Schmidtberg B, Johnson JD, Kia C, et al. Flexor Hallucis longus transfer improves Achilles tendon load to failure in surgery for non-insertional tendinopathy: a biomechanical study. J Bone Joint Surg Am. 2019;101(16):1505–12.

43. Lui TH, Lo CY, Siu YC. Minimally invasive and endoscopic treatment of Haglund syndrome. Foot Ankle Clin. 2019;24(3):515–31.

44. Leitze Z, Sella EJ, Aversa JM. Endoscopic decompression of the retrocalcaneal space. J Bone Joint Surg Am. 2003;85(8):1488–96.

45. Alessio-Mazzola M, Russo A, Capello AG, et al. Endoscopic calcaneoplasty for the treatment of Haglund's deformity provides better clinical functional outcomes, lower complication rate, and shorter recovery time compared to open procedures: a systematic review. Knee Surg Sports Traumatol Arthrosc. 2020;29:2462.

46. Zadek I. An operation for the cure of Achilloburistis. Am J Surg. 1939;43(2):542–6.

47. López-Capdevila L, Santamaria Fumas A, Dominguez Sevilla A, et al. Dorsal wedge calcaneal osteotomy as surgical treatment for insertional Achilles tendinopathy. Rev Esp Cir Ortop Traumatol. 2020;64(1):22–7.

48. Georgiannos D, Lampridis V, Vasiliadis A, Bisbinas I. Treatment of insertional Achilles pathology with dorsal wedge calcaneal osteotomy in athletes. Foot Ankle Int. 2017;38(4):381–7.

49. Maffulli N, Gougoulias N, D'Addona A, Oliva F, Maffulli GD. Modified Zadek osteotomy without excision of the intratendinous calcific deposit is effective for the surgical treatment of calcific insertional Achilles tendinopathy. Surgeon. 2020;19:e344.

50. Nordio A, Chan JJ, Guzman JZ, Hasija R, Vulcano E. Percutaneous Zadek osteotomy for the treatment of insertional Achilles tendinopathy. Foot Ankle Surg. 2020;26(7):818–21.

51. Abraham E, Pankovich AM. Neglected rupture of the Achilles tendon. Treatment by V-Y tendinous flap. J Bone Joint Surg Am. 1975;57(2):253–5.

52. Staggers JR, Smith K, de Netto CC, Naranje S, Prasad K, Shah A. Reconstruction for chronic Achilles tendinopathy: comparison of flexor hallucis longus (FHL) transfer versus V-Y advancement. Int Orthop. 2018;42(4):829–34.

53. Wagner E, Gould JS, Kneidel M, Fleisig GS, Fowler R. Technique and results of Achilles tendon detachment and reconstruction for insertional Achilles tendinosis. Foot Ankle Int. 2006;27(9):677–84.

54. Tallerico VK, Greenhagen RM, Lowery C. Isolated gastrocnemius recession for treatment of insertional Achilles tendinopathy: a pilot study. Foot Ankle Spec. 2015;8(4):260–5.

55. Nawoczenski DA, DiLiberto FE, Cantor MS, Tome JM, DiGiovanni BF. Ankle power and endurance outcomes following isolated gastrocnemius recession for Achilles tendinopathy. Foot Ankle Int. 2016;37(7):766–75.

56. Gurdezi S, Kohls-Gatzoulis J, Solan MC. Results of proximal medial gastrocnemius release for Achilles tendinopathy. Foot Ankle Int. 2013;34(10):1364–9.

57. Chimenti RL, Cychosz CC, Hall MM, Phisitkul P. Current concepts review update: insertional Achilles tendinopathy. Foot Ankle Int. 2017;38(10):1160–9.

58. Wiegerinck JI, Kerkhoffs GM, van Sterkenburg MN, Sierevelt IN, van Dijk CN. Treatment for insertional Achilles tendinopathy: a systematic review. Knee Surg Sports Traumatol Arthrosc. 2013;21(6):1345–55.

59. Irwin TA. Current concepts review: insertional achilles tendinopathy. Foot Ankle Int. 2010;31(10):933–9.

Part IV

Management of Acute and Chronic Achilles Complications

Reconstruction of Chronic Achilles Tendon Ruptures

17

Karl M. Schweitzer Jr and Rishin J. Kadakia

Introduction

Achilles tendon tears are a common injury encountered by a wide variety of healthcare providers. The reported incidence of acute Achilles tendon ruptures ranges from 5.5 to 18 per 100,000 individuals [1]. These injuries most commonly occur in younger, male patients and are typically sustained during recreational sporting activities. A recent study evaluating the epidemiology of Achilles tendon ruptures found that the incidence is rising, even for older patients [2]. The largest rise was seen in patients 40 to 59 years old [2]. This could be attributable to a more active, maturing population.

Despite being a common injury, Achilles tears are reportedly missed or diagnosed late in 25% of cases [3]. Misdiagnosis may be attributable to a failure of proper physical examination techniques and to understand anatomy. Plantarflexion, albeit weaker in a patient with a chronic Achilles rupture, is still maintained to some degree due to the action of other ankle flexor tendons. Furthermore, a palpable gap is not always present in the chronic setting.

While there is an ongoing controversy regarding the optimal management of acute Achilles tendon ruptures, chronic ruptures, however, are typically managed surgically using a variety of treatment options. A chronic Achilles rupture is typically defined as an untreated tear at least 4–6 weeks out from the initial injury [4, 5]. However, as some of these injuries are able to undergo a successful primary repair, a more practical definition may be a tendon rupture that requires additional or secondary measures in order to reapproximate the tendon ends [6].

Patients with chronic Achilles ruptures complain of persistent swelling, diminished push-off strength, gait abnormalities, and balance issues. A recent Swedish cost analysis and outcome study determined that the mean health care costs were notably higher for patients undergoing the surgical management of chronic Achilles tendon ruptures versus the costs associated with either the nonoperative or surgical management of acute tears [4]. Those patients undergoing reconstruction of their chronic Achilles rupture had improved ankle function at 1 year postoperatively. All of this demonstrates that missed or neglected Achilles tendon ruptures have both

K. M. Schweitzer Jr
Department of Orthopaedic Surgery, Duke University Medical Center, Duke Orthopaedics of Raleigh, Raleigh, NC, USA
e-mail: karl.schweitzer@duke.edu

R. J. Kadakia (✉)
Department of Orthopaedic Surgery, Emory University School of Medicine, Atlanta, GA, USA
e-mail: Rishin.j.kadakia@emory.edu

functional and economic consequences for patients and the health system [4].

While bracing and physical therapy may be the appropriate management option for some patients with chronic Achilles ruptures (e.g., patients determined to be poor surgery candidates or of lower functional demand), most patients with chronic Achilles ruptures undergo a surgical reconstruction with the goal of improving strength, balance, gait, and function. There are a host of described surgical procedures for use in these patients, depending on factors such as tendon gap size, tendon quality, the location of the rupture, and surgeon preference.

Diagnosis

The presentation of a patient with a chronic Achilles tendon rupture can differ dramatically from that of a patient with an acute tendon injury. Acute Achilles tendon tears present with a recent injury mechanism, patient discomfort, and a fairly discernable set of positive examination findings. Patients presenting with chronic ruptures have minimal discomfort but have more functional complaints. In the chronic setting, the patient's exam findings can be blunted, emphasizing the importance of maintaining a high index of suspicion for this diagnosis on the part of the evaluating provider.

Patients with chronic Achilles tendon ruptures complain of gait abnormalities, including difficulty and weakness with push-off. On examination, the rupture site may be palpable with retracted tendon stump ends, but in some patients, this defect can fill in with intervening scar tissue leading to an overall thickening to the normal Achilles tendon contour and the loss of the palpable gap sign. There is intact but weak ankle plantarflexion as there are functioning, secondary ankle plantarflexors, such as the peroneal, posterior tibialis, flexor hallucis longus, and flexor digitorum longus tendons. However, due to this relative loss of gastrocnemius-soleus strength, there is a reduced or loss of ability to perform repeated single-limb heel raises. There is notable calf atrophy with the loss of the normal gastrocnemius muscle contour, which can be compared to the normal contralateral side.

When there is suspicion of a chronic Achilles tendon rupture, further imaging can be important for clarifying the diagnosis. Standard ankle radiographs can be helpful, particularly a lateral view (Fig. 17.1) to demonstrate a loss in the normal posterior soft tissue density in the area of the Achilles tendon, consistent with an Achilles injury (i.e., loss in the definition of the Kager triangle [6, 7]). Additionally, it is not uncommon to see changes consistent with calcific tendinitis about the posterior heel, including a Haglund's prominence, calcifications along the course and/or insertion of the Achilles tendon, and perhaps sequelae from insertional or sleeve avulsion injuries leading to proximally migrated ossific fragments within the tendon [6, 7] (Fig. 17.2).

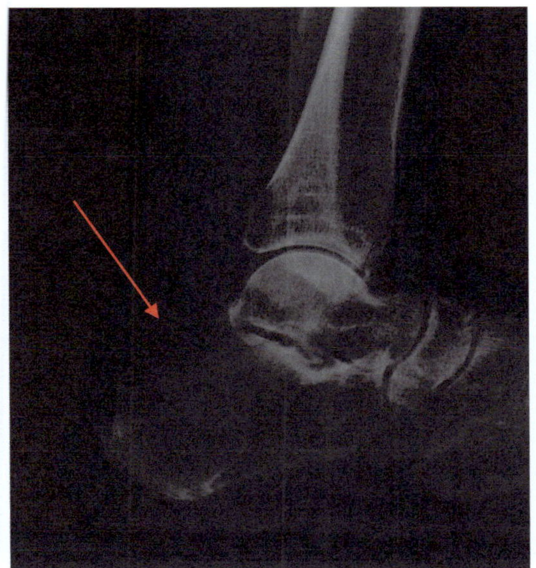

Fig. 17.1 Lateral ankle radiograph of a patient with a chronic Achilles rupture, demonstrating the loss of the normal posterior ankle soft tissue contours and shadowing (red arrow), commonly referred to as Kager's triangle. This area is typically sharply defined posteriorly by the anterior border of the Achilles tendon, anteriorly by the posterior border of the FHL tendon and muscle belly, and inferiorly by the dorsal aspect of the posterior calcaneus

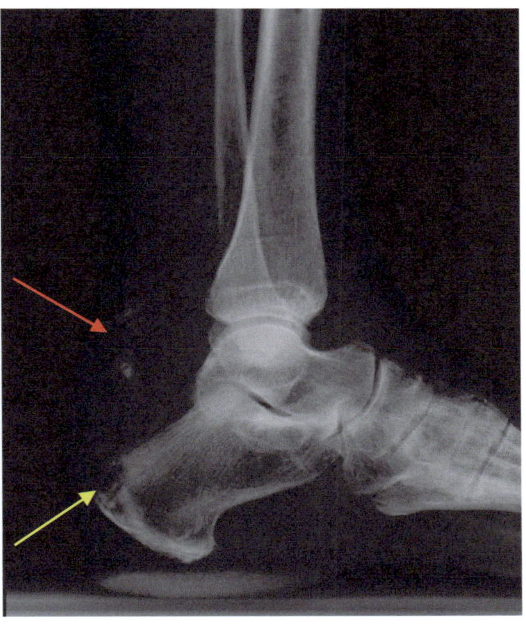

Fig. 17.2 Lateral ankle radiograph of a patient with a chronic, insertional Achilles rupture. Shown proximally are ossific, avulsion fragments (red arrow) from the posterior calcaneus, where there are baseline enthesopathic changes (yellow arrow), including spurring and calcific changes, along with a Haglund's prominence

Ultrasound can also be utilized to demonstrate abnormal tendon morphology and vascularity consistent with chronic tendon injury [8]. Magnetic resonance imaging (MRI), particularly the sagittal and axial sequences, provides a high level of detail regarding the tendon rupture site/pattern, the size of the rupture gap, and tendon quality—all of which are imperative for preoperative planning purposes (Fig. 17.3).

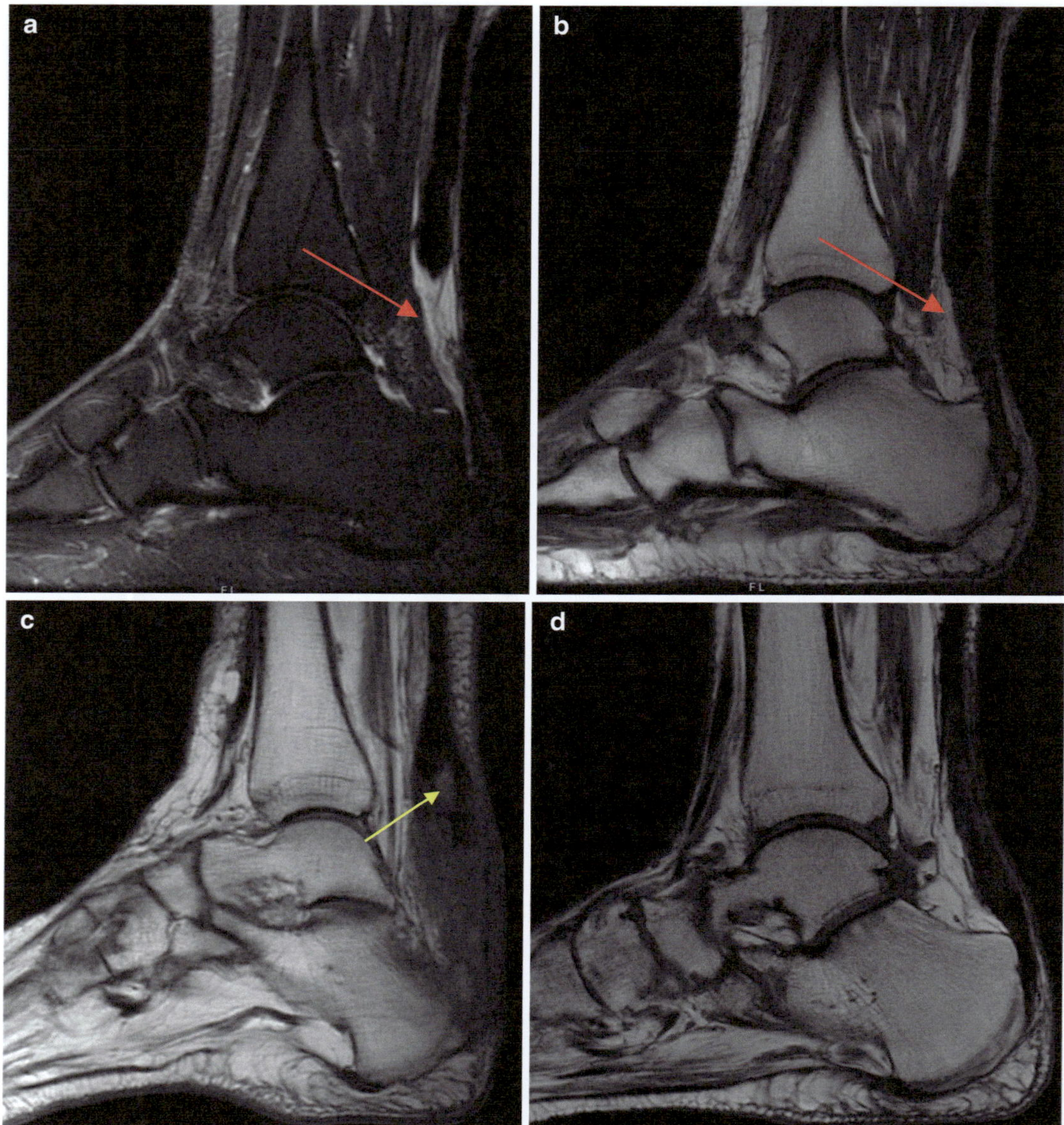

Fig. 17.3 MRI appearance of various chronic Achilles ruptures. Sagittal T2 FS (**a**) and T1 (**b**) sequences of the patient with a chronic, insertional Achilles rupture, with intervening scar tissue formation (red arrow) between the proximal Achilles tendon stump and residual distal tendon stump fibers. Sagittal T1 sequence (**c**) of the patient with a chronic, insertional Achilles rupture with avulsion fragment (yellow arrow), with proximal thickened Achilles stump and enthesopathic changes distally at the posterior calcaneus. Sagittal T1 sequence (**d**) of the patient with a chronic Achilles midsubstance rupture with a bridging scar between Achilles tendon stumps

Nonoperative Management

The surgical management of acute Achilles tendon ruptures remains a controversial topic as nonoperative care with accelerated functional rehabilitation has been shown to have good outcomes in certain populations. On the other hand, for reasonable surgical candidates, chronic Achilles tendon ruptures are best managed operatively. There are some cases, however, where nonoperative treatment may be preferred. Patients who present with significant risk factors for procedural failure, such as those with poor vascularity or soft tissue condition, current tobacco use, or other comorbidities that would preclude a safe surgical reconstructive effort, are best managed conservatively. Furthermore, those with lower functional demands may be most optimally treated in this manner as well. Functional bracing with an ankle foot orthosis and intensive physical therapy can often help these patients through improvements in strength, balance, gait, and overall function.

Surgical Management

Acknowledging the relative increased risks of surgical complications compared to nonoperative management, surgical treatment is generally considered the best means of treating patients with chronic Achilles ruptures. These injuries tend to have less predictable postoperative outcomes when compared to patients undergoing acute Achilles repairs. There are a host of described techniques for treating these chronic injuries. Surgical management depends primarily upon the tendon gap size and the health of the residual tendon, but other criteria are considered as well, such as patient factors and rupture site location. While the tendon gap can be estimated based on sagittal MRI sequences, the exact defect size is typically measured intraoperatively after an appropriate tendon stump debridement [6]. Thus, it is imperative for treating surgeons to have a working plan of attack for the surgery and, even more importantly, to have a strong working knowledge of when and how to perform the various reconstructive procedures based on intraoperative findings (Fig. 17.4), allowing appropriate adjustment of the plan as the surgeon sees fit. The majority of surgical management options can be grouped into four categories—direct repair, fascial rearrangement/advancement flaps, tendon transfers, and grafts (auto-, allo-, synthetic).

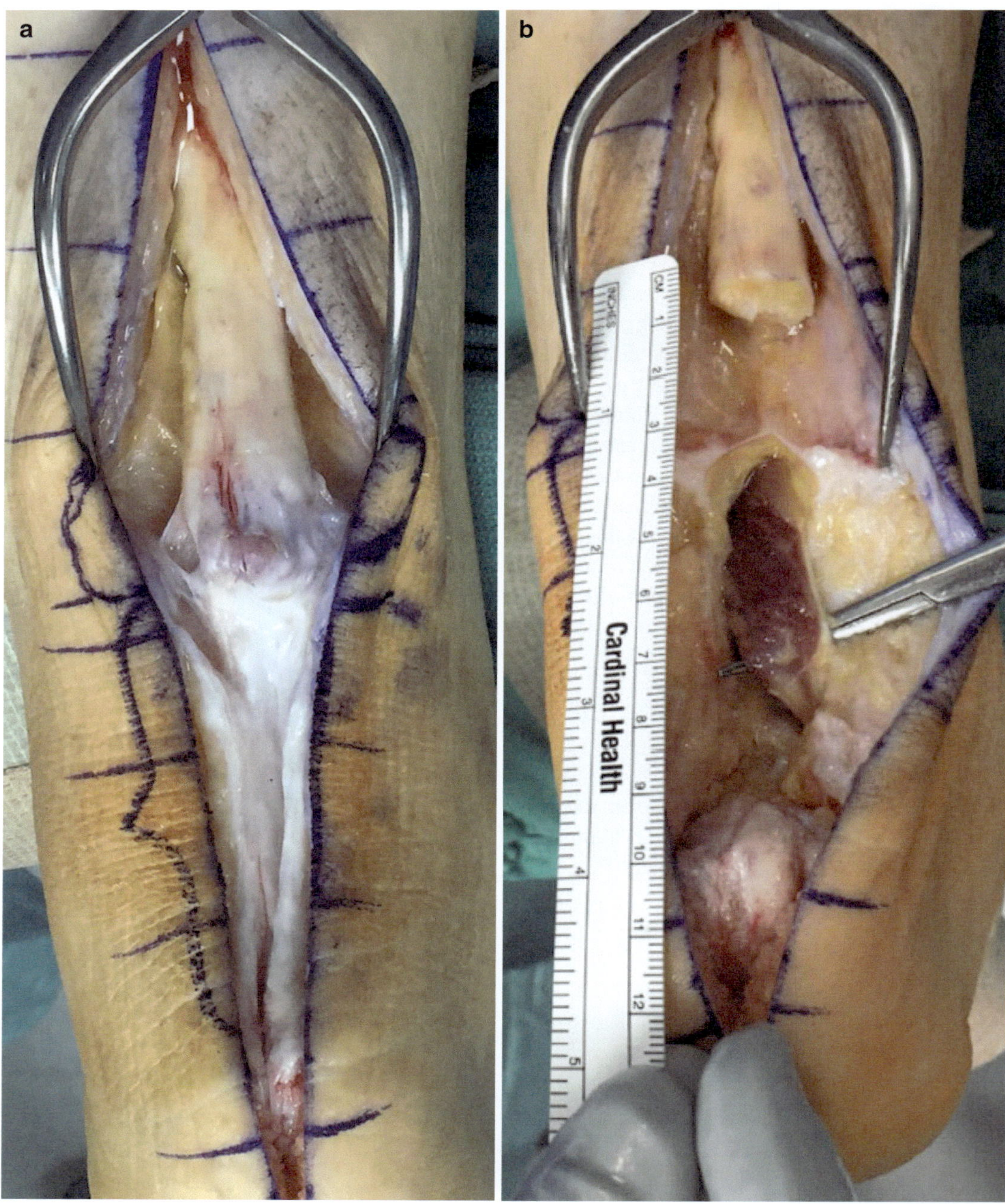

Fig. 17.4 Intraoperative photographs of a patient with a chronic insertional Achilles tendon rupture, seen both prior to (**a**) and after (**b**) tendon stump debridement. There is an ossific, avulsion fragment (a, red arrow) seen, with native Achilles tendon stump proximal to this and intervening scar tissue distally. The postdebridement, intraoperative Achilles tendon defect is shown, which is measured between the distal aspect of the proximal stump and the superior portion of the calcaneus, given the lack of a substantial distal tendon stump with this particular injury pattern. The FHL muscle belly and tendon are seen deep within the surgical wound (over the curved hemostat)

Direct Repair

The primary repair of chronic Achilles tendon ruptures is rarely performed as the gap size tends to be too large to allow for end-to-end apposition via the mobilization of the contracted tendon ends; however, a few techniques have been reported in the literature with success using direct repair. If the tendon ends can be mobilized to a defect of around 2–2.5 cm or less, a repair can be performed [7, 9]. Scar tissue that forms between the tendon stumps is sharply debrided back to healthy margins. Adhesions to surrounding fascia and muscle must be bluntly released to allow for more effective mobilization. The posterior compartmental fascia can be released as well, which can additionally help with paratenon mobilization and closure at the conclusion of the case. An Allis clamp or passing a heavy stay suture through the proximal tendon stump in order to pull some steady traction on the proximal musculotendinous segment to allow for further tendon gap reduction. The Achilles tendon stumps are then repaired in a traditional end-to-end fashion using heavy nonabsorbable sutures (Fig. 17.5). Proper tension must be ensured. The repair is performed with the ankle in approximately 20 to 30 degrees of plantarflexion [9].

There are limited reported outcomes following primary repair for chronic Achilles ruptures. Yasuda et al. [10] performed a direct repair technique using interposed scar tissue resection and tendon stump reduction and repair on six patients with chronic Achilles ruptures at a mean time of 22 weeks out from initial injury. Preoperative T2-weighted MRI sequences on all patients revealed a diffusely thickened Achilles tendon with associated high-signal bands along the length of the tendon. Intraoperative rupture gaps were 3 to 5 cm, and 2 to 3 cm of scar tissue was routinely excised. They reported significantly improved AOFAS scores at a mean follow-up of 31 mo. There were no reruptures, all patients reported no difficulty walking or climbing stairs, and all patients returned to their preinjury level of function [10].

Porter et al. [11] reported their results using a similar technique, with the exception that a minimal incision of the scar tissue was performed with the goal of imbricating this tissue into the primary repair. Eleven recreational athletes with chronic Achilles ruptures that were 4 to 12 weeks from injury were treated with a mean follow-up of 3.5 years. There were no reruptures, and all patients were able to return to their preinjury level of activity at a mean of 5.8 months.

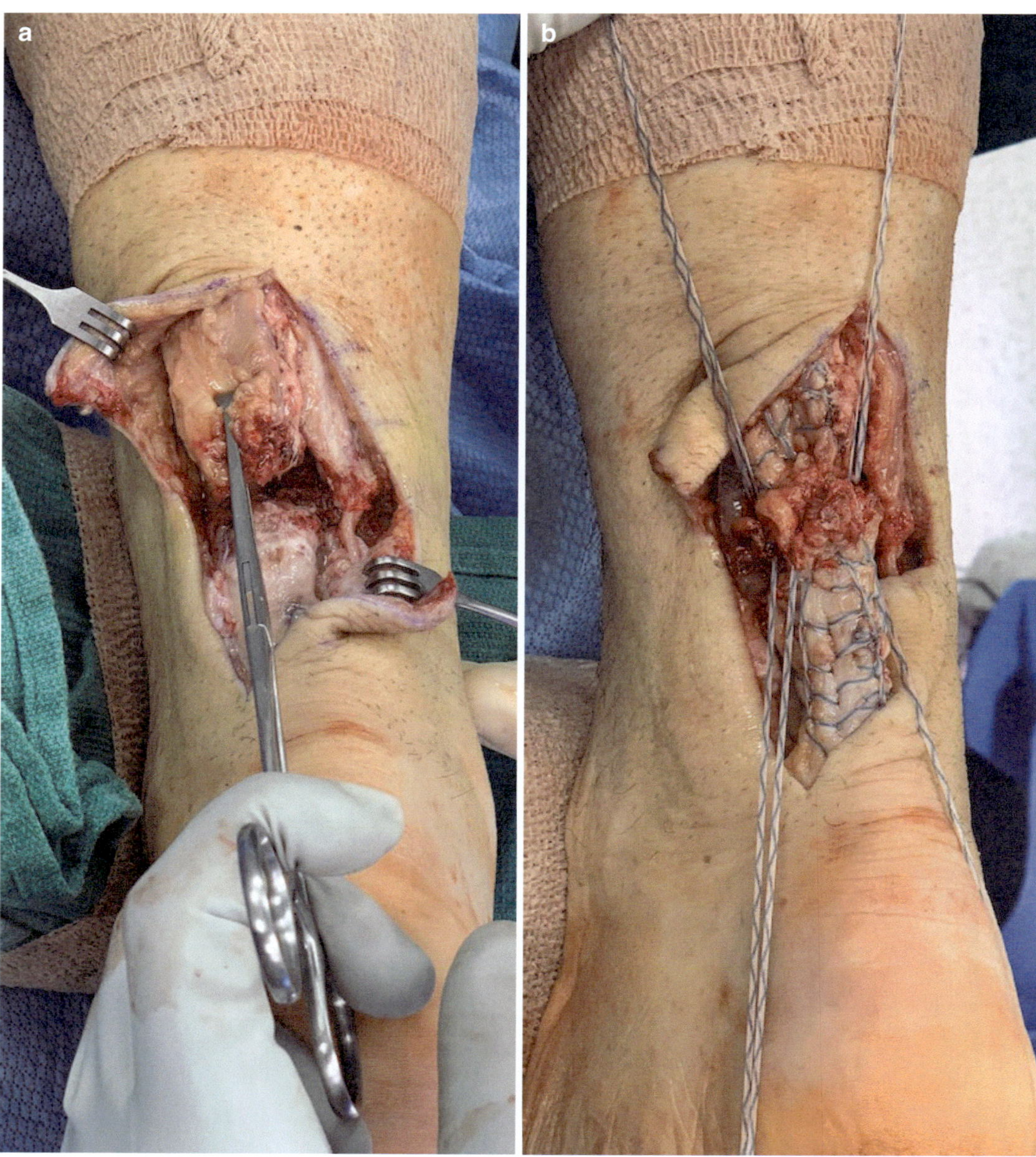

Fig. 17.5 Intraoperative photographs of a patient who underwent a mini-open Achilles repair 3 months prior, with construct failure due to reinjury in the early phase of rehabilitation. At the revision procedure, the prior short horizontal incision was extended in a Z fashion proximally and distally. Tendon stumps were identified, debrided, and mobilized using blunt dissection and longitudinal traction with an Allis clamp (**a**). Once the tendon stump ends were reducible, an open direct repair was performed using a four-strand Krackow-type construct using nonabsorbable flat-braided sutures (**b**)

Gastrocnemius Fascial Advancement/Rearrangement Flaps

Some of the earliest described techniques for reconstructing chronic Achilles ruptures were a V-Y advancement of the aponeurosis [12] and Achilles tendon turndown [13] in order to reduce the chronic tendon gap, depending on defect size. Other proposed less invasive solutions have included gastrocnemius recession, which can reduce distal tendon defect but to a lesser extent than the former advancement procedures.

V-Y Advancement Flap

In cases where the tendon defect size remains greater than 2 cm even after mobilization techniques, the next surgical option is generally a gastrocnemius fascial advancement flap. These procedures are typically reserved for chronic Achilles ruptures with intraoperative tendon gaps of 2 to 5 cm [6, 14–16]. There are a variety of techniques published, and most of these procedures are performed in conjunction with local tendon transfers [16, 17].

A V-Y advancement flap is performed by making an inverted V-shaped incision in the proximal aponeurosis, preserving the underlying soleus muscle attachment (Fig. 17.6a). The gap defect determines the length of each arm of the V, with each arm made between 1.5 and 2 times the length of the gap [14]. The arms of the V are advanced and repaired, resulting in a Y-shaped configuration. Distally, this allows for a primary repair of the Achilles tendon stumps using non-absorbable suture.

Guclu et al. [17] reported on the long-term outcomes of their patients who underwent a V-Y fascial advancement combined with a fascial turndown distally in 17 patients with a chronic Achilles rupture with a mean follow-up of around

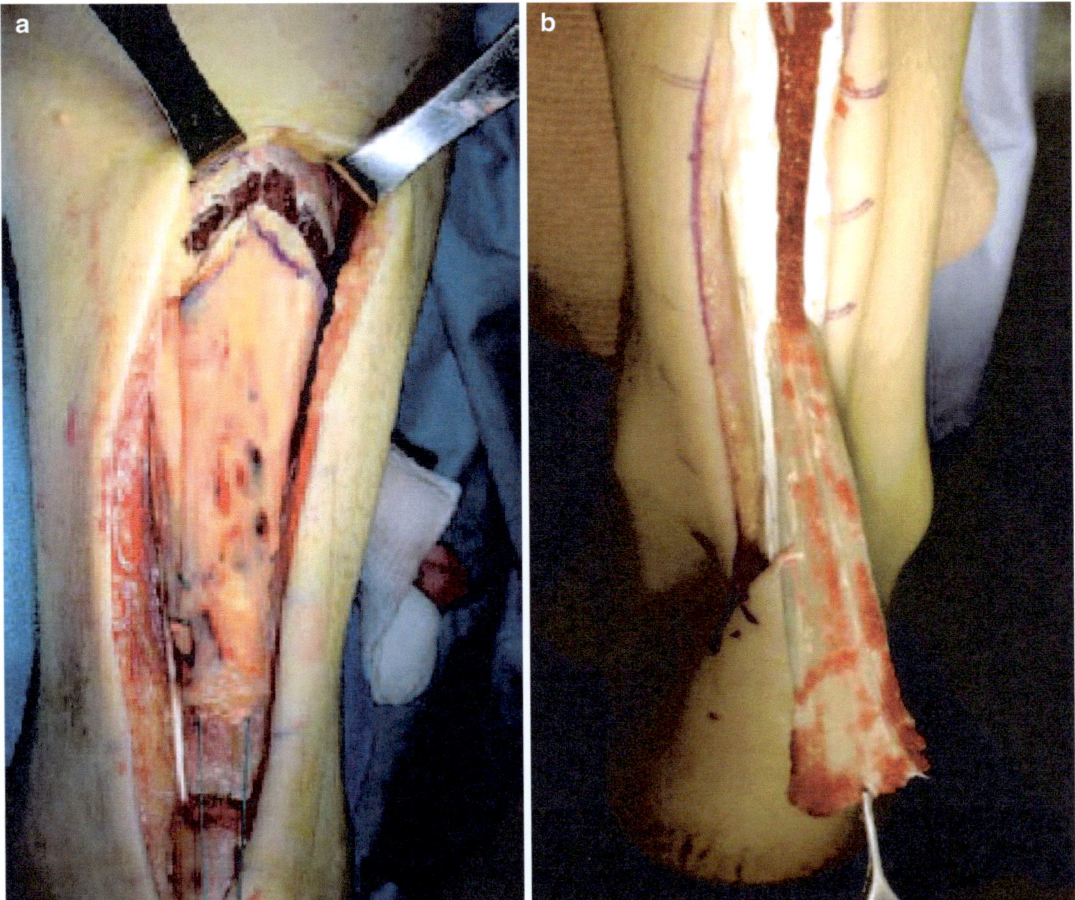

Fig. 17.6 Intraoperative photographs of a V-Y gastrocnemius fascial advancement (**a**) and an Achilles turndown flap (**b**) being used to reconstruct chronic Achilles ruptures

16 years. Patients had a mean tendon gap size of 6 cm and had surgery at a mean of 7 months from injury. Significant improvements in AOFAS scores were reported, along with other functional improvements and no reruptures [17].

Lin et al. [18] studied 20 patients who underwent a V-Y advancement at a mean follow-up of 32.8 months with mean tendon operative gaps of 5 cm. Low complication rates were reported with good functional results as all patients were able to return to their preinjury level, perform repeated single-limb heel raises, and ambulate without a limp. Furthermore, reported advantages of this procedure were described, such as it being a simple and cost-effective technique, thus avoiding the costs of synthetic materials or allograft tendons [18].

Achilles Turndown Flap

The concept for an Achilles turndown flap is similar to that of a V-Y fascial advancement. This technique is recommended for cases where the operative Achilles defect size is 2–5 cm; however, some also advocate for its use in tendon gaps greater than 5 cm [19]. There are variations in the exact surgical technique. In general, a central tendon flap is harvested from the proximal stump and flipped down distally to be sewn to the distal tendon stump to span the tendon gap (Fig. 17.6b). Much of the published literature on the outcomes following turndown flaps involves this technique being performed in conjunction with other concomitant procedures [20, 21].

Koh et al. [21] retrospectively reviewed a cohort of 49 patients over a 10-year period with chronic Achilles ruptures that were at least 4 weeks out from injury, who underwent repair with either a flexor hallucis longus (FHL) tendon transfer alone or FHL tendon transfer combined with a turndown flap. Both groups had similar and significant improvements in outcome scores (AOFAS, VAS, and SF-36). The operative time was significantly longer by a mean of 27 min for the FHL transfer with the turndown group compared to the FHL transfer alone. The former also had two patients with soft tissue complications, compared to no such complications in the latter group. Neither group had a rerupture. In considering both of these procedures, Koh et al. [21] concluded that the FHL tendon transfer technique alone should be used in the reconstruction of chronic Achilles ruptures due to shorter operative times, low rates of complications, and similar outcome scores.

Local Tendon Transfers

While V-Y fascial advancement flaps and turndown procedures have demonstrated good outcomes, they are not without their own shortcomings. These procedures can result in decreased plantarflexion strength, alter the biomechanics of the gastrocnemius complex, and require large surgical approaches and operative times [6]. In contrast, the use of local tendon transfers in the reconstruction of chronic Achilles ruptures, whether alone or in conjunction with other procedures, can preserve the natural biomechanics of the gastrocnemius complex, result in reduced surgical times and exposures, and augment the overall plantarflexion strength of the construct. Historically, there are a variety of tendon transfers described for this purpose; however, the FHL tendon transfer is most commonly employed, followed less commonly by the peroneus brevis (PB) and flexor digitorum longus (FDL) tendons [5–7, 14, 19].

Flexor Hallucis Longus (FHL) Tendon Transfer

Generally speaking, the FHL tendon transfer is considered the "workhorse" for Achilles tendon pathology, whether for chronic rupture or chronic tendinopathy/tendinosis settings, with short (posteromedial ankle at the fibro-osseous tunnel) and long (at or distal to the knot of Henry) harvests utilized, depending on the length of the tendon required [6, 19]. The basis for the utility of the FHL tendon transfer in the setting of chronic

Achilles ruptures goes back to basic tendon transfer principles—that is, the FHL tendon is stronger than other potential tendon candidates (i.e., FDL, PB, and plantaris tendons), the axis of musculotendinous pull and its phase are similar to those of the Achilles tendon, the FHL tendon is in close proximity to the Achilles tendon, and the associated muscle belly of the FHL tendon may enhance the vascularity of the injury site to promote healing [22].

As alluded to, there is a wide variety of techniques published on this tendon transfer with variations in both the harvesting of the tendon (short/proximal and long/distal harvests) and the method of incorporation and fixation into the final reconstruction [5–7, 19] (Fig. 17.7). In reference to the short harvest, it is imperative to ensure that the structure identified is in fact the FHL tendon as the tibial nerve also courses posteromedially at the ankle [23]. Nerve injury and sequelae thereof can also potentially occur with the longer midfoot FHL harvest as the medial and lateral plantar nerves are near the knot of Henry [23].

Abubeih et al. [24] reported on a prospective case series of 21 patients who underwent FHL tendon transfers for chronic Achilles ruptures, utilizing a short harvest at the fibro-osseous tunnel. At a mean follow-up of 15 months, they reported that patient AOFAS scores improved from 57.4 preoperatively to 95.3 postoperatively with no loss in great toe function and only one superficial infection, and all patients were satisfied with their outcome [24].

Alhaug et al. [25] evaluated retrospective outcomes after a two-incision (midfoot harvest) FHL tendon transfer in 21 patients with chronic Achilles ruptures. The distal FHL stump was tenodesed to the FDL tendon, and the harvested FHL tendon was tensioned, transferred to the calcaneus, and then via bone tunnel routed cephalad and tenodesed to the proximal Achilles tendon stump.

The maximal strength of the affected side following FHL transfer was nearly equal to that of the uninjured side but with notably lower endurance testing results. Nearly 50% of the patients in this series sustained at least one com-

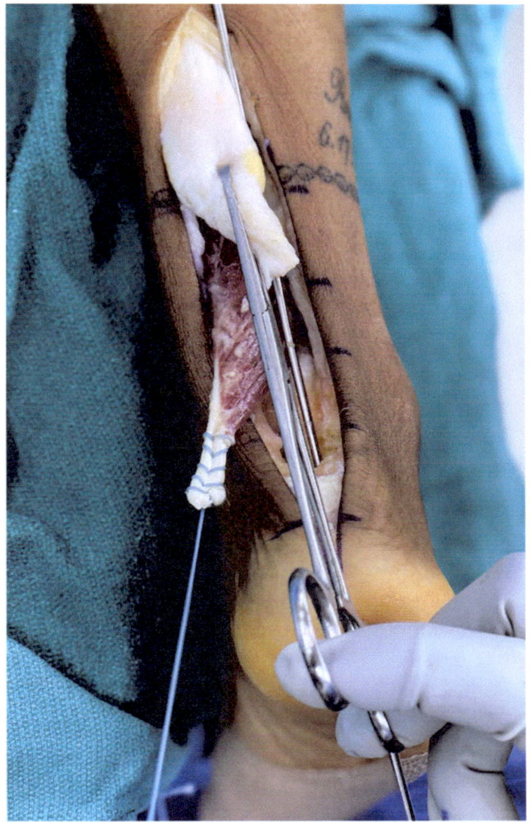

Fig. 17.7 Intraoperative photograph demonstrating a patient with a chronic Achilles rupture with an Allis clamp on the proximal Achilles stump, along with a short harvest of the FHL tendon shown after nonabsorbable suture placement. Note the large and vascular FHL muscle belly present. A guidewire is shown through the posterior calcaneus that will be used for FHL tendon transfer after overreaming

plication, most commonly infection and loss of sensibility, usually in the sural nerve distribution [25]. This increased complication risk could be attributable due to the long harvest technique, which requires more dissection and a two-incision approach.

In part as an effort to reduce complications associated with open FHL tendon transfer techniques for chronic Achilles ruptures, endoscopic FHL tendon transfer techniques have also been developed and outcomes studied. Vega et al. [26] reported on their series of 22 patients treated with an endoscopic, short FHL tendon harvest and transfer to the calcaneus at a mean follow-up of

30.5 months. AOFAS scores improved from 55 preoperatively to a mean of 91 postoperatively. All patients had reported good functional outcomes with a complete return to the preinjury level of activity, without any symptomatic hallux flexion deficits or major reported complications [26]. It is worth noting that in this study, and other reporting on minimally invasive approaches for reconstructing chronic Achilles ruptures, that tangibly reconnecting the Achilles tendon ends was not necessary in order to restore patient function and strength [26–28].

Peroneal Brevis (PB) Tendon Transfer

PB tendon transfer for the management of chronic Achilles tendon ruptures has also been reported with good outcomes. In its original description, the technique involved harvesting the PB tendon distally from the base of the fifth metatarsal, passing it through a transverse calcaneal drill hole, and tenodesing it to the proximal Achilles tendon stump [29]. Later modification of this technique involved routing the harvested PB tendon instead through the distal Achilles tendon stump [30].

A biomechanical study using 17 fresh-frozen human cadavers compared the FHL and PB tendon transfers and found no difference in stiffness and energy-to-peak load between the two techniques [31]. Interestingly, the PB tendon transfer group did have a higher mean load to failure. In all cases, construct failure occurred where the tendon transfer was sewn to either the proximal or distal Achilles stump, emphasizing the importance of creating a secure tendon-to-tendon attachment or even considering tendon-to-bone fixation in preventing pullout and overall construct failure [31].

The PB tendon transfer utilized in patients with chronic Achilles ruptures has proven successful in the long term as well—Maffulli et al. [32] reported on 16 patients with a mean follow-up of 15.5 years and found that patients did well with no issues in performing daily activities. Patients did have a decrease in calf circumference and plantarflexion strength; however, they did not report being functionally limited as a result of these findings.

As with any tendon transfer, consideration needs to be given to the potential functional losses that may be associated with "robbing Peter to pay Paul." The potential concern is the disruption of normal anatomy and the overall effect on foot and ankle muscle balance/function resulting from sacrificing the tendon. The PB tendon transfer can result in weaker eversion, with a resulting loss of the normal ankle inversion-eversion balance relationship, and the PB tendon transfer does not possess some of the same inherent biomechanical advantages noted with the FHL tendon transfer.

Flexor Digitorum Longus (FDL) Tendon Transfer

An alternative tendon to consider for use in chronic Achilles reconstructions is the FDL tendon transfer. The FDL tendon transfer, as originally reported by Mann et al. [33] in seven patients with overall good to excellent results at a mean follow-up of 39 months, was viewed as superior to the PB tendon transfer for several reasons. This rationale included the following points: the FDL medial line of pull more closely matches the Achilles tendon axis, the FDL harvest does not impact the inversion-eversion balance at the ankle, and there is no loss of lesser toe flexion due to tenodesis of the distal FDL stump to the intact FHL tendon at the knot of Henry.

De Cesar Netto et al. [34] reported on 15 patients (17 feet) at a mean follow-up of 27.5 months, who underwent an FDL tendon transfer for the treatment of chronic Achilles tendinopathy utilizing a three-incision approach. Of note, this also included patients with chronic Achilles issues outside of chronic rupture pathology. A significant improvement in VAS, SF-36, and LEFS scores was realized, with 86% of patients returning to their prior recreational sports activity level, as applicable. One patient complained of weakness in the plantarflexion of the lesser toes without impact on gait. There were three superficial infections and two deep infections, for which surgical debridement was required in the latter cases. The authors concluded this to be a safe alternative to FHL transfer with minimal complications and negligible morbidity associated with FDL tendon harvest, particularly in patients with prior failed FHL tendon transfers or in athletes where there is a desire to minimize any potential weakness with hallux flexion and push-off strength through the harvest of the FHL tendon [34].

Grafts

Chronic Achilles ruptures with large tendon defects (> 5 cm) that cannot be solved through other techniques, such as fascial advancement, turndowns, or local tendon transfers alone, generally require the use of free tendon autograft or allograft for reconstruction [6, 7]. While there are several studies on both types of grafts, there are no comparative analyses between free autograft and allograft tendon reconstruction for chronic Achilles ruptures. Both have their theoretic advantages and disadvantages, and based on patient factors and both surgeon preference and experience, auto- or allograft may be deemed most appropriate for use in the setting of a chronic Achilles rupture with a large tendon gap. Various synthetic grafts have been reported on as well, and in certain situations, these might be useful in chronic Achilles reconstructive surgery. For each of these graft options, open, limited-open, and endoscopic approaches have been described, the exact use of which can be tailored based on patient and surgeon factors.

Free Autograft Tendon

The use of free tendon autograft in the reconstruction of chronic Achilles ruptures with large tendon defects was first described with hamstring (e.g., gracilis and semitendinosus) and quadriceps tendon harvests [35–40]. These graft harvest techniques are well described and studied in the sports medicine literature as they are commonly performed for ligamentous reconstructions typi-

cally in the knee, avoid sacrifice and the potential creation of an agonist/antagonist imbalance of the tendons around the foot and ankle, and offer greater length and more tissue than local ankle tendon harvest options for large gaps (or when local ankle tendon transfers are not possible). These free autograft techniques have been advanced to the point where they can be performed in a minimal-invasive fashion [37, 38], avoiding larger dissections in patients who may be prone to wound-healing issues or infection.

Maffulli et al. [35, 36] reported their results using a free gracilis tendon autograft for large chronic Achilles tendon defects using a 12 to 15 cm incision and looping the gracilis tendon graft through both Achilles tendon stumps. The mean tendon gap size was 6.8 cm, and they reported no reruptures or harvest site complications around the knee [35]. Five out of 21 patients had a superficial wound infection at the Achilles reconstruction site with this early, more invasive approach [35]. At a mean follow-up of 10.9 years, patients demonstrated good functional outcomes, although they had calf muscle atrophy and ankle plantarflexion weakness on strength testing [36].

Maffulli et al. developed and reported their outcomes of treating patients with chronic Achilles ruptures using a minimally invasive approach with a free semitendinosus tendon graft for reconstruction, either as a woven tendon loop [37] or calcaneal bone tunnel with an interference screw fixation [38] construct. In using smaller incisions to gain access to the chronic tendon stumps and thus avoid a longitudinal incision over the chronic tendon rupture site, which can be prone to contracture and wound issues, they realized dramatically lower wound infection rates (7.7% and 0%) [37, 38] while maintaining excellent functional outcomes.

Allograft Tendon

In a similar fashion to free tendon autograft reconstruction, allograft tendon techniques have been described for chronic Achilles reconstructive surgeries with large tendon defects [41–43]. Allograft tendon is commonly utilized in various orthopedic surgery applications, including the foot and ankle. Potential advantages to allograft use include the elimination of the surgical time and exposure required for autograft tendon harvest, no associated harvest site morbidity, and the ability to select optimal tendon sizing (i.e., length and diameter) for the specifically intended indication. The theoretic disadvantages of allograft use (relative to autograft use) include potential host-mediated immune response, disease transmission, slower reincorporation and remodeling rate, and higher associated costs of allograft tissue [6, 41, 43].

In general, the relative advantages of allograft use tend to outweigh the potential disadvantages, and the safe and efficacious use of allograft tendons for various reconstructions throughout the foot and ankle is well established [44–46]. A hamstring allograft tendon can be used in a similar fashion to a free hamstring autograft tendon in chronic Achilles reconstructions [6]. A semitendinosus or gracilis allograft tendon can be either woven through both debrided Achilles tendon stumps and tensioned with the ankle in plantarflexion or can be woven through the proximal Achilles stump and then passed into a transverse calcaneal bone tunnel with interference screw fixation at an appropriate tension [6, 41–43] (Fig. 17.8).

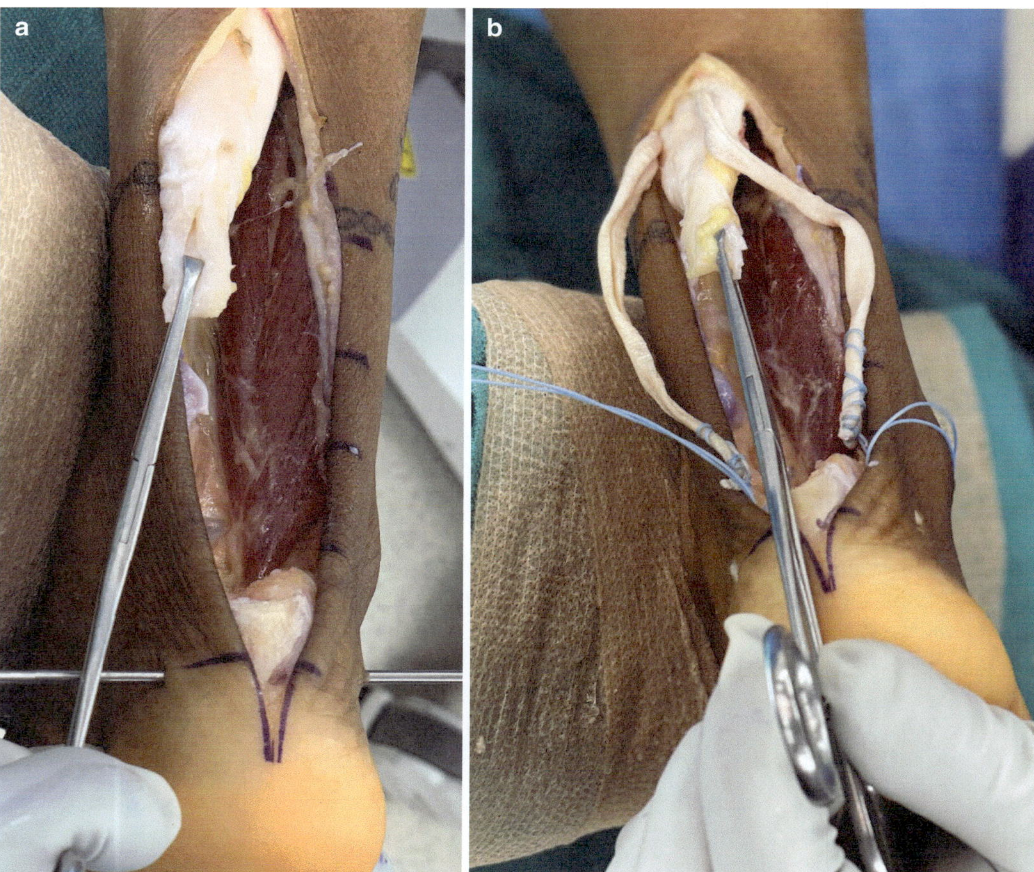

Fig. 17.8 Case example of semitendinosus allograft reconstruction with FHL tendon transfer in a patient with a chronic Achilles tendon rupture. FHL muscle belly (**a**) seen after tendon transfer into the posterior calcaneus, along with transverse guide wire placement for an eventual bone tunnel for allograft passage. The semitendinosus allograft has been passed through the proximal Achilles tendon stump with suture limbs passed in an opposing fashion through the transverse calcaneal drill tunnel (**b**). After allograft limb passage through the bone tunnel, they are tensioned and then fixated with a tenodesis screw (**c**) to create the final construct (**d**). Lateral ankle radiograph demonstrating the vertical FHL and transverse semitendinosus allograft tendon-bone tunnels (**e**)

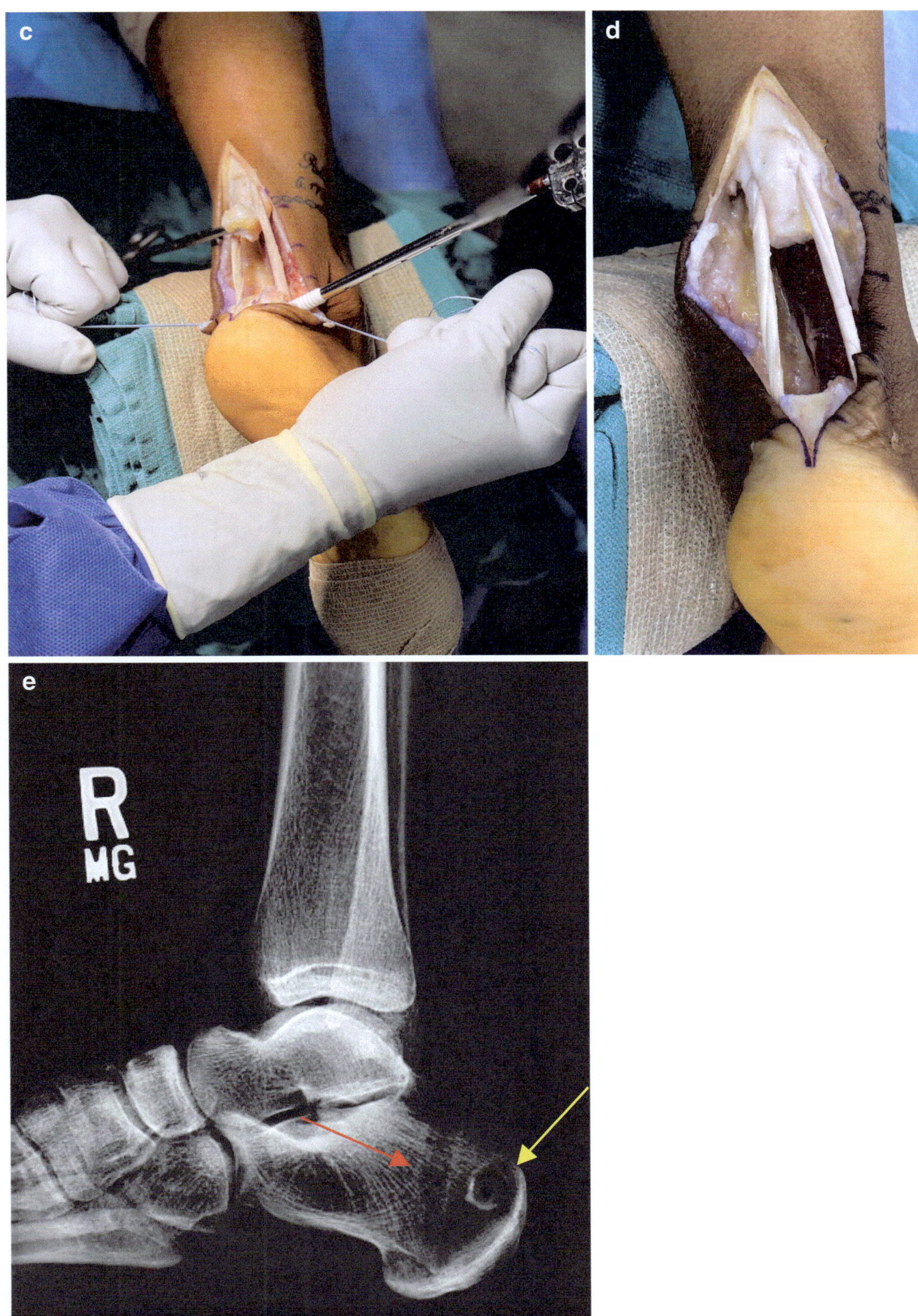

Fig. 17.8 (continued)

Song et al. [42] reported satisfactory results with significant improvements in clinical and functional outcomes, with no reruptures or infections, using a semitendinosus allograft in 33 patients with chronic Achilles tendon ruptures with large defects (range: 4–10 cm following debridement with the ankle in a neutral position), at a mean follow-up of 53 months.

In the case of poor quality or quantity of distal Achilles tendon stump, such as chronic insertional Achilles tendon ruptures, another option for reconstruction is the use of an Achilles tendon-bone block allograft (Fig. 17.9). This technique achieves tendon-to-tendon and bone-to-bone healing or incorporation proximally and distally, respectively [6, 41, 43, 47, 48]. In this technique, the allograft bone block is inserted into a trough of a similar shape created in the patient's native posterior calcaneus to reestablish the Achilles tendon insertion, which is typically fixated with two cancellous screws. The attached allograft Achilles tendon is then sewn into the native proximal Achilles tendon stump at an appropriate tension [6, 47, 48].

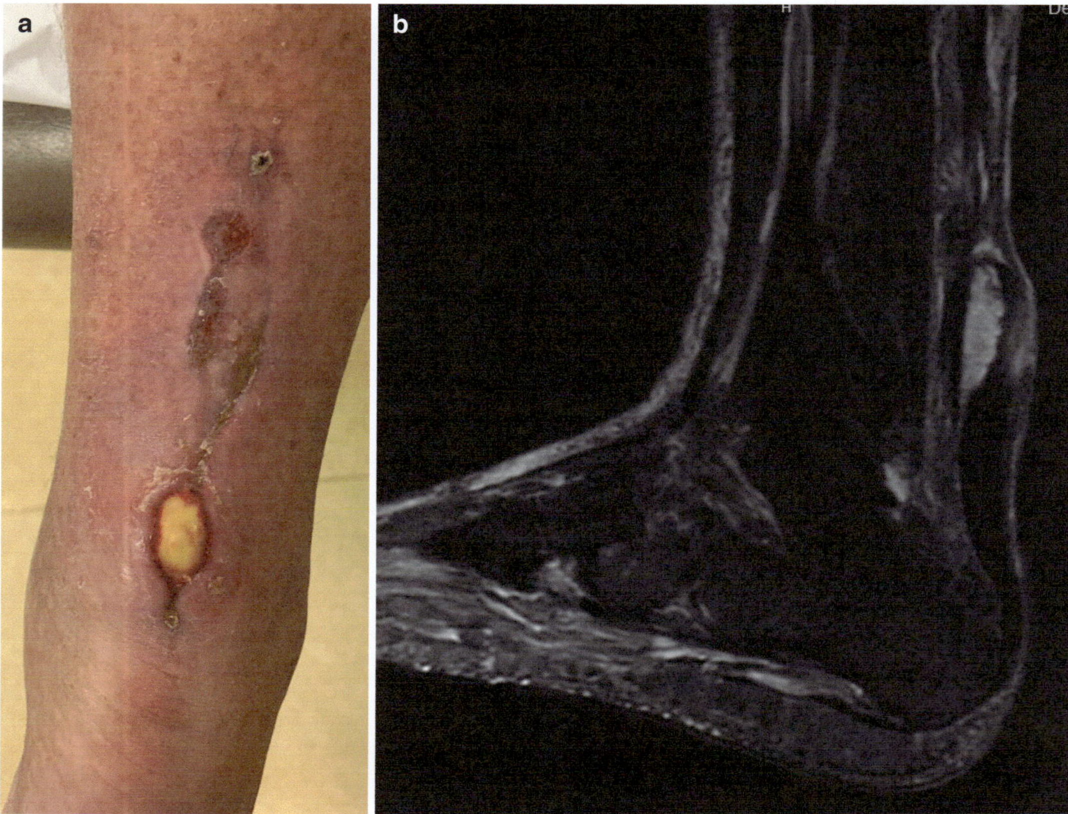

Fig. 17.9 Clinical photograph (**a**) and sagittal FSE IR MRI sequence (**b**) of a patient presenting status-post several failed Achilles surgeries, with a resulting open wound and an exposed Achilles tendon with associated deep infection. A large portion of the involved Achilles tendon was resected, followed by the insertion of an antibiotic-impregnated cement spacer (**c**) that would also serve as a soft tissue expander for eventual reconstruction. Around 2.5 months later, once the infection was clinically cleared and soft tissues healed, the second stage procedure involved spacer removal and reconstruction with a bone block Achilles tendon allograft and FHL tendon transfer (**d**). Intraoperative photograph (**e**) of the final construct and postoperative lateral radiograph showing the incorporated bone block into the native calcaneus with screw fixation and vertical drill tunnel used for the FHL tendon transfer (**f**)

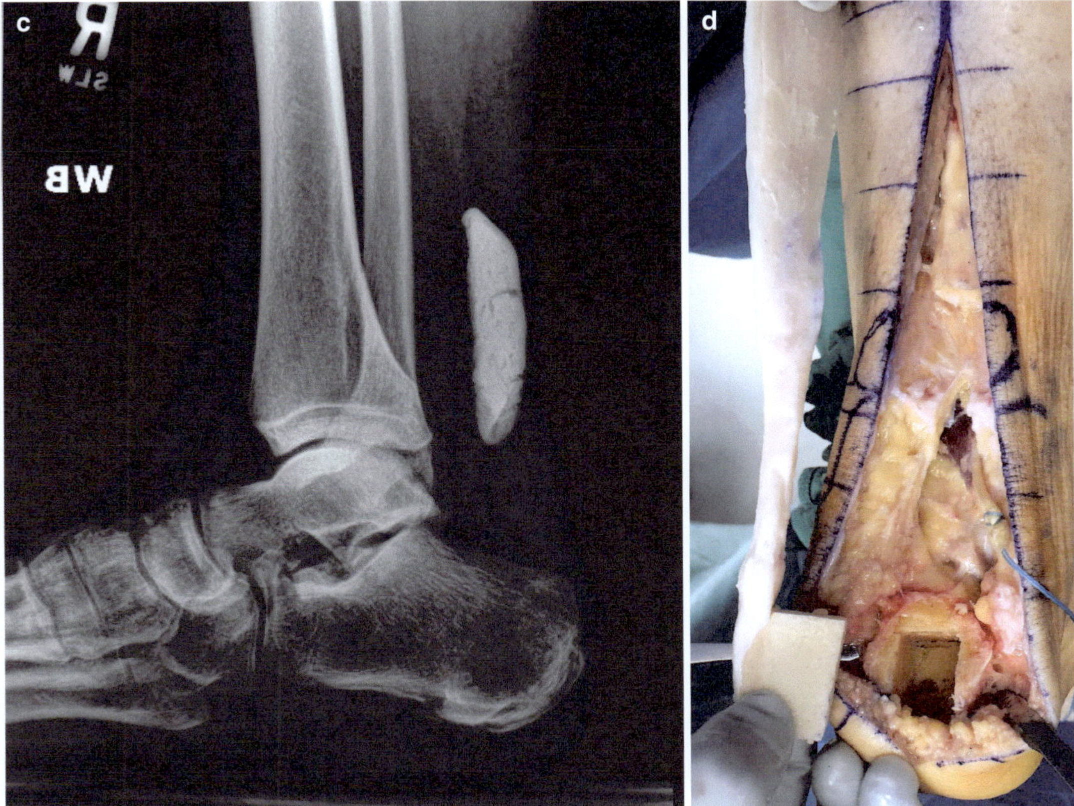

Fig. 17.9 (continued)

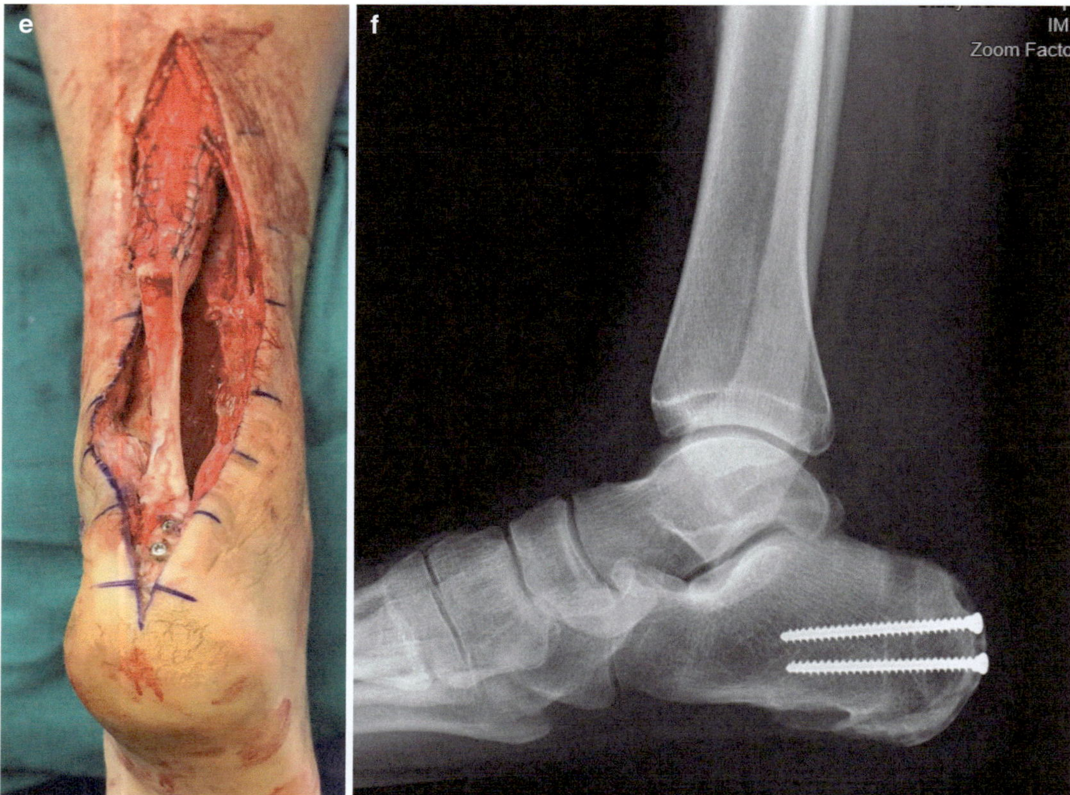

Fig. 17.9 (continued)

Synthetic Materials

Various synthetic materials have been described in case series for use in chronic Achilles reconstructions, which can help avoid the need for local or free tendon harvesting to span chronic tendon defects. Examples of these materials include but are not limited to carbon fiber, Marlex mesh, Dacron vascular graft, polyester tape, GraftJacket matrix, and Artelon [6, 7, 9]. Most proponents of these types of materials tout the augmented strength of the reconstruction at time zero, which can facilitate and expedite the postoperative recovery and rehabilitation process. Ultimately, long-term outcome data for the use of these materials in patients undergoing chronic Achilles tendon reconstructions are lacking. Furthermore, many of these materials are nonabsorbable, with concerns over their use in an area that is prone to wound breakdown and infection. As such, these may not be the best choice for reconstructive purposes in this specific usage.

References

1. Suchak AA, Bostick G, Reid D, Blitz S, Jomha N. The incidence of Achilles tendon ruptures in Edmonton, Canada. Foot Ankle Int. 2005;26:932–6.
2. Lemme NJ, Li NY, DeFroda SF, Kleiner J, Owens BD. Epidemiology of Achilles tendon ruptures in the United States: athletic and nonathletic injuries from 2012 to 2016. Orthop J Sports Med. 2018;6:2325967118808238.
3. Scheller AD, Kasser JR, Quigley TB. Tendon injuries about the ankle. Orthop Clin North Am. 1980;11:801–11.
4. Nilsson N, Helander KN, Senorski EH, Holm A, Karlsson J, Svensson M, Westin O. The economic cost and patient-reported outcomes of chronic Achilles tendon ruptures. J Exp Orthop. 2020;7:60.

5. Padanilam TG. Chronic Achilles tendon ruptures. Foot Ankle Clin. 2009;14:711–28.

6. Schweitzer KM Jr, Dekker TJ, Adams SB. Chronic Achilles ruptures: reconstructive options. J Am Acad Orthop Surg. 2018;26:753–63.

7. Maffulli N, Ajis A. Management of chronic ruptures of the Achilles tendon. J Bone Joint Surg Am. 2008;90:1348–60.

8. de Vos RJ, Weir A, Cobben LP, Tol JL. The value of power Doppler ultrasonography in Achilles tendinopathy: a prospective study. Am J Sports Med. 2007;35:1696–701.

9. Chen C, Hunt KJ. Open reconstructive strategies for chronic Achilles tendon ruptures. Foot Ankle Clin. 2019;24:425–37.

10. Yasuda T, Shima H, Mori K, Kizawa M, Neo M. Direct repair of chronic Achilles tendon ruptures using scar tissue located between the tendon stumps. J Bone Joint Surg Am. 2016;98:1168–75.

11. Porter DA, Mannarino FP, Snead D, Gabel SJ, Ostrowski M. Primary repair without augmentation for early neglected Achilles tendon ruptures in the recreational athlete. Foot Ankle Int. 1997;18:557–64.

12. Abraham E, Pankovich AM. Neglected rupture of the Achilles tendon: treatment by V-Y tendinous flap. J Bone Joint Surg Am. 1975;57:253–5.

13. Christensen I. Rupture of the Achilles tendon: analysis of 57 cases. Acta Chir Scand. 1953;106:50–60.

14. Myerson MS. Achilles tendon ruptures. Instr Course Lect. 1999;48:219–30.

15. Kraeutler MJ, Purcell JM, Hunt KJ. Chronic Achilles tendon ruptures. Foot Ankle Int. 2017;38:291–929.

16. Elias I, Besser M, Nazarian LN, Raikin SM. Reconstruction for missed or neglected Achilles tendon rupture with V-Y lengthening and flexor hallucis longus tendon transfer through one incision. Foot Ankle Int. 2007;28:1238–48.

17. Guclu B, Basat HC, Yildirim T, Bozduman O, Us AK. Long-term results of chronic Achilles tendon ruptures repaired with V-Y tendon plasty and fascia turndown. Foot Ankle Int. 2016;37:737–42.

18. Lin YJ, Duan XJ, Yang L. V-Y tendon plasty for reconstruction of chronic Achilles tendon rupture: a medium-term and long-term follow-up. Orthop Surg. 2019;11:109–16.

19. Den Hartog BD. Surgical strategies: delayed diagnosis or neglected Achilles tendon ruptures. Foot Ankle Int. 2008;29:456–63.

20. Us AK, Bilgin SS, Aydin T, Mergen E. Repair of neglected Achilles tendon ruptures: procedures and functional results. Arch Orthop Trauma Surg. 1997;116:408–11.

21. Koh D, Lim J, Chen JY, Singh IR, Koo K. Flexor hallucis longus transfer versus turndown flaps augmented with flexor hallucis longus transfer in the repair of chronic Achilles tendon rupture. Foot Ankle Surg. 2019;25:221–5.

22. Wapner KL, Pavlock GS, Hecht PJ, Naselli F, Walther R. Repair of chronic Achilles tendon rupture with flexor hallucis longus tendon transfer. Foot Ankle. 1993;14:443–9.

23. Mulier T, Rummens E, Dereymaeker G. Risk of neurovascular injuries in flexor hallucis longus tendon transfers: an anatomic cadaver study. Foot Ankle Int. 2007;28:910–5.

24. Abubeih H, Khaled M, Saleh WR, Said GZ. Flexor hallucis longus transfer clinical outcome through a single incision for chronic Achilles tendon rupture. Int Orthop. 2018;42:2699–704.

25. Alhaug OK, Berdal G, Husebye EE, Hvaal K. Flexor hallucis longus tendon transfer for chronic Achilles tendon rupture: a retrospective study. Foot Ankle Surg. 2019;25:630–5.

26. Vega J, Vilá J, Batista J, Malagelada F, Dalmau-Pastor M. Endoscopic flexor hallucis longus transfer for chronic noninsertional Achilles tendon rupture. Foot Ankle Int. 2018;39:1464–72.

27. Lui TH, Chan WC, Maffulli N. Endoscopic flexor hallucis longus tendon transfer for chronic Achilles tendon rupture. Sports Med Arthrosc Rev. 2016;24:38–41.

28. Maffulli N, Oliva F, Maffulli GD, Del Buono A, Gougoulias N. Surgical management of chronic Achilles tendon ruptures using less invasive techniques. Foot Ankle Surg. 2018;24:164–70.

29. Pérez TA. Traumatic rupture of the Achilles tendon: reconstruction by transplant and graft using the lateral peroneus brevis. Orthop Clin North Am. 1974;5:89–93.

30. Turco VJ, Spinella AJ. Achilles tendon ruptures: peroneus brevis transfer. Foot Ankle. 1987;7:253–9.

31. Sebastian H, Datta B, Maffulli N, Neil M, Walsh WR. Mechanical properties of reconstructed Achilles tendon with transfer of peroneus brevis or flexor hallucis longus tendon. J Foot Ankle Surg. 2007;46:424–8.

32. Maffulli N, Spiezia F, Pintore E, Longo UG, Testa V, Capasso G, Denaro V. Peroneus brevis tendon transfer for reconstruction of chronic tears of the Achilles tendon: a long-term follow-up study. J Bone Joint Surg Am. 2012;94:901–5.

33. Mann RA, Holmes GB Jr, Seale KS, Collins DN. Chronic rupture of the Achilles tendon: a new technique of repair. J Bone Joint Surg Am. 1991;73:214–9.

34. de Cesar NC, Chinanuvathana A, Furtado da Fonseca L, Dein EJ, Tan EW, Schon LC. Outcomes of flexor digitorum longus (FDL) tendon transfer in the treatment of Achilles tendon disorders. Foot Ankle Surg. 2019;25:303–9.

35. Maffulli N, Leadbetter WB. Free gracilis tendon graft in neglected tears of the Achilles tendon. Clin J Sport Med. 2005;15:56–61.

36. Maffulli N, Spiezia F, Testa V, Capasso G, Longo UG, Denaro V. Free gracilis tendon graft for reconstruction of chronic tears of the Achilles tendon. J Bone Joint Surg Am. 2012;94:906–10.

37. Maffulli N, Del Buono A, Spiezia F, Maffulli GD, Longo UG, Denaro V. Less-invasive semitendinosus tendon graft augmentation for the reconstruction

of chronic tears of the Achilles tendon. Am J Sports Med. 2013;41:865–71.

38. Maffulli N, Loppini M, Longo UG, Maffulli GD, Denaro V. Minimally invasive reconstruction of chronic Achilles tendon ruptures using the ipsilateral free semitendinosus tendon graft and interference screw fixation. Am J Sports Med. 2013;41:100–1107.

39. Mudgal CS, Martin TL, Wilson MG. Reconstruction of Achilles tendon defect with a free quadriceps bone-tendon graft without anastomosis. Foot Ankle Int. 2000;21:10–3.

40. Jiang WJ, Shen JJ, Huang JF, Tong PJ. Reconstruction of Myerson type III chronic Achilles tendon ruptures using semitendinosus tendon and gracilis tendon autograft. J Ortho Surg. 2019;27:1–6.

41. Song YJ, Hua YH. Tendon allograft for treatment of chronic Achilles tendon rupture: a systematic review. Foot Ankle Surg. 2019;25:252–7.

42. Song YJ, Chen G, Jia SH, Xu WB, H YH. Good outcomes at mid-term following the reconstruction of chronic Achilles tendon rupture with semitendinosus allograft. Knee Surg Sports Traumatol Arthrosc. 2020;28:1619–24.

43. Gross CE, Nunley JA. Treatment of neglected Achilles tendon ruptures with interpositional allograft. Foot Ankle Clin N Am. 2017;22:735–43.

44. Mook WR, Parekh SG, Nunley JA. Allograft reconstruction of peroneal tendons: operative technique and clinical outcomes. Foot Ankle Int. 2013;34:1212–20.

45. Huh J, Boyette DM, Parekh SG, Nunley JA. Allograft reconstruction of chronic tibialis anterior tendon ruptures. Foot Ankle Int. 2015;36:1180–9.

46. Pelligrini MJ, Glisson RR, Matsumoto T, Schiff A, Laver L, Easley ME, Nunley JA. Effectiveness of allograft reconstruction vs tenodesis for irreparable peroneus brevis tears: a cadaveric model. Foot Ankle Int. 2016;37:803–8.

47. Haraguchi N, Bluman EM, Myerson MS. Reconstruction of chronic Achilles tendon disorders with Achilles tendon allograft. Tech Foot Ankle Surg. 2005;4:154–9.

48. Hanna T, Dripchak P, Childress T. Chronic Achilles rupture repair by allograft bone block fixation: technique tip. Foot Ankle Int. 2014;35:168–74.

Soft Tissue Reconstruction of Achilles-Tendon-Associated Wounds

18

Nicholas C. Oleck, Ronnie L. Shammas, and Suhail K. Mithani

Introduction

The Achilles is the most frequently injured tendon in the lower extremity, making up 20% of all tendon injuries [1, 2]. While excellent functional outcomes are frequently achieved with operative repair, rates of postoperative wound-healing complications approach 7–13% [3]. Soft tissue defects overlying the Achilles tendon pose a distinct challenge for reconstructive surgeons due to tenuous blood supply, a paucity of local tissue, and shearing forces associated with shoe wearing and ambulation that may impair wound healing. Stable soft tissue coverage of Achilles wounds is essential for proper tendon excursion, the avoidance of desiccation, and the provision of durable tissue for ambulation.

Patient Evaluation

As with all defects, the successful reconstruction of a wound that overlies the Achilles tendon begins with a thorough history and physical examination. The mechanism of injury is of particular importance in these cases as trauma or prior surgical intervention may limit the availability of local tissue for soft tissue reconstruction. A careful pulse examination and assessment for the stigmata of peripheral vascular disease are also warranted to determine if inadequate tissue perfusion is a contributing factor to wound complication. Additionally, antibiotic therapy for infection and adequate debridement of any devitalized tissue are essential to determine the true extent of the wound that requires reconstruction. Complex injuries may require both tendinous and soft tissue reconstruction either concurrently or with a staged approach. In addition, a thorough medical history should take into consideration medical comorbidities such as diabetes mellitus, tobacco use, and chronic steroid therapy, each of which have been identified as independent risk factors that predispose patients to wound complications following an open Achilles tendon repair [3]. These risk factors may also impact the algorithmic approach to soft tissue reconstruction.

Wound Etiology

As previously discussed, wound breakdown is a well-documented risk of Achilles tendon reconstruction, with upward of 7–13% of patients experiencing some form of wound complication after surgical repair [3]. Common causes of wound breakdown in this population include vascular insufficiency, infection, and suture foreign body reaction. In terms of vascular insufficiency,

N. C. Oleck · R. L. Shammas · S. K. Mithani (✉)
Division of Plastic, Maxillofacial, and Oral Surgery, Department of Surgery, Duke University Health System, Durham, NC, USA
e-mail: nicholas.oleck@duke.edu;
ronnie.shammas@duke.edu;
suhail.mithani@duke.edu

the posterior ankle is particularly susceptible to postoperative wound-healing complications due to the tenuous blood supply of this region. Patient-specific factors contributing to regional vascular compromise such as smoking and diabetes mellitus have been identified as independent risk factors for superficial wound necrosis [3]. In particular, tobacco usage has been shown to have a deleterious effect on the regional microvasculature of the lower extremity, disrupting both wound and bone healing in this region [4].

Surgical site infection following Achilles tendon repair is a particularly devastating complication and a significant predisposing factor for wound breakdown. Infection rates of 3–5% have been reported in the literature, with *staphylococcus aureus* as the most commonly identified organism [3, 5, 6]. Deep wound space infection necessitating surgical debridement may lead to an additional deficiency of already limited skin and subcutaneous tissue [6]. The excision of infected and devitalized tissue may include the resection of the Achilles tendon itself, leading to a complex, composite defect.

Another factor likely contributing to wound breakdown is the foreign body reaction associated with high-strength orthopedic sutures commonly used in Achilles tendon repair [7]. These sutures are made up of polymers, such as ultra-high molecular weight polyethylene, and are often coated with additional substances to enhance malleability and handling characteristics [8]. Differential rates of inflammatory response and foreign body capsule formation have been demonstrated between commonly used sutures in both animal models and radiographic studies [7, 8]. This inflammatory reaction and potential for bacterial adherence to suture material may contribute to the relatively high rates of wound complications seen in this patient population.

Nonoperative Management

Superficial defects with minimal tendon exposure and adequate vascularity may be amenable to treatment by a nonoperative approach, including local wound care, compression wrapping, and negative pressure vacuum-assisted closure (VAC) (Fig. 18.1). Negative pressure vacuum therapy is a useful adjunct in preparing these wounds for eventual closure by decreasing edema, increasing vascularity, and promoting wound bed granulation [9]. VAC therapy may also serve as a bridge to definitive closure with a split-thickness skin graft (STSG) in select cases [1, 10].

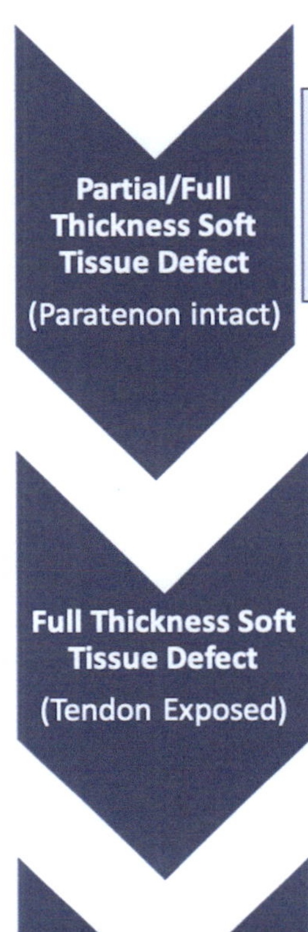

Fig. 18.1 Algorithmic approach to the management of Achilles-tendon-associated wounds. *VAC* vacuum-assisted therapy, *MSAP* medial sural artery perforator flap, *SCIP* superficial circumflex iliac artery perforator flap

Compression Is Critical

Superficial wounds of the Achilles and ankle region are often seen in patients with chronic venous insufficiency. Venous stasis is primarily a disorder of valve incompetence resulting in venous hypertension and skin changes, as well as endothelial damage and the release of inflammatory cytokines. These changes to both the macro- and microvenous circulation result in a characteristic wound appearance of shallow ulcers with irregularly shaped edges, granulation and fibrinous tissue at the base, and yellow/white exudates [11]. External compression therapy is the mainstay of venous stasis ulcer management. The Unna boot is a traditional method of compression therapy that was originally introduced in the nineteenth century and continues to be implemented today. It consists of a low-compression gauze bandage containing 10% zinc oxide paste, gelatin, glycerin, and water and applied to the affected lower extremity [12]. The boot is applied to the affected lower extremity and changed every 3–7 days. It has been shown to be effective in maintaining a moist environment conducive to wound healing, reducing wound healing time, and improving overall patient quality of life [13]. Compression therapy with the Unna boot is certainly a cornerstone of nonoperative management of superficial wounds of the Achilles region.

Dermal Substitutes and Skin Grafts

The utility of STSG for complex Achilles wounds with exposed tendon or bone exposure is relatively limited; however, several reports of successful STSG reconstruction exist [14, 15]. The avascular nature of exposed tendons without paratenon may inhibit STSG take. In order to address this deficiency, dermal regeneration templates such as Integra (Integra Life Sciences, Plainsboro, NJ) have been employed to provide a well-vascularized surface for skin graft placement that will not adhere to the underlying Achilles tendon. This dermal substitute consists of bovine tendon collagen and chondroitin-6-sulfate, facilitating fibroblast migration, neovascularization, and wound remodeling/maturation [16]. Several studies have demonstrated that even with an exposed Achilles tendon, Integra has the potential to fully incorporate and provide a vascularized wound bed that is amenable to skin grafting [17–19]. While these reports are promising, additional investigation is warranted in order to determine the true utility of dermal substitutes in wounds with exposed Achilles tendons, and a sufficient degree of facility with the limits of these devices is key to their successful use.

Local and Regional Options

Local reconstructive options for Achilles wounds are relatively limited due to limited tissue excursion, tenuous blood supply, and potential concomitant injuries; however, several local options have been previously described [2].

Bipedicle Fasciocutaneous Flap

Adjacent tissue transfer utilizing a bipedicle fasciocutaneous flap is a local option that has been

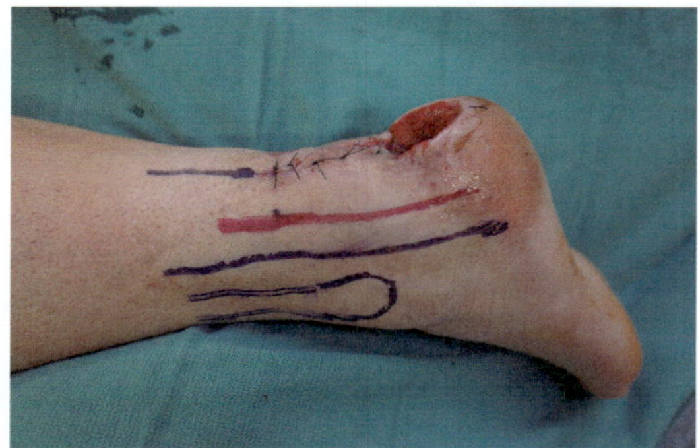

Fig. 18.2 Clinical photograph depicting operative markings for a bipedicle fasciocutaneous flap for the coverage of an Achilles-tendon-associated wound

previously described in detail by the senior author [2]. This flap is advantageous as the surgical technique is straightforward and the operative time is relatively short. Flap design and elevation involve a longitudinal incision lateral to the defect, subfascial dissection, and flap transposition [20]. The flap is based on the lateral calcaneal artery, a reliable branch of the peroneal artery. The incision is made posterior to the lateral malleolus and anterior to the sural nerve and peroneal artery, which can be identified by Doppler (Fig. 18.2). The flap is elevated in a subfascial plane to the lateral border of the wound edge and is then transposed to close the posterior defect. The resulting donor site defect is often closed with a split-thickness skin graft. The bipedicle fasciocutaneous flap has excellent vascularity and limited donor-site morbidity. Additionally, this single-stage approach is particularly beneficial in a community hospital setting without the capabilities necessary for free tissue transfer [2]. Its use is limited to relatively small defects and requires relatively robust adjacent tissue perfusion, making this flap not an ideal one for patients with significant comorbid peripheral vascular disease.

Propeller Flap

Perforator-based propeller flaps are another local option for the reconstruction of soft tissue Achilles defects. The fasciocutaneous propeller flap is an extremely versatile reconstructive option that was initially described in the distal lower extremity and has since been employed for a wide range of defects throughout the body [21]. The flap is designed with two "propeller blades" of unequal length extending outward from a perforator, which serves as the flap pivot point [21, 22]. Microvascular perforator dissection helps facilitate up to 180 degrees of flap rotation, making these flaps ideal for small and medium-sized defects of the distal third of the lower extremity. For Achilles defects, in particular, propeller flaps based on perforating branches of the peroneal and posterior tibial arteries have been described [21]. Previous studies have demonstrated that a peroneal artery perforator identified within 3–7 cm of an Achilles defect allows a flap of up to 23 cm in length to be designed. While the data are relatively limited, existing studies have demonstrated complication rates of up to 40% with peroneal artery perforator propeller flaps. Venous congestion is the most commonly cited complication, which is thought to be attributable to the kinking of the vena comitantes during rotation. However, preliminary data suggest that flap dimension and the arc of rotation are not significantly associated with an increased risk of venous congestion [23]. Previous studies have advocated for the use of perforators of at least 1 mm in diameter, additional intramuscular dissection to minimize vessel kink, and careful patient selection in order to minimize complication risk [22]. While one must remain cognizant of these risks, the perforator-based propeller flap is an important tool in the armamentarium of the reconstructive surgeon, particularly in patients who may not be candidates for free tissue transfer.

Free Tissue Transfer

While isolated soft tissue Achilles defects may be amenable to a more conservative option, large composite defects involving the tendon itself often require a more complex reconstructive approach. Free tissue transfer allows for the transfer of skin, soft tissue, fascia, tendon, and muscle on a single vascular pedicle. Many composite flaps have been described for the reconstruction of complex Achilles defects, with some of the most common being the radial forearm, the anterolateral thigh, and the lateral arm flaps [1, 24]. More recently, isolated perforator flaps, such as the superficial circumflex iliac artery and medial sural artery perforator flaps, have been utilized.

Radial Forearm Free Flap

The radial forearm free flap is the procedure of choice for many complex Achilles defects requiring free tissue transfer. This well-vascularized, reliable, fasciocutaneous flap is highly versatile and is particularly well suited for defects of the Achilles region [24, 25]. The flap is supplied by the radial artery, necessitating a preoperative Allen's test to confirm adequate hand perfusion via the ulnar artery. Venous drainage occurs through a deep system of paired venae comitantes, and the cephalic vein—if included—drains the superficial system. The donor site may be closed primarily in smaller flaps measuring <4 cm in diameter, with larger flaps requiring split-thickness skin grafting. The thin, pliable nature of the flap makes it an ideal choice for defects of the Achilles region, providing durable soft tissue coverage and tendon excursion without compromising shoe wearing and ambulation [24].

Composite Achilles defects involving soft tissues and tendons may also be addressed with the radial forearm free flap. Vascularized tendon grafts from the palmaris longus or flexor carpi radialis may be harvested in conjunction with the fasciocutaneous flap with careful preservation of the perforating branches to these respective structures [23, 24]. Excellent functional outcomes have been demonstrated with this technique, including the restoration of the physiologic gait and the significant recovery of the range of motion [23].

Lateral Arm Flap

The free lateral arm flap is another commonly cited option for Achilles reconstruction. Similar to the radial forearm free flap, this is a thin and pliable fasciocutaneous flap well suited for small to medium-sized defects [26]. Unlike the radial forearm free flap, however, the lateral arm flap does not compromise a major blood vessel to the hand. The flap is based on the posterior radial collateral artery (PRCA) and its septocutaneous perforators emerging from the lateral intermuscular septum. Flap dimensions of up to 20 × 14 cm may be achieved, and those with a diameter of 6 cm or less may be closed primarily [25]. If a sensate flap is desired, the lower lateral cutaneous nerve of the arm may be included during elevation.

Tendon reconstruction with a composite lateral arm flap has also been described utilizing a portion of the triceps tendon. Tendon harvest is typically limited to one third of the triceps tendon in order to minimize donor site deficit and the loss of forearm extension. The tendon may be "rolled up" prior to inset in order to match the defect size and improve tensile strength [26, 27]. Commonly cited disadvantages of the lateral arm flap include a relatively short pedicle, a small artery, and limited flap size. Dissection of the vascular pedicle is particularly tedious due to intimate association with the radial nerve. Care must be taken during dissection to avoid nerve compression and damage [25].

Anterolateral Thigh Flap

The anterolateral thigh flap (ALT) is another preferred option for both isolated soft tissue and composite defects of the Achilles region. The ALT is a workhorse perforator flap with utility in a variety of traumatic and oncologic defects throughout the body. This is a particularly favorable option for Achilles defects due to a large flap area, minimal donor site morbidity, and the ability to harvest a composite flap with multiple tissue types on a single vascular pedicle. Arterial supply to the flap is derived from the descending branch of the lateral circumflex femoral artery—a branch of the profunda femoris—as it courses between the rectus femoris and vastus lateralis. Perforating branches are reliably found along a line drawn from the anterior superior iliac spine (ASIS) to the lateral knee. If desired, a sensate flap may be elevated with the inclusion of the lateral femoral cutaneous nerve, increasing the likelihood of the recovery of protective sensation [28]. For composite defects involving the Achilles tendon, a vascularized portion of the tensor fascia lata (TFL) may be harvested, along with the soft tissue of the ALT. Significant improvements in both objective functional assessment and patient-reported outcomes have been demonstrated with the use of the composite ALT/TFL flap [28].

A limitation of the ALT flap is its relative bulkiness. Interestingly, a higher body mass index (BMI) has been shown to negatively correlate with both functional and patient-reported outcome measures due to the bulkier nature of the transferred flap [28]. ALT flap "thinning"— either in a subsequent procedure or concurrently during the index operation—has emerged as a technique to address this deficiency. Several techniques such as suprafascial flap elevation and microdissection have also been described, with no clear data to favor one technique over another [29].

Isolated Perforator Flaps and Other Options

Recent advancements in microsurgical techniques have led to several additional options for thin and pliable flaps amenable to the coverage of soft tissue Achilles defects. The "ultrathin'' superficial circumflex iliac artery perforator (SCIP) flap has been described for lower third extremity reconstruction. This flap has been touted as similar in character to the native tissue of the distal third of the lower extremity in terms of relative thickness and durability. Dissection in the suprascarpal plane—between the fibrous suprascarpal fat and loose globular subscarpal fat—allows up to a 50% reduction in relative flap thickness [30]. Similarly, the medial sural artery perforator (MSAP) flap is another thin, yet durable, option for the soft tissue coverage of the Achilles region [31].

Conclusion

Options for the soft tissue reconstruction of Achilles tendon defects exist along the entire spectrum of the reconstructive ladder. Stable soft tissue coverage facilitates proper tendon excursion, prevents desiccation, and provides durable tissue for shoe wearing and ambulation. Superficial soft tissue defects may be amenable to nonsurgical management. Dermal substitutes in conjunction with skin grafting can be utilized in a clean well-vascularized wound even in the setting of tendon exposure. Propeller and bipedicle advancement flaps are excellent options for slightly larger and deeper soft tissue defects. Free tissue transfer may be required for larger or composite defects with tendon loss or injury. The radial forearm, ALT, and lateral arm flap are frequently employed in these cases, and more recently, ultrathin and isolated perforator flaps have emerged as viable reconstructive options.

References

1. Marchesi A, Pc P, Brioschi M, et al. Soft-tissue defects of the Achilles tendon region: management and reconstructive ladder. Review of the literature. Injury. 2016;47:S147–53. https://doi.org/10.1016/j.injury.2016.07.053.
2. Dekker TJ, Avashia Y, Mithani SK, Matson AP, Lampley AJ, Adams SB. Single-stage Bipedicle local tissue transfer and skin graft for Achilles tendon surgery wound complications. Foot Ankle Spec. 2017;10(1):46–50. https://doi.org/10.1177/1938640016669796.
3. Bruggeman NB, Turner NS, Dahm DL, et al. Wound complications after open Achilles tendon repair: an analysis of risk factors. Clin Orthop Relat Res. 2004;427:63–6. https://doi.org/10.1097/01.blo.0000144475.05543.e7.
4. Ishikawa SN, Murphy GA, Richardson EG. The effect of cigarette smoking on Hindfoot fusions. Foot Ankle Int. 2002;23(11):996–8. https://doi.org/10.1177/107110070202301104.
5. Bhandari M, Guyatt GH, Siddiqui F, et al. Treatment of acute Achilles tendon ruptures a systematic overview and metaanalysis. Clin Orthop Relat Res. 2002;400:190–200. https://doi.org/10.1097/00003086-200207000-00024.
6. Pajala A, Kangas J, Ohtonen P, Leppilahti J. Rerupture and deep infection following treatment of total achilles Tendon rupture. J Bone Joint Surg Am. 2002;84(11):2016–21. https://doi.org/10.2106/00004623-200211000-00017.
7. Cho J, Kim H-J, Lee JS, et al. Comparing absorbable and nonabsorbable suture materials for repair of Achilles tendon rupture: a magnetic resonance imaging-based study. Diagnostics. 2020;10(12):1085. https://doi.org/10.3390/diagnostics10121085.
8. Carr BJ, Ochoa L, Rankin D, Owens BD. Biologic response to orthopedic sutures: a histologic study in a rabbit model. Orthopedics. 2009;9:828. https://doi.org/10.3928/01477447-20090922-11.
9. Argenta LC, Morykwas MJ. Vacuum-assisted closure: a new method for wound control and treatment: clinical experience. Ann Plast Surg. 1997;38(6):563–76. discussion 577.
10. Repta R, Ford R, Hoberman L, Rechner B. The use of negative-pressure therapy and skin grafting in the treatment of soft-tissue defects over the Achilles Tendon. Ann Plast Surg. 2005;55(4):367–70. https://doi.org/10.1097/01.sap.0000181342.25065.60.
11. Raffetto JD. Pathophysiology of chronic venous disease and venous ulcers. Surg Clin N Am. 2018;98(2):337–47. https://doi.org/10.1016/j.suc.2017.11.002.
12. Luz BSR, Araujo CS, Atzingen DANCV, dos Anjos Mendonça AR, Mesquita Filho M, de Medeiros ML. Evaluating the effectiveness of the customized Unna boot when treating patients with venous ulcers. An Bras Dermatol. 2013;88(1):41–9. https://doi.org/10.1590/s0365-05962013000100004.
13. Cullen GH, Phillips TJ. Clinician's perspectives on the treatment of venous leg ulceration. Int Wound J. 2009;6(5):367–78. https://doi.org/10.1111/j.1742-481X.2009.00626.x.
14. Boyce A, Atherton DD, Tang R, Jawad M. The use of Matriderm® in the management of an exposed Achilles tendon secondary to a burns injury. J Plast Reconstr Aesthet Surg. 2010;63(2):e206–7. https://doi.org/10.1016/j.bjps.2009.02.054.
15. Attinger CE, Ducic I, Hess CL, Basil A, Abbruzzesse M, Cooper P. Outcome of skin graft versus flap surgery in the salvage of the exposed Achilles tendon in diabetics versus nondiabetics. Plast Reconstr Surg. 2006;117(7):2460–7. https://doi.org/10.1097/01.prs.0000219345.73727.f5.
16. Singer M, Korsh J, Predun W, et al. A novel use of integraTM bilayer matrix wound dressing on a pediatric scalp avulsion: a case report. Eplasty. 2015;15:e8.
17. Hulsen J, Diederich R, Neumeister MW, Bueno RA. Integra® dermal regenerative template application on exposed tendon. Hand (New York, NY). 2014;9(4):539–42. https://doi.org/10.1007/s11552-014-9630-1.

18. Lee LF, Porch JV, Spenler W, Garner WL. Integra in Lower Extremity Reconstruction after Burn Injury. Plast Reconstr Surg. 2008;121(4):1256–62. https://doi.org/10.1097/01.prs.0000304237.54236.66.

19. Shores JT, Hiersche M, Gabriel A, Gupta S. Tendon coverage using an artificial skin substitute. J Plast Reconstr Aesthet Surg. 2012;65(11):1544–50. https://doi.org/10.1016/j.bjps.2012.05.021.

20. Makhlouf MV, Obermeyer Z. Bipedicle flap for wounds following Achilles tendon repair. Plast Reconstr Surg. 2008;121(4):235e–6e. https://doi.org/10.1097/01.prs.0000305395.82008.96.

21. Teo TC. The propeller flap concept. Clin Plast Surg. 2010;37(4):615–26. https://doi.org/10.1016/j.cps.2010.06.003.

22. Jakubietz RG, Jakubietz MG, Gruenert JG, Kloss DF. The 180-degree perforator-based propeller flap for soft tissue coverage of the distal, lower extremity: A new method to achieve reliable coverage of the distal lower extremity with a local, fasciocutaneous perforator flap. Ann Plast Surg. 2007;59(6):667–71. https://doi.org/10.1097/SAP.0b013e31803c9b66.

23. Innocenti M, Menichini G, Baldrighi C, Delcroix L, Vignini L, Tos P. Are there risk factors for complications of perforator-based propeller flaps for lower-extremity reconstruction? Clinical Orthop Relat Res. 2014;472(7):2276–86. https://doi.org/10.1007/s11999-014-3537-6.

24. Moyer K, Levin LS. Free tissue reconstruction. In: Nunley JA, editor. The Achilles tendon. New York: Springer; 2008. p. 131–41. https://doi.org/10.1007/978-0-387-79205-7_12.

25. Wei F-C, Mardini S. Flaps and reconstructive surgery. Amsterdam: Elsevier; 2017.

26. Kim C-H, Tark M-S, Choi C-Y, Kang S-G, Kim Y-B. A single-stage reconstruction of a complex Achilles wound with modified free composite lateral arm flap. J Reconstr Microsurg. 2008;24(2):127–30. https://doi.org/10.1055/s-2008-1076090.

27. Smit JM, Darcy CM, Audolfsson T, Hartman EHM, Acosta R. Multilayer reconstructions for defects overlying the Achilles tendon with the lateral-arm flap: long-term follow-up of 16 cases: lateral arm flap for Achilles tendon defects. Microsurgery. 2012;32(6):438–44. https://doi.org/10.1002/micr.21972.

28. Jandali Z, Lam M, Merwart B, et al. Predictors of clinical outcome after reconstruction of complex soft tissue defects involving the Achilles tendon with the composite anterolateral thigh flap with vascularized fascia Lata. J Reconstr Microsurg. 2018;34(08):632–41. https://doi.org/10.1055/s-0038-1660830.

29. Agostini T, Lazzeri D, Spinelli G. Anterolateral thigh flap thinning: techniques and complications. Ann Plast Surg. 2014;72(2):246–52. https://doi.org/10.1097/SAP.0b013e31825b3d3a.

30. Nalamlieng MD, Gould DJ, Patel KM. Ultrathin free flaps to the foot and ankle: new options for optimal soft tissue coverage and functional contour. J Foot Ankle Surg. 2019;58(4):802–6. https://doi.org/10.1053/j.jfas.2018.11.014.

31. Fitzgerald O'Connor E, Ruston J, Loh CYY, Tare M. Technical refinements of the free medial sural artery perforator (MSAP) flap in reconstruction of multifaceted ankle soft tissue defects. Foot Ankle Surg. 2020;26(2):233–8. https://doi.org/10.1016/j.fas.2019.02.003.

Orthobiologic Augmentation of Achilles Tendinitis and Tendon Repairs

19

Richard Danilkowicz and Samuel B. Adams

Introduction

Orthobiologics is a growing field of treatment modalities that can be used independently or as adjuncts with other treatments to cover an array of pathologies. The term covers a wide spectrum of products, from molecular growth factors and decellularized physical scaffolds to various blood and cell-based therapies and whole tissues. The source of these products also varies from patient specific to allogenic donor material to engineered. Within the field of foot and ankle surgery, the most commonly used orthobiologics include injectable additives such as platelet-rich plasma (PRP), platelet-derived growth factor (PDGF), and bone and marrow aspirate concentrate (BMAC), among others. The Achilles tendon is a prime target for the use of orthobiologics as pathologies of this tendon are often seen in active people who want to try nonoperative treatments to avoid the prolonged recovery of surgical procedures. When considering Achilles tendon injuries specifically, orthobiologics have been used along the treatment continuum in various forms for both nonoperative and operative management with promising results. The purpose of this chapter is to outline the use of orthobiologics in the treatment of Achilles tendon injuries.

R. Danilkowicz · S. B. Adams (✉)
Department of Orthopaedic Surgery, Duke University Medical Center, Durham, NC, USA
e-mail: Richard.danilkowicz@duke.edu; Samuel.
adams@duke.edu

Overview of Orthobiologics Used for Achilles Tendon Pathology

In order to understand the role that orthobiologics may play in Achilles pathology, it is important to appreciate the mechanisms of the individual modalities. As previously mentioned, the most commonly utilized orthobiologics used for Achilles tendon pathology are autologous injectables. While each is similar in utilizing a patient's own biology to stimulate a local healing response, they vary enough to elicit potentially differing outcomes with their use.

PRP is a widely utilized preparation created from autologous plasma that produces a supraphysiologic concentration of platelets about five times that of the whole blood. Known to contain over 300 proteins that are bioactive, the platelets in PRP are thought to assist in the healing of tissues with poor blood supply, such as the Achilles tendon, by providing high concentrations of these factors locally [1]. More specifically, the alpha granules of platelets are a rich source of essential growth factors and cytokines that aid the body's own healing process by inducing cellular proliferation, matrix formation, and collagen synthesis as part of the regenerative process [2]. The concentrated solution is injected directly into the site of injury and provides a local response, with studies showing the secretion of active metabolites within an hour of clotting [3]. There continues to be research on the ideal preparation and uses of PRP as variations in procurement, preparation, and consistency in interpreting concentrations have all been sources of study and controversy. Additionally, there is much work being done to investigate the effects of platelet concentration in the sample, leucocyte concentration, the volume of injected PRP, and patient-specific factors, including injury location and type in regard to how one may respond to a PRP injection [2]. As part of the before-mentioned alpha granules of platelets, PDGF is a molecule recognized to stimulate the migration, multiplication, and also differentiation of different cell types that are involved in the healing process [4]. PDGF has been isolated, and a recombinant form of PDGF (recombinant human PDGF (rhPDGF)) is approved by the United States Food and Drug Administration (FDA) for multiple uses, including for fusions of the ankle and hindfoot [5].

Concentrated bone marrow aspirate (CBMA) is one of the few FDA-approved methods for obtaining mesenchymal stem cells, cytokine and growth factors, and other progenitor cells that can be later injected back locally into the patient [6]. CBMA is reported to have high concentrations of various growth factors, which include interleukin-1 receptor antagonist (IL-1RA), interleukin-8 (IL-8), PDGF, transforming growth factor-β (TGF-β), BMPs 2 and 7, and vascular endothelial growth factor (VEGF), which have all been shown to have anti-inflammatory properties [7]. While not currently studied in Achilles tendon pathology, CBMA has been shown to have a positive effect in animal and small human cohorts with rotator cuff tendon healing [8, 9]. Additionally, CBMA is a source of both hematopoietic stem cells (HSCs) and mesenchymal stem cells (MSCs), which can aid in the tendon healing process by either direct action or stimulating a host response of cellular and growth factor infiltration [7].

Nonoperative Orthobiologic Supplementation of Achilles Tendinopathy

Nonoperative Achilles tendinopathy has a range of presentations and may require alternative means of treatment based on the location and severity of the injury. Based largely on the inherent lack of a regenerative capacity of the tendon, the use of injectable biologics has been a popular area of study in order to enhance a patient's ability to heal without the need for surgical intervention. While the bulk of current literature exists for biologics and noninsertional Achilles tendinopathy, there is some evidence for their use with insertional tendinopathy as well.

Noninsertional Achilles tendinopathy is an increasingly common overuse disorder of the posterior ankle, which encompasses up to 65% of Achilles injuries and continues to rise as the aging population strives to remain active [10]. The pathology is a process of inflammation leading to degeneration that occurs proximal to the Achilles insertion, which is traditionally treated with conservative means. Due to the primarily nonoperative nature of the disease process, injectable biologics have provided an intriguing adjunct to assist in the recruitment of local host factors to assist in this notoriously difficult area to heal. PRP has been shown to be effective in multiple retrospective studies for chronic noninsertional Achilles tendinopathy, although the results have not been unanimously touted in level I randomized control trials [11, 12]. Owens Jr. et al. retrospectively evaluated a single injection of PRP for chronic midsubstance Achilles tendinopathy with multiple PROs and MRI data and found that of the eight patients, the average SF-8 score increased from 24.9 to 30.0, the average FAAM score increased from 55.4 to 65.8, and the average FAAMS score increased from 14.8 to 17.4. There was only one patient who showed MRI improvement in the cohort. [13] Similarly, Murawski et al. retrospectively evaluated 32 patients with chronic midsubstance Achilles tendinopathy who received a single PRP injection with clinical and MRI evaluation at 6 months postinjection. Of the 32 patients, 25 (78%) were asymptomatic at follow-up and were able to resume activities and sports, while the remaining seven progressed to surgery. There were minimal changes observed at 6 months postinjection MRI, with only four patients observing an improvement in swelling; however, no Achilles progressed to a full intrasubstance tear [14]. A 2020 systematic review on treatments for noninsertional Achilles tendinopathy included six studies on PRP and found improvement in VISA-A scores in four; however, the one included randomized controlled trial did show no difference from placebo, leaving the authors to note that higher quality evidence is needed before recommending PRP as a treatment for noninsertional Achilles tendinopathy [12]. One additional systematic review and meta-analysis and a second meta-analysis echoed these recommendations, with each pooling 170 patients and finding no differences between PRP and placebo saline plus eccentric strength training exercises [15, 16]. Similarly, in a large RCT comparing PRP vs placebo saline injection, de Vos et al. found no difference at 1-year follow-up in VISA-A scores between the cohorts [17]. Along similar lines to PRP, the use of an adipose-derived stromal vascular fraction (SVF) has been investigated as a potential treatment for noninsertional chronic Achilles tendonitis as it is a source of MSCs, which are theorized to play a role in tendon regeneration immunomodulation [18].

Girolamo et al. investigated the effects of PRP vs SVF in the treatment of noninsertional Achilles tendonitis as part of a randomized controlled trial (RCT), with VAS pain scale, VISA-A, AOFAS Ankle-Hindfoot Score, and the SF-36 form as primary outcome measures. Additionally, patients were evaluated by ultrasound and magnetic resonance pre and postinjection. The primary results of this study were significant improvements in outcome scores for both cohorts compared to baseline preinjection; however, the SVF group was able to achieve a significant improvement of VAS, AOFAS, and VISA-A by 15 days postinjection [19]. Interestingly, an in vitro analysis of the SVF samples showed only a minor concentration of MSCs; nevertheless, they were able to differentiate and propagate. Usuelli et al. published their results on the same methodology 2 years later, finding similar results. They showed that both groups significantly improved scores above baseline; however, VAS, AOFAS, and VISA-A were significantly better at 15 and 30 days postinjection in the SVF cohort. These differences were not seen, however, at later time points of 60, 120, and 180 days postinjection [20].

Orthobiologic Supplementation of Acute Achilles Tendon Rupture

In cases of acute Achilles rupture, biologics have been utilized as augments in both operative and nonoperative treatments. While many of the same injectables outlined previously for nonoperative tendinopathy also have been studied in acute rupture management, additional biologic modalities exist as supplementation for surgical management. The groundwork for the use of biologics stems from basic science and animal model projects; however, there have also been a number of level 1 studies that attempt to bridge the gap from bench to bedside [21]. The indications for the nonoperative vs operative management of acute Achilles rupture management are beyond the scope of this chapter; however, the results have shown equivocal outcomes in randomized controlled trials between the two [22].

Nonoperative management for acute Achilles tears has been established as a first-line treatment; however, the role of biologic augmentation is still a topic of much interest and research. The goal of biologics in acute nonoperative Achilles tear management is to assist in a more timely and robust healing response that allows for the regeneration of strong tissues that are protective against reruptures using many of the same injectables previously mentioned. PRP has been most extensively studied to this point; however, the evidence for its use has been equivocal, with multiple randomized controlled trials finding no benefit over its use vs placebo. Boesen et al. recently conducted a double-blinded RCT of 40 patients comparing PRP vs saline injections to acute Achilles ruptures and found no difference at any time points along the 12-month follow-up in Achilles tendon Total Rupture Scores (ATRS), heel-rise work, heel-rise height, tendon elongation, calf circumference, and the range of motion for ankle dorsiflexion [23]. Similar findings had previously been reported in an RTC of 230 patients by Keene et al., who similarly compared PRP to a dry needle placebo and also found no significant difference in muscle-tendon function or biopsy results at 24 weeks follow-up [24]. Despite the equivocal outcomes reported to this point in the nonoperative arena, the heterogeneity of PRP preparations and the continuing work done to perfect the methodology have left the door open for continued research [25].

Biologics have arguably played a larger role in the augmentation of surgically repaired acute Achilles ruptures. Zou et al. studied PRP injection to the paratenon sheath in addition to an end-to-end modified Krackow suture repair in 36 patients as part of a prospective randomized trial. The primary results of this study showed that the PRP group achieved greater SF-36 and Leppilahti scores at both the 6- and 12-month time points, while the ankle range of motion was improved at 24 months [26]. Stein et al. studied the use of CBMA in combination with open repair in a series of 28 tendons and concluded excellent results with no reruptures and early mobilization; however, there was no comparative arm to their study [27]. They found that 92% (25 of 27) of patients returned to sports in 5.9 months with a mean Achilles tendon Total Rupture Score (ATRS) at final follow-up of 91/100 [27]. The evidence for PDGF and acute Achilles tears is limited to this point in the literature, with only one case report available for review. Morimoto et al. reported on a basketball athlete who was treated surgically for an acute Achilles tear but also subsequently underwent a PDGF injection to the prior site of injury at 4 weeks postoperatively. This patient was able to return to full pain-free activity at 3 months postop and had sustained pain-free activity with no rerupture at 2 years [28]. Outside of injectables, the role of biomaterials in acute Achilles rupture augmentation is still being explored. Limited case series have presented the use of biomaterials from PCL-based polyurethane urea as an augment to the primary repair of local tissue in both chronic and acute surgically repaired Achilles ruptures. In one case of acute repair with augment, the patient returned to full weight-bearing at 8 weeks without complications and with a rapid return to function, while a series of seven patients who underwent repair of chronic injuries with residual postdebridement gaps had a good result with no graft-related complications [29, 30]. However, there are also reports of impaired healing necessitating revision

surgery after the use of these biomaterials as well. [31] Further research is indicated before any definitive recommendations can be made.

Conclusions

Biologic augmentation of Achilles tendon repair is an evolving field. Studies have investigated injectable autologous preparations, including PRP, PDGF, and CBMA, as well as the application of entire biologic tissues as a means of supplementing local tissue repair, to this point with mixed results in case series and little reported efficacy in randomized trials, systematic reviews, and meta-analyses. Future research is needed to solidify the correct preparations and techniques needed to optimize the outcomes of biologic use in the treatment of Achilles tendon repair.

References

1. Lin SS, Montemurro NJ, Krell ES. Orthobiologics in foot and ankle surgery. J Am Acad Orthop Surg. 2016;24(2):113–22. https://doi.org/10.5435/jaaos-d-14-00155.
2. Alsousou J, Thompson M, Hulley P, Noble A, Willett K. The biology of platelet-rich plasma and its application in trauma and orthopaedic surgery: a review of the literature. J Bone Joint Surg. 2009;91(8):987–96. https://doi.org/10.1302/0301-620x.91b8.22546.
3. Marx RE. Platelet-rich plasma: evidence to support its use. J Oral Maxillofac Surg. 2004;62(4):489–96. https://doi.org/10.1016/j.joms.2003.12.003.
4. Claesson-Welsh L. Mechanism of action of platelet-derived growth factor. Int J Biochem Cell Biol. 1996;28(4):373–85. https://doi.org/10.1016/1357-2725(95)00156-5.
5. Hollinger JO, Hart CE, Hirsch SN, Lynch S, Friedlaender GE. Recombinant human platelet-derived growth factor: biology and clinical applications. J Bone Joint Surg Am. 2008;90(Suppl 1):48–54. https://doi.org/10.2106/jbjs.G.01231.
6. Chahla J, Mannava S, Cinque ME, Geeslin AG, Codina D, LaPrade RF. Bone marrow aspirate concentrate harvesting and processing technique. Arthrosc Tech. 2017;6(2):e441–5. https://doi.org/10.1016/j.eats.2016.10.024.
7. Harford JS, Dekker TJ, Adams SB. Bone marrow aspirate concentrate for bone healing in foot and ankle surgery. Foot Ankle Clin. 2016;21(4):839–45. https://doi.org/10.1016/j.fcl.2016.07.005.
8. Mazzocca AD, McCarthy MB, Chowaniec DM, Cote MP, Arciero RA, Drissi H. Rapid isolation of human stem cells (connective tissue progenitor cells) from

the proximal humerus during arthroscopic rotator cuff surgery. Am J Sports Med. 2010;38(7):1438–47. https://doi.org/10.1177/0363546509360924.

9. Liu XN, Yang CJ, Kim JE, et al. Enhanced tendon-to-bone healing of chronic rotator cuff tears by bone marrow aspirate concentrate in a rabbit model. Clin Orthop Surg. 2018;10(1):99–110. https://doi.org/10.4055/cios.2018.10.1.99.

10. Pearce CJ, Tan A. Non-insertional Achilles tendinopathy. EFORT Open Rev. 2017;1(11):383–90. https://doi.org/10.1302/2058-5241.1.160024.

11. Filardo G, Kon E, Di Matteo B, et al. Platelet-rich plasma injections for the treatment of refractory Achilles tendinopathy: results at 4 years. Blood Transfus. 2014;12(4):533–40. https://doi.org/10.2450/2014.0289-13.

12. Jarin I, Bäcker HC, Vosseller JT. Meta-analysis of noninsertional Achilles tendinopathy. Foot Ankle Int. 2020;41(6):744–54. https://doi.org/10.1177/1071100720914605.

13. Owens RF Jr, Ginnetti J, Conti SF, Latona C. Clinical and magnetic resonance imaging outcomes following platelet rich plasma injection for chronic midsubstance Achilles tendinopathy. Foot Ankle Int. 2011;32(11):1032–9. https://doi.org/10.3113/fai.2011.1032.

14. Murawski CD, Smyth NA, Newman H, Kennedy JG. A single platelet-rich plasma injection for chronic mid-substance achilles tendinopathy: a retrospective preliminary analysis. Foot Ankle Spec. 2014;7(5):372–6. https://doi.org/10.1177/1938640014532129.

15. Nauwelaers A-K, Van Oost L, Peers K. Evidence for the use of PRP in chronic midsubstance Achilles tendinopathy: a systematic review with meta-analysis. Foot Ankle Surg. 2020;27:486. https://doi.org/10.1016/j.fas.2020.07.009.

16. Zhang YJ, Xu SZ, Gu PC, et al. Is platelet-rich plasma injection effective for chronic Achilles tendinopathy? A meta-analysis. Clin Orthop Relat Res. 2018;476(8):1633–41. https://doi.org/10.1007/s11999.0000000000000258.

17. de Vos RJ, Weir A, van Schie HT, et al. Platelet-rich plasma injection for chronic Achilles tendinopathy: a randomized controlled trial. JAMA. 2010;303(2):144–9. https://doi.org/10.1001/jama.2009.1986.

18. Schu S, Nosov M, O'Flynn L, et al. Immunogenicity of allogeneic mesenchymal stem cells. J Cell Mol Med. 2012;16(9):2094–103. https://doi.org/10.1111/j.1582-4934.2011.01509.x.

19. de Girolamo L, Grassi M, Viganò M, Orfei CP, Montrasio UA, Usuelli F. Treatment of Achilles tendinopathy with autologous adipose-derived stromal vascular fraction: results of a randomized prospective clinical trial. Orthop J Sports Med. 2016;4:2325967116S0012. https://doi.org/10.1177/2325967116S00128.

20. Usuelli FG, Grassi M, Maccario C, et al. Intratendinous adipose-derived stromal vascular fraction (SVF) injection provides a safe, efficacious treatment for Achilles tendinopathy: results of a randomized controlled clinical trial at a 6-month follow-up. Knee Surg Sports Traumatol Arthrosc. 2018;26(7):2000–10. https://doi.org/10.1007/s00167-017-4479-9.

21. Okamoto N, Kushida T, Oe K, Umeda M, Ikehara S, Iida H. Treating Achilles tendon rupture in rats with bone-marrow-cell transplantation therapy. J Bone Joint Surg Am. 2010;92(17):2776–84. https://doi.org/10.2106/jbjs.I.01325.

22. Willits K, Amendola A, Bryant D, et al. Operative versus nonoperative treatment of acute Achilles tendon ruptures: a multicenter randomized trial using accelerated functional rehabilitation. J Bone Joint Surg Am. 2010;92(17):2767–75. https://doi.org/10.2106/jbjs.I.01401.

23. Boesen AP, Boesen MI, Hansen R, et al. Effect of platelet-rich plasma on nonsurgically treated acute Achilles tendon ruptures: a randomized, double-blinded prospective study. Am J Sports Med. 2020;48(9):2268–76. https://doi.org/10.1177/0363546520922541.

24. Keene DJ, Alsousou J, Harrison P, et al. Platelet rich plasma injection for acute Achilles tendon rupture: PATH-2 randomised, placebo controlled, superiority trial. BMJ. 2019;367:l6132. https://doi.org/10.1136/bmj.l6132.

25. Kreuz PC, Krüger JP, Metzlaff S, et al. Platelet-rich plasma preparation types show impact on Chondrogenic differentiation, migration, and proliferation of human subchondral mesenchymal progenitor cells. Arthroscopy. 2015;31(10):1951–61. https://doi.org/10.1016/j.arthro.2015.03.033.

26. Zou J, Mo X, Shi Z, et al. A prospective study of platelet-rich plasma as biological augmentation for acute Achilles tendon rupture repair. Biomed Res Int. 2016;2016:9364170. https://doi.org/10.1155/2016/9364170.

27. Stein BE, Stroh DA, Schon LC. Outcomes of acute Achilles tendon rupture repair with bone marrow aspirate concentrate augmentation. Int Orthop. 2015;39(5):901–5. https://doi.org/10.1007/s00264-015-2725-7.

28. Morimoto S, Iseki T, Nakayama H, et al. Return to the original sport at only 3 months after an Achilles tendon rupture by a combination of intra-tissue injection of freeze-dried platelet-derived factor concentrate and excessively early rehabilitation after operative treatment in a male basketball player: a case report. Regen Ther. 2021;18:112–6. https://doi.org/10.1016/j.reth.2021.05.002.

29. Petranto RD, Lubin M, Floros RC, et al. Soft tissue reconstruction with Artelon for multiple foot and ankle applications. Clin Podiatr Med Surg. 2018;35(3):331–42. https://doi.org/10.1016/j.cpm.2018.02.008.

30. Shoaib A, Mishra V. Surgical repair of symptomatic chronic achilles tendon rupture using synthetic graft augmentation. Foot Ankle Surg. 2017;23(3):179–82. https://doi.org/10.1016/j.fas.2016.04.006.

31. Mohamed A, Oliva F, Nardoni S, Maffulli N. Failed synthetic graft after acute Achilles tendon repair. Muscles Ligaments Tendons J. 2017;7(2):396–402. https://doi.org/10.11138/mltj/2017.7.2.396.

Index

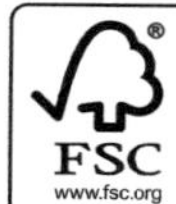

MIX
Papier aus verantwortungsvollen Quellen
Paper from responsible sources
FSC® C105338

If you have any concerns about our products,
you can contact us on
ProductSafety@springernature.com

In case Publisher is established outside the EU,
the EU authorized representative is:
Springer Nature Customer Service Center GmbH
Europaplatz 3, 69115 Heidelberg, Germany

Printed by Libri Plureos GmbH
in Hamburg, Germany